# The 80/10/10 Diet

"For people who want to create balance in their lives and reach and sustain the level of health they deserve, I highly recommend this book."

*—Kimberly Mac, The "Naked" Vegan,*
*radio talk show host and live-food chef*

"When I stick with Dr. Graham's 80/10/10 diet program, I am full of energy and vitality. I am able to live life to the fullest and enjoy every moment. As an added bonus, I start to lose extra weight and I feel healthy. I don't want for anything when I can eat all the strawberries and watermelon that I desire."

*—Rachel Johnson, author of Wake Up Running!*

"I have been following Dr. Graham's 80/10/10 diet and lifestyle for seven years, and it is the best thing I have ever done. His program has allowed me to fine tune my eating habits so that I'm functioning at my best. For me, the benefits of this lifestyle include high energy, disappearance of all ailments, cessation of depression, more patience, a reverence for life, and much more."

*—Gary Orlando, author of Beyond Raw eBook*

"The 80/10/10 diet as explained and advocated by Dr. Graham in his book, is in my opinion, the greatest breakthrough ever made in the field of nutrition. Read it, study it, and apply it as if your life depended on it—because it does."

*—Frederic Patenaude, author of The Raw Secrets*

"Armed with data drawn from the latest scientific research, Dr. Graham convincingly makes the case that humans are essentially frugivorous and that we should all be living on a fruit-based diet. The 80/10/10 Diet is a courageous, thoroughly researched work. In a field that is beset by hucksters and charlatans, this new book establishes Dr. Graham as the undisputed voice of authority and wisdom."

*—Rynn Berry, author of*
*Food for the Gods: Vegetarianism and the World's Religions*
*and historical advisor to the North American Vegetarian Society*

# The 80/10/10 Diet

**Balancing Your Health, Your Weight, and Your Life One Luscious Bite at a Time**

Dr. Douglas Graham

Published by:
FoodnSport Press
609 N. Jade Drive
Key Largo, FL 33037 U.S.A.

Printed in the United States of America

Logo Design by Janie Gardener
Peach Photo by Carina Honga
Back Cover Portrait by StrickfadenPhoto.com

10 9 8 7 6 5 4 3 2 1
Publisher's Cataloging-in-Publication
(Provided by Quality Books, Inc.)

Graham, Douglas N.
The 80/10/10 diet : balancing your health, your weight, and your life one luscious bite at a time / by Douglas N. Graham ; foreword by Ruth Heidrich.
p. cm.
Includes bibliographical references.
ISBN-13: 978-1-893831-24-7
ISBN-10: 1-893831-24-8

1. High-carbohydrate diet. 2. Low-fat diet. 3. Raw foods. 4. Nutrition. I. Title. II. Title: Eighty ten ten diet. III. Title: Balancing your health, your weight, and your life one luscious bite at a time.

RM237.59.G73 2006 613.2'83
QBI06-600292

**Trademark Statement**

Since my graduation from chiropractic college in 1983, I have performed considerable research and have lectured extensively on the subjects of health, diet, and athletics to tens of thousands of people in the United States and around the world. The essence of my life's work has been summed up in the related phrases **80/10/10** and **80/10/10rv**, and their corresponding shorthand **811** and **811rv**. While **80/10/10** originally referred to a nutritional ratio, followers of my work know that it has come to mean much more. Over the decades, I have strived to imbue the **80/10/10** concept with the additional meanings of adequate sleep, exercise, positive outlook on life, and many other health-promoting factors. As a result, I am formally asserting trademark rights to **80/10/10**, **80/10/10rv**, **811**, and **811rv** in order to maintain the high standards they have come to represent in the public mind and to protect the public's association of these concepts with me and my work. I hope everyone in the health/nutrition field will honor and respect these marks, using them only when licensed or authorized or, if without specific authorization, with proper acknowledgment and notice in accordance with law and custom.

**Disclaimer**

*The information contained in* The 80/10/10 Diet *is provided for your general information only. It is not intended as a substitute for any treatment that may have been prescribed by your doctor. Dr. Douglas Graham does not give medical advice or engage in the practice of medicine. Under no circumstances does Dr. Graham recommend particular treatment for specific individuals, and he recommends in all cases that you consult your physician or a qualified practitioner before pursuing any course of treatment or making any changes to your diet or medications.*

— Douglas N. Graham, DC

## Dedication

With fondest respect,
I dedicate this book to my friend and mentor,
the late T.C. Fry.

When I gave the eulogy at Terry's memorial service, I promised that his memory would live on. My life, and this book, are testaments to that intention. May his work continue to influence people for the better until living healthfully becomes a normal and natural part of every person's life.

# Acknowledgments

I wish to offer my gratitude to the many people who made this book possible. It is not possible to name them all, as so many folks played an important part in its creation.

First, my special thanks go to the following people, each of whom worked with me and helped me to clarify my thoughts on the subject matter in this book: Gail Davis, Dave Klein, Ken Lyle, Laurie Masters, Tim Trader, Laurie Clifford, Robert Sniadach, Bruce Brazis, David Rodenbucher, Catherine Galipeau, and John Pierre.

Contributions came in many forms, from information to editing, from research to relief. Some of you provided me with the necessary sounding board that I needed, others asked the questions that brought clarity to some aspect of this project or another. Some folks provided help simply by sharing the details of their program with me, including the problems and solutions they had discovered along the way. I wish all of you could know how important your influence really was.

For their behind-the-scenes contributions, I would like to especially thank Dennis Nelson, David Taylor, Justin Lelia, Josh Steinhauser, Tom Cushwa, Gideon and Jackie Graff, Nancy Parlette, Todd Ewen, Dr. Deborah Wood, Charlie Mort, Craig Bishop, Coby Siegenthaler, Suzanne Slusser, and Shari Leiterman.

I wish to thank John Robbins and Michael Greger for giving me their kind permission to reprint some of their previously published work, and also Antonia Horne for allowing me the privilege of including excerpts from her late husband Ross Horne's work.

Many people simply pushed for me to put this body of work into print, as they wanted to show it to their dear ones. Each of you contributed in your own special way, giving something that made it possible for me to get on with my work. For this I thank you. It means a great deal to me that you would think my work so valuable as to be willing to take the energy to prod me into writing this book. Those of you who actually gave up your precious time in order for me to move forward with this project provided invaluable support.

Many people helped with the creation of the Frequently Asked Questions section, providing questions and, in many instances, appropriate responses. My appreciation goes to Randall Phelps, Janie Gardener, and Jack Whitley for their help with editing the FAQs.

Marr Nealon, your efforts to help me promote this cause were (and continue to be) stupendous, thank you.

To my niece, Shyella Joy Mayk, thank you for all your fitness motivation, support, and your endless help with my website. And to Liati Natanya Mayk, her sister, thank you for keeping me intellectually honest and helping me maintain my perspective through the relaxation of music.

To Gail Davis, my publicist, thank you for the long nights of proofreading and your continual input on how to illuminate this book and my business so that they would evolve into everything I knew they could be.

The hours just kept speeding by while I worked on The 80/10/10 Diet. I often lost track of time, and sometimes also lost track of commitments, appointments, meals, my personal needs for physical activity, and even sleep.

Fortunately, I am extremely blessed, in that I have a personal angel in my life who makes it her full-time job to look after me. I wish to thank my beautiful wife Rozi, for her selfless and endless attention while I worked on this book. Without her constant help and support, I would never have been able to have made time for this book. Even if I had been forced to try, I do not think I would have successfully or healthfully been able to complete it without her.

Thank you, Rozi, for paying attention to so many of life's little and big details. I would have let them slip in pursuit of finishing this task. I can only hope that you feel as rewarded by me as I do by you, and as supported.

I am forever indebted to my loving parents, Marty and Bea, who have always taught me how to be a successful adult by their shining example. My wish is that in raising my own child, Faychesca, I am able to employ the same parenting skills that they have shown me, with at least a modicum of their competence and grace.

## Special Thanks

I would especially like to extend sincere appreciation to my editor, Laurie Masters of Precision Revision (www.GreenSongPress.org) and to Carina Honga, whose position is as varied as all the tasks we have encountered. The time these wonderful women have devoted to researching, editing, and organizing this book amounts to years. Their dedication, writing skills, and teamwork have taken this book to a new level.

Laurie, thank you for keeping me honest through your amazing research skills and for distilling my writing down to what I was actually trying to say. Your signature knack for "rototilling" a disjointed manuscript and turning it into a coherent book has once again proven invaluable. I am forever grateful for your steadfast commitment to me and to this project and for your tenacity in keeping its zillion details on track. Thank you in particular for your personal contributions to this book (notably Chapter 8 and Appendix D.). I am convinced you are the best editor this side of the universe.

Carina, adding you to our team was one of the best things I have ever done. Thank you for your tireless efforts to complete any and every thing that was asked of you with incredible speed and skill.

## Also by Douglas N. Graham

Grain Damage
Nutrition and Athletic Performance
Perpetual Health Calendar
The High Energy Diet Recipe Guide

For Articles, Recorded Seminars,
& online discussion group visit
http://foodnsport.com

# Table of Contents



# Sidebars and Tables

## Foreword

As an Ironman triathlete, ultramarathoner, and holder of nearly 1,000 race first places, I know how important the right diet is. It dismays me to see how much dietary misinformation is being spread with the main goal being to make money. Because so many people are misinformed about the proper diet, obesity is at the highest rates in history, and as more people buy into these money-making schemes, obesity and its associated diseases are going to continue to increase at horrendous rates.

Over and over again, I hear people saying they've tried "everything" to lose weight—low fat, high fat, low carb, high carb, low protein, high protein, all kinds of pills, shots, powders, and shakes—you name it and they say they've tried it. The main cause of their failure is misinformation.

There are reasons for each of these dietary failures. What they were told was "low fat," usually 30%, actually is not low fat at all, and they have no idea how to get to an effective low-fat 10% as described in this book. High-fat diets can be dangerous and put you at risk for the diseases that most Westerners die from prematurely. Low-carb diets are also dangerous, and most people have no idea that the ideal diet consists of 80% carbs. But, it must be the right carbs.

High-protein diets lead to osteoporosis, kidney disease, and lack of energy for exercise. Most people think that low protein diets will never work, having been convinced by the meat and dairy industries that the more protein you eat, the better—and nothing could be further from the truth.

As for pills, shots, powders, and shakes, these gimmicks will never give people the health they really seek. What they don't realize is that obesity is actually a symptom of eating the wrong diet. The same is true of most of the other diseases we suffer from, for example, heart disease, cancer, stroke, diabetes, arthritis, colitis, constipation, osteoporosis, acne, erectile dysfunction, dementia, and even vision and hearing problems. These are all symptoms of the diseases of consuming the wrong diet.

You are holding in your hands the book that will give you the dietary information we all need to have. You don't have to be an Ironman triathlete or even want to be one, but you owe it to yourself to read *The 80/10/10 Diet!*

Ruth E. Heidrich, PhD
Author, *A Race For Life*
www.ruthheidrich.com

## Preface

This was not an easy book to write. I tried to create The 80/10/10 Diet on several occasions in the past, but it has proven to be a daunting project riddled with false starts. For some reason, nothing about this particular piece of work has been easy. I can only assume that it must be like the old saying, "nothing worthwhile is ever easy." I believe that this is the most worthwhile book that I have written to date.

In writing The 80/10/10 Diet, I found myself constantly enmeshed in a deep inner debate, wondering how to most effectively reach the largest number of people:

- Will I reach more people through appeals to their heads or their hearts? Will quoting numbers, current research, scientific studies, and textbook facts bolster their willingness to make dietary changes?

- Will such minutiae cause readers to lose interest, or can each bit of data build upon the previous ones until it forms a convincing and solid information base?

- How deep need I go in order to get my point across? Will it suffice to say that all the animals built like us eat fruits and vegetables and very little fat, therefore we should too?

- Will stories and testimonials about high levels of health, boundless energy, unexpected healing, effortless weight loss, spiritual awakening, and newfound enthusiasm for life be viewed as hyperbole or truthful inspiration?

And perhaps most worrisome …

- If I leave something out, will I get a second chance?

The research for this book often left me studying for several days in order to write just one or two sentences. The more I learned, the more there was to learn, it seemed. I eventually had to choose between writing a book and becoming a full-time reader of other people's work.

I gathered a tremendous amount of information, but a great deal of what I learned proved simply not to be relevant to the creation of this book. I can only hope it will be valuable material for future works.

## Who Should Read This Book?

I wrote this book for anyone who believes that appropriate body weight and vibrant well-being are their birthright as well as their responsibility—anyone willing to keep striving for the physique and the health they desire.

The 80/10/10 plan is not an all-or-nothing proposition. It allows you to work toward a goal, rather than simply follow a diet. You do not have to eat primarily vegetarian or raw foods to benefit from the 80/10/10 program.

If you eat a relatively typical American diet, 80/10/10 is a program that allows you to continue eating the foods you are used to, while beginning to introduce the new foods that will lead you toward your goal. Direction, not speed, is the most important aspect of learning to succeed with 80/10/10.

If you have already transitioned your diet to vegetarian, vegan, or raw foods, you will still find the principles in this book to be a step forward for you. In fact, this book represents the brass ring for raw fooders. I feel ecstatic that I finally have succeeded in writing about the program I have taught for years in the raw and vegetarian communities.

Discouraged by their inability to succeed on raw food and confused by the opposing information they hear from other teachers, raw food enthusiasts have pleaded with me: "I bet I am eating high-fat raw, but I don't know how to figure it out, and I need more information on what to do about it."

Now, with the sample calculations in hand, I stand before the raw food community with clear evidence of the dangerously high fat consumption common in our ranks—and with a clearly articulated plan for those who wish to raise the bar a notch and reach for the ultimate low-fat plan for raw health.

## The Results Speak for Themselves

The principles I share in this book represent more than twenty-five years of research and almost two decades of assisting people with their health, nutrition, and athletic performance in private consultation. During that time, I have used the 80/10/10 program myself—and with thousands of clients who are consistently delighted with their newfound health, vigor, and physical appearance.

I have seen the sickest of the sick regain high levels of health and vitality, simply by making intelligent food and lifestyle modifications. I have watched people pronounced "terminally ill" by the medical establishment heal themselves using the program described in this book. I have watched former world-class athletes rejuvenate themselves to the degree that they are once again achieving "personal best" performances. Truly, 80/10/10 is not only a "diet" but a success formula. And it just keeps getting better.

In Appendix C, I have compiled a collection of testimonials from healthy, happy, and successful practitioners of the 80/10/10 way of life. Their inspiring stories speak for themselves.

Wherever you are on your journey to ever-greater well-being, I hope that you enjoy reading The 80/10/10 Diet and find it valuable, insightful, and motivating. It is my sincerest belief that you will find within these pages the nutritional guidance you need to attain, regain, and maintain the radiant, trim body of your dreams and an even a higher level of health than you have ever dared to strive for.

## Let All Find Their Own Path

While in my experience, consuming a 100% raw version of the 80/10/10 diet is optimal, other low(er)-fat plant-centered diet programs also offer substantial health benefits … and many people find them to be the right choice for their lives. If you find yourself judging others for not choosing all raw, all low-fat, or even all vegan foods, I implore you to take a BIG step backward and recognize that all of us must make our own choices, and no one path is best for all people.

I have been saddened and dismayed by the number of people who tell me that an enthusiastic 80/10/10 supporter has stopped talking to his or her family, or has taken on a holier-than-thou fundamentalist attitude with friends who do not "see the light."

Friends, if you stop connecting with your loved ones over the food you eat, you have missed the point! Healthful living includes healthy relationships and compassion for your fellow humans. If you wish to contribute to your loved ones, accept them where they are, and then lead by example, with an open heart … you will have far greater success if you do.

## A Tribute to T.C. Fry

The late T.C. Fry (1926–1996), a world-renowned and much-loved health educator, was a mentor for me. He helped me sort the trash from the treasures in the world of health and nutrition. He never told me what to think, but he often instructed me in how to think … to refine the process of thinking so that I could come up with truth for myself. He loved to pursue a line of thought through to its logical and often only valid conclusion.

T.C. (he told me on several occasions that T. was his full name, but that his friends often called him Terry) and I lectured in hundreds of cities together, giving weekend seminars throughout much of the 1980s and into the early '90s. We sold no products, just education. The topics were almost always different, but always about some aspect of health.

I once asked Terry why we didn't simply come up with a format of lecture topics that we could stick to, one we could take to all the different cities on our tour.

"I am training you," he said, proffering his irresistible smile. I like to think he did a good job.

Terry was not perfect, by any stretch of the imagination. He openly admitted his flaws. He had minimal formal education. At the age of 45, with his health failing terribly due to an intensely abusive lifestyle characterized by its excessiveness, he turned his life around. The doctors had already told him that he didn't have much longer to live. A change in diet coupled with attention to many of the other necessities of healthful living gave Terry another twenty-five years.

In the end, his intensity got the better of him. He simply worked himself to death in an effort to spread the health message to as many people as possible. His work was not in vain. His students have had a profound effect upon the current health movement, and are continuing to do so. Most notable is the work of Harvey and Marilyn Diamond with their groundbreaking book, *Fit for Life*. Many of Terry's other students have authored books. I am proud to be among them.

When he was alive, Terry often visited my home. On more than one visit he had proclaimed that his writing was for the public, that he wanted it to go to good use. He generously made the offer that I should reprint his writing wherever I saw fit.

This is one of those occasions. I have incorporated several short pieces of Terry's writing into The 80/10/10 Diet. His comparative anatomy assessment of the natural diet for humans, which I have included in a somewhat revised form as Chapter 1, is the longest of them.

# Introduction

Americans have been told for more than forty years that we are eating too much fat, yet our consumption of this nutrient has remained essentially unchanged during that time.[1] We have made no headway in eating less fat, despite massive educational programs, the carbohydrate-loading craze, leaner meats, low-fat fiber-filled cereals and bars, and low-fat desserts, dairy products, and entrées.

## We Are Fatter (and Sicker) Than Ever

Meanwhile, as a nation, we have become the fattest people on Earth and are still getting fatter. Two-thirds of all Americans are overweight, half of them obese. Because obesity is so common, few of us realize that our current view of "normal" body fat levels has been skewed to allow for several dozen extra pounds. Sadly, morbid obesity is rapidly moving up in the ranks of "causes of preventable death" statistics in our nation. Consider the following:

### Nearly One-Third of the Calories

**by Sarah Yang, Media Relations | 01 June 2004**[2]

*U. C. Berkeley News*

Gladys Block, professor of epidemiology and public health nutrition at the University of California, Berkeley, published a study in the June 2004 issue of the *Journal of Food Composition and Analysis.*

The study reveals that three food groups—sweets and desserts, soft drinks and alcoholic beverages—comprise almost 25 percent of all calories consumed by Americans. Salty snacks and fruit-flavored drinks make up another five percent, bringing the total energy contributed by nutrient-poor foods to at least 30 percent of the total calorie intake.

"What is really alarming is the major contribution of 'empty calories' in the American diet," said Block. "We know people are eating a lot of junk food, but to have almost one-third of Americans' calories coming from those categories is a shocker. It's no wonder there's an obesity epidemic in this country."

| What Americans Eat[3] | | | |
|---|---|---|---|
| **Rank** | **Food Group** | **% of Total Energy** | **Cumulative %** |
| 1 | Sweets, desserts | 12.3 | 12.3 |
| 2 | Beef, pork | 10.1 | 22.3 |
| 3 | Bread, rolls, crackers | 8.7 | 31.0 |
| 4 | Mixed dishes | 8.2 | 39.2 |
| 5 | Dairy | 7.3 | 46.5 |
| 6 | Soft drinks | 7.1 | 53.6 |
| 7 | Vegetables | 6.5 | 60.1 |
| 8 | Chicken, fish | 5.7 | 65.8 |
| 9 | Alcoholic beverages | 4.4 | 70.2 |
| 10 | Fruit, juice | 3.9 | 74.2 |

The standard American diet (SAD) is a sad testament to the rampant physical and mental decay of the most prosperous nations on Earth. As our consumption of junk foods, animal products, chemical additives, toxic pesticides, and genetically modified organisms have increased, our health has plummeted. The numbers are staggering:

**Obesity:** In 2000, poor diet including obesity and physical inactivity caused more than 320,000 U.S. deaths and numbered among the top preventable causes of disease.[4] Obesity is the leading cause of all three of our top killers: heart disease, cancer, and stroke.[5]

**Heart disease:** Although the first recorded heart attack is said to have appeared in British medical literature just over a hundred years ago (1878), more than one in five Americans now suffers from some form of cardiovascular disease, and more than 2,500 Americans die from it each day.[6] In 2001, just under 700,000 Americans died of heart disease.[7]

**Cancer:** Just a generation or two ago, cancer was a grandparents' disease. Today, we have entire cancer hospitals for children. Some 1.3 million new cancer cases were expected to be diagnosed and nearly 564,000 cancer deaths were predicted in 2004.[8]

**Diabetes:** More than 18 million Americans have diabetes, the sixth most frequent cause of death in North America. The number of U.S. adults with diagnosed diabetes has increased 61% since 1991 and is projected to more than double by 2050, afflicting one in three Americans born in 2000. Today, diabetes claims more than 200,000 lives each year.[9]

## Mixed Messages

It is crazy to think that we can keep doing what we have been doing while expecting the outcome to be any different than it has been. If we truly want healthy results, we are going to have to start living more healthfully. But exactly what changes should we make?

Daily, we encounter an endless barrage of contradictory opinions and opposing interpretations of practically every aspect of nutritional science. Nutrition is so rife with conflicting theories that the so-called "hard scientists," the physicists, mathematicians, physical chemists, and others, frequently denigrate nutrition as "not a real science."

Confusion seems to be the only constant in weight management. A new diet craze comes into vogue almost every week, each one hyped as "the answer" to our waistline woes. Some advisors tell us to minimize fat, while others assert that eating fat does not make us fat and in fact brings us greater health. Some vilify carbohydrates, while others show convincing evidence that whole grains should be our staple. We have to wonder: Which of these conflicting theories are true? Which are hogwash? Could there be some middle ground?

Worse yet, if you desire not only a trim physique but also vibrant health, the waters become even muddier. One self-proclaimed "expert" tells you that minerals are the most important aspect of nutrition, while another claims that structured water will cure all that ails you. Hordes of scientists, nutritionists, doctors, "healers," and lay people fill the bookstores and crowd the lecture circuit with convincing tales of the indispensable virtues of vitamins, essential fatty acids, antioxidants, enzymes, or some other silver bullet that is sure to ameliorate all of your health, aging, and weight issues.

All of these parties defend their turf with a vengeance. And understandably so. Most of them have deep economic ties to their particular nutritional approach, complete with programs, supplements, superfoods, motivational seminars, prepackaged meals, and a wide assortment of accessories.

That confusion was not lost on me. Over the years I have tried more diets than most people have even heard of. This is especially true because I was seeking an optimal plan for health, athletic performance, and body-weight management—all at the same time. I got tired of trying one new approach after another, but what else was there to do? I had to keep looking for something that worked for me, on all levels.

## The Science of Health

For me, the fog began to lift in the late 1970s. I remember the sense of thrill and relief I felt, after years of fumbling around with diets and health fads, to finally alight upon a diet that works—in all the ways I sought—and the clear and incontrovertible evidence to back it up. In this book, I share with you some salient bits from the body of knowledge called "Natural Hygiene" (literally, the science of health), information that changed my life and allowed me to coach thousands of people to attain the well-being, vitality, and physique they have always wanted.

The dietary approach I recommend, especially with its emphasis on fresh fruits and vegetables, may sound radical, particularly in light of the prevailing attitude held by doctors, supplement vendors, and fad-diet hawkers, who all would have you believe that the keys to health and fitness most certainly do not grow on trees.

I invite you, however, to withhold judgment, and stick with me as we examine the natural simplicity of living a high-produce, low-fat lifestyle—truly the one for which Nature designed us.

## Pitfalls of Fragmented Thinking

The Natural Hygiene approach to diet and nutrition is markedly different than the fragmented perspective that is common among health seekers and diet promoters. The fragmented view does not so much look at foods as it does their component parts. It also fails to distinguish true well-being from merely looking good, feeling good, or removing symptoms of dis-ease—a grave error, indeed.

The fragmented approach extols the virtues of certain nutrients in a "pick-and-choose" fashion—the kind used in infomercial sales pitches. Excellently geared toward selling a specific product, this viewpoint never considers the full story, always omitting material that would give a more balanced view of the situation.

Like a person who makes a decision after listening to only one side in a debate, the fragmented thinker relies on skewed information, and the resulting incomplete picture provides a misunderstanding of nutrition that can only spiral out of control.

Below is one version of a famous Indian legend. The story pointedly illustrates the confusion that results when we mistake a fragmented view for the whole picture.

### The Blind Men and the Elephant[10]

**It was six men of Indostan**
To learning much inclined,
Who went to see the Elephant
(Though all of them were blind),
That each by observation
*Might satisfy his mind.*

**The First approached the Elephant,**
And happening to fall
Against his broad and sturdy side,
At once began to bawl:
"God bless me! but the Elephant
*Is very like a wall!"*

**The Second, feeling of the tusk**
Cried, "Ho! what have we here,
So very round and smooth and sharp?
To me `tis mighty clear
This wonder of an Elephant
*Is very like a spear!"*

**The Third approached the animal,**
And happening to take
The squirming trunk within his hands,
Thus boldly up he spake:
"I see," quoth he, "the Elephant
*Is very like a snake!"*

**The Fourth reached out an eager hand,**
And felt about the knee:
"What most this wondrous beast is like
Is mighty plain," quoth he;
"'Tis clear enough the Elephant
*Is very like a tree!"*

**The Fifth, who chanced to touch the ear,**
Said: "E'en the blindest man
Can tell what this resembles most;
Deny the fact who can,
This marvel of an Elephant
*Is very like a fan!"*

**The Sixth no sooner had begun**
About the beast to grope,
Than, seizing on the swinging tail
That fell within his scope.
"I see," quoth he, "the Elephant
*Is very like a rope!"*

**And so these men of Indostan**
Disputed loud and long,
Each in his own opinion
Exceeding stiff and strong,
Though each was partly in the right,
And all were in the wrong!

**Moral**

So oft in theologic wars,
The disputants, I ween,
Rail on in utter ignorance
Of what each other mean,
And prate about an Elephant
Not one of them has seen!

As with the blind men's wildly divergent assessments of the same elephant, the misinformation coming from most diet and nutrition "experts" who teach from their fragmented perspectives may be correct, in some sense—but none of it leaves its recipients properly informed.

Using the fragmented approach, if I were concerned about calcium, I would seek out foods high in calcium. I would not likely consider the foods that cause me to lose calcium, or even those that interfere with calcium uptake. I would not research the lifestyle factors that result in calcium losses, nor those that enhance calcium absorption.

Alternatively, I might choose to take calcium supplements, a prime example of fragmented thinking. It is unlikely that I would inquire about any possible adverse effects of consuming too much calcium. Nor would I tend to educate myself about the bioavailability of one form of calcium versus another. Perhaps most important, I would not know to question the wisdom of thinking in terms of isolated nutrients in the first place.

In nature, calcium (and all other nutrients) come packaged in a very precise combination in plant foods, accompanied by hundreds, even thousands, of other micronutrients that are designed to be consumed together. We cannot improve upon Nature's pristine design by extracting and refining one or even a few dozen nutrients—removing them from the cofactors they naturally accompany—and produce a positive result.

What is more, I have heard estimates that scientists today may have discovered only 10% of the nutrients in existence, particularly the so-called phytonutrients (plant nutrients). In light of this, we might stop for a moment to wonder: How can any of us claim to have zeroed in on some specific nutrient deficiency and take informed action toward correcting it? It cannot be done intelligently, in my opinion.

## Whole Foods, First and Only

Despite our technological advances, nutrition is a young science. We lack both the knowledge and the technology to reproduce in a laboratory the brilliant balance of nutrients found in whole plant foods.

*Anything short of whole plant foods—be they green juices, "healthy" oils, dehydrated "whole-food" supplements, or white-powdered pharmaceutical-grade "superfoods"—always misses the mark, guaranteed.*

- All we can hope to accomplish through eating refined, fractional foods is satiation and compromised nutrition.
- All we can hope to achieve through supplementation with isolated nutrients is to relieve symptoms while creating further imbalances.

People tell me that hearing this discussion confuses them, for they often experience welcome increases in energy and apparent reversal of health challenges through supplementation. I find that these results come, however, at great cost. If these individuals distance themselves from the supplement-vendor hype and slow their quest for quick relief, they usually notice that their life has become an endless shell game, in which they shift symptoms but never reach true health, homeostasis, and peace.

## Health and Feeling Good Are *Not* the Same

This analogy sometimes helps people understand the difference between creating health (the big picture) and treating symptoms (the fragmented view):

**Employment example:** Suppose you work in a dreary office for too little pay and endure daily verbal abuse from a tyrannical employer. If you quit that job and break free, would you now say that you have just the perfect job, the work of your dreams? Of course not. What you have is nothing … no job at all. True, your newfound liberation may bring welcome relief from the abuse, but alleviating your pain is a far cry from the target—if your true desire is for fulfilling, rewarding work. Without positive action toward a better job, you may sit idle for a very long time, having traded in one set of problems (an oppressive work environment) for another (unemployment).

**Health example:** Similarly, many people use treatments, pharmaceuticals, or "natural" drugs to suppress symptoms such as overweight, candida, allergies, or headaches, or even to eliminate tumors and other forms of severe breakdown. Once they experience relief—the headaches subside, the allergic wheezing abates, the tumor shrinks—they proclaim themselves "cured" and believe that they have regained health. They may look and feel better, but their newfound absence of dis-ease is just that—a void. Again, this is a vast improvement over pain and suffering. But it is nothing close to the vibrant energy and well-being that many of us desire.

People are incredulous when they first hear this: *"You mean, if I get rid of my seizures* (or tumors, or migraines, or candida, or lupus, or …), *that doesn't mean I'm healthy?"*

The answer is, unequivocally, no. If they continue the cycle of living in ways that created their health issues in the first place—and then attacking the inevitable symptoms with remedies and treatments—they set in motion the aforementioned shell game, repeatedly trading in one set of health complaints for another seemingly unrelated complex of maladies, never getting closer to the goal of lasting, radiant health.

In both examples, the new liberation represents a zero point, a neutral position from which health or recurring disease (satisfying work or ongoing unemployment) can emerge. The person who is free of symptoms is no more healthy than the unemployed person is professionally fulfilled.

To attain the (big-picture) goal of gratifying work or lasting well-being, we must take positive action toward our desired result, not just negative action away from the condition we do not want (a fragmented solution at best). When we use remedies and therapies to eliminate symptoms, we do nothing to address their original cause, hence nothing to create health. We must educate ourselves about the causes of health (not disease) and include these in our daily routine.

### Your Doctor Cannot Help Here ...

*Many drugs, diets, and supplements are sold with an admonition to "consult your physician" before consuming them. But is there value in looking to the medical profession for nutritional advice? Consider this sobering tidbit:*

"In a medical journal article entitled 'Bizarre and Unusual Diets,' the authors warn that the Atkins Diet had such questionable safety that it should 'only be followed under medical supervision.' But what do doctors know about nutrition? Even though the United States Congress mandated that nutrition become an integrated component of medical education, as of 2004, less than half of all U.S. medical schools have a single mandatory course in nutrition. That explains the results of a study published in the *American Journal of Clinical Nutrition* that pitted doctors against patients head to head in a test of basic nutrition knowledge. The patients won."[11]

Since doctors generally have nothing to offer us once we shift our focus from treating disease to causing wellness, it is important to familiarize yourself with the elements of health. The following list of thirty-two key contributors to human well-being is a good start. Though there is no official order or ranking, I would venture to say that the first ten are actually indispensable—essential—for even a moderate level of true health.

## Fundamental Elements of Health
### Are You Thriving or Surviving?

Rate yourself, from zero to ten, in each of the following areas.

| Rating | No. | Element |
|---|---|---|
| 5 | **1.** | Clean, fresh air |
|  | **2.** | Pure water |
| 10 | **3.** | Foods for which we are biologically designed |
| 6 | **4.** | Sufficient sleep |
| 10 | **5.** | Rest and relaxation |
| 6 | **6.** | Vigorous activity |
| 9 | **7.** | Emotional poise and stability |
| 7 | **8.** | Sunshine and natural light |
| 10 | **9.** | Comfortable temperature |
| 10 | **10.** | Peace, harmony, serenity, and tranquility |
| 2 | **11.** | Human touch |
| 7 | **12.** | Thought, cogitation, and meditation |
| 2 | **13.** | Friendships and companionship |
| 4 | **14.** | Gregariousness (social relationships, community) |
| 4 | **15.** | Love and appreciation |
| 6 | **16.** | Play and recreation |
| 8 | **17.** | Pleasant environment |
| 5 | **18.** | Amusement and entertainment |
| 4 | **19.** | Sense of humor, mirth, and merriment |
| 8 | **20.** | Security of life and its means |
| 5 | **21.** | Inspiration, motivation, purpose, and commitment |
| 4 | **22.** | Creative, useful work (pursuit of interests) |
| 8 | **23.** | Self-control and self-mastery |
| 10 | **24.** | Individual sovereignty |
| 0 | **25.** | Expression of reproductive instincts |
| 9 | **26.** | Satisfaction of the aesthetic senses |
| 8 | **27.** | Self-confidence |
| 6 | **28.** | Positive self-image and sense of self-worth |
| 10 | **29.** | Internal and external cleanliness |
| 8 | **30.** | Smiles |
| 6 | **31.** | Music and all other arts |
| 7 | **32.** | Biophilia (love of nature) |

The big-picture approach that I espouse is based on this simple concept: "It is always better to correct a problem—to remove its cause—than it is to supplement or suppress it." Nutrition is a very complex field of endeavor, and it is easily misunderstood and misinterpreted, just as the forest can become invisible when looking at individual trees.

With 80/10/10, I endeavor to give a new interpretation of nutritional information, one that is not designed to incite fear in an attempt to stimulate product sales. By putting the parts together into one simple but complete package, I hope that nutrition will become a less daunting subject. True health is within everyone's grasp, but it is necessary to see the big picture.

This radically different view is unpopular, because it does not generate any revenue. The 80/10/10 approach uses no repeat products, no supplements, no high-priced, elitist "superfoods." 80/10/10 uses a simple grocery-store approach to nutrition that brings this program easily into the grasp of everyone.

## Weight Watching: The Ultimate in Shortsightedness

Shifting this discussion to body weight, I think of how sad I feel when I see people who are obsessed with losing (or gaining) weight, to the exclusion of their well-being and vitality. Myopically focused on body image, they consume all manner of nutritional experiments, with little if any regard for possible consequences.

Despite our wishful thinking—and advertising to the contrary—our digestive system is more than just a pleasure tube that eventually eliminates whatever indigestible concoction we filled it with. Our bodies replace the vast majority of our cells within seven years or less. Some, such as the cells that line the mouth and digestive tract, are replaced daily. In a very real sense, the foods we eat are constantly in the process of becoming "us."

***What would be the point of losing weight while compromising your health?***

Given this fact, wouldn't you want to ensure that every bite you take is made of the highest-quality raw materials (pun intended) from which to build the "you" that you are becoming? What would be the point of following a diet that compromises your health in the process? Is it worth ruining your kidneys, heart, or liver just to lose or gain weight, especially when you can achieve your goal without causing such damage?

Youth is forgiving; we can eat practically any abomination for some period of decades with no apparent adverse effects. But eventually, the statistics say, virtually all of us have to admit to ourselves that the gig is up. Eating garbage to look thin, consuming fat to gain weight, stimulating ourselves to artificial highs through supplements that give us "energy," and relieving one discomfort while unknowingly creating another, simply have not gotten us where we wanted to go.

Herein lies the paradox: losing weight, feeling good, even ridding ourselves of intractable diseases, does not necessarily mean we have become healthier. Heroin users feel good. So do coffee drinkers. So too do superfood evangelists. Junk-food-eating entertainers, anorexic runway models, and supplement-pounding body builders may look good...but are any of these people nourishing their bodies on a cellular level? Are they eating whole, unrefined foods in the quantities and proportions on which their bodies were designed to thrive? Absolutely not.

## Where Diet and Health Meet

I struggled with how to position this book, debating with several colleagues whether 80/10/10 referred to a weight-management plan or a healthy eating guideline. As you may have guessed, it's really a bit of both.

I have spent the last several pages driving home the differences between fragmented thinking and the big-picture perspective for one purpose: to cement in your mind the obvious and inextricable relationship between the goals of weight management and healthful living.

If you picked up this book looking for guidance in losing or gaining weight, rest assured, you have come to the right place. Yet I hope I have succeeded in persuading you that a perfect-looking body is not really all you want. Shifting your focus to your health will speed you toward optimal body weight, I promise ... but chances are you will feel so great that your appearance will take backseat—a mere sideshow to the vital main event your life has become. Eating healthfully does not represent deprivation; having our health destroyed—literally taken away by the mouthful—that is deprivation. People say, "Everything in moderation." I suggest that foods that are good for us are good only in moderation, but that the foods that are harmful to us should be avoided, regardless of the dose.

***Whole foods are always more nutritious than their refined counterparts. This includes all supplements.***

Some say, "It is a sickness to try to eat too well." I suggest that it is a sickness to intentionally do anything that is self-destructive. I believe it is time that we all started loving ourselves a lot more, and that we demonstrate that love by nourishing our bodies with foods that love us back.

My goal in writing this book is to provide a definitive resource for those who want to reach for the sky. I am committed to having it all in life, and I want that for my loved ones, my clients, and my audiences, as well.

In these pages, I define healthful nutrition and summarize some relevant information about carbohydrates, proteins, and fats and their roles in our bodies. I describe the 80/10/10 diet, my low-fat, low-protein program based on eating whole, fresh, ripe, raw, organic, plant-based foods. I teach how to improve your diet in a gradual, easy way. Finally, I share numerous testimonials from people who have transformed their lives by following this program.

Rather than coming out against fat or any other dietary choice, my intention is to give voice to what has proven to be the healthiest choice in the world of food and nutrition. I am convinced that the 80/10/10 plan meets human nutritional needs as well as can be hoped for in our modern world.

# Chapter 1
# Determining Our True Dietary Nature

How does one determine the correct food for any given creature? Let us suppose that you were given a baby animal and you had no idea what it was or what it was supposed to eat. Perhaps it was a gift from a foreign land. How would you know what to feed it?

The answer is relatively simple. All you would have to do is offer the creature different types of foods in their whole, natural state. That which it was designed for, it would eat. It would likely ignore all the other items, not even considering them as food. I have done this successfully with orphaned animals that I have saved.

The same technique would work with a human child. Put the child in a room with a lamb and a banana. Sit back and watch to see which he plays with and which he eats. We can be fairly sure of the outcome. Try again with fats versus fruits by offering a choice of (natural, raw, unsalted) nuts, seeds, avocados, or olives on the one hand and any fresh sweet fruit on the other. Again, we can safely predict that the child will choose the sweet fruit.

## Aren't We Carnivores?

Our anatomy, physiology, biochemistry, and psychology all indicate that we are not carnivores. To say that carnivores eat carnage or flesh does not accurately portray such creatures. Animals that live on other animals usually eat raw meat, straight from the carcass, with relish. Carnivores consume most of the animal, not merely the flesh, eating the muscle meat as well as the organs and lapping up the warm, fresh blood and other bodily fluids with gusto. They delight in the guts and their partially digested contents. They even crush, split, and eat the smaller bones and their marrow and gristle (collagen or cartilage).

Dogs, for instance, require far more calcium than humans, for animal flesh is extremely acid forming. The calcium (an alkaline mineral) in blood and bones offsets the acidic end materials of flesh foods. They also require much more protein than humans do.[12] When you note the vigor with

***Humans do not enjoy devouring bones, gristle, entrails, raw fat and flesh, and bits of hair and vermin.***

which dogs devour whole animals, you can be sure that what carnivores need for their nourishment is quite delicious to them.

Most of us love animals as fellow creatures on Earth. We do not salivate at the idea of crushing the life out of a rabbit with our bare hands and teeth, and the thought of eating one in a freshly killed state is repulsive. We certainly do not enjoy chewing on bones, gristle, entrails, chunks of raw fat and flesh, and the hair and vermin that inevitably accompany them. We can not imagine slurping hot blood, getting it all over our faces, hands, and bodies. These behaviors are alien to our natural disposition and are actually sickening.

***Put a child in a room with a lamb and a banana. Note which one he plays with and which one he eats.***

The sights and smells of the slaughterhouse and even the butcher shop are those of death. Many people find them unspeakably abhorrent. Slaughterhouses are so objectionable to most people that no one is allowed to visit. Even the employees find slaughterhouse conditions impossible to make peace with. Slaughterhouses have the highest employee turnover rate of any industry. Meat eating does not fit in with our concepts of kindness or compassion. There is no humane way to kill another creature.

We kill our animals by proxy, finding the actual carcass or corpse to be a thing of disgust. The vast majority of adults agree that if they had to kill the animals in order to eat, they would not eat meat ever again. We disguise animal flesh by eating only small cuts of the muscle and some organ meats. Even then, we prefer to cook them and camouflage them with condiments.

We disguise the reality of meat by changing the names of the foods from what they really are to something more acceptable. We do not eat cow, pig, or sheep, but rather eat mutton, pork, ham, beef, steak, and veal. We do not speak of eating blood or lymph, but we salivate at the thought of a "juicy" steak. We distort reality even further by giving animal qualities to our natural foods. Hence we refer to the "skin" of the fruit, eat its "flesh," dig out the "meat" of the nut, and even slice the "cheeks" or "shoulders" off fruit when we cut two sides away from the pit. These animal allusions minimize the horror of eating true flesh, but those of us who have not been desensitized are still aware of it.

## The Evidence

When we weigh the evidence, we see that too many considerations exist in physiology, anatomy, aesthetic disposition, and psychology for us to even seriously entertain the notion that we were designed to eat flesh. By the time you finish this chapter (substantially derived from the writings of T.C. Fry), I think you will agree that human beings simply are not equipped to be carnivores.

| **Humans vs. Carnivores**<br>The following is an incomplete list of the major differences between humans and carnivorous creatures. | |
|---|---|
| **Walking** | We have two hands and two feet, and we walk erect. All of the carnivores have four feet and perform their locomotion using all fours. |
| **Tails** | Carnivores have tails. |
| **Tongues** | Only the truly carnivorous animals have rasping (rough) tongues. All other creatures have smooth tongues. |
| **Claws** | Our lack of claws makes ripping skin or tough flesh extremely difficult. We possess much weaker, flat fingernails instead. |
| **Opposable thumbs** | Our opposable thumbs make us extremely well equipped to collect a meal of fruit in a matter of a few seconds. Most people find the process effortless. All we have to do is pick it. The claws of carnivores allow them to catch their prey in a matter of seconds as well. We could no more catch and rip the skin or tough flesh of a deer or bear barehanded than a lion could pick mangos or bananas. |
| **Births** | Humans usually have children one at a time. Carnivores typically give birth to litters. |
| **Colon formation** | Our convoluted colons are quite different in design from the smooth colons of carnivorous animals. |
| **Intestinal length** | Our intestinal tracts measure roughly 12 times the length of our torsos (about 30 feet). This allows for the slow absorption of sugars and other water-borne nutrients from fruit. In contrast, the digestive tract of a carnivore is only 3 times the length of its torso. This is necessary to avoid rotting or decomposition of flesh inside the animal. |

| | |
|---|---|
| | The carnivore depends upon highly acidic secretions to facilitate rapid digestion and absorption in its very short tube. Still, the putrefaction of proteins and the rancidity of fats is evident in their feces. |
| **Mammary glands** | The multiple teats on the abdomens of carnivores do not coincide with the pair of mammary glands on the chest of humans. |
| **Sleep** | Humans spend roughly two thirds of every 24-hour cycle actively awake. Carnivores typically sleep and rest from 18 to 20 hours per day and sometimes more. |
| **Microbial tolerance** | Most carnivores can digest microbes that would be deadly for humans, such as those that cause botulism. |
| **Perspiration** | Humans sweat from pores on their entire body. Carnivores sweat from the tongues only. |
| **Vision** | Our sense of vision responds to the full spectrum of color, making it possible to distinguish ripe from unripe fruit at a distance. Meat eaters do not typically see in full color. |
| **Meal size** | Fruit is in scale to our food requirements. It fits our hands. A few pieces of fruit is enough to make a meal, leaving no waste. Carnivores typically eat the entire animal when they kill it. |
| **Drinking** | Should we need to drink water, we can suck it with our lips, but we cannot lap it up. Carnivores' tongues protrude outward so they can lap water when they need to drink. |
| **Placenta** | We have a discoid-style placenta, whereas the carnivores have zonary placentas. |
| **Vitamin C** | Carnivores manufacture their own vitamin C. For us, vitamin C is an essential nutrient that we must get from our food. |
| **Jaw movement** | Our ability to grind our food is unique to plant eaters. Meat eaters have no lateral movement in their jaws. |

| | |
|---|---|
| **Dental formula** | Mammalogists use a system called the "dental formula" to describe the arrangement of teeth in each quadrant of the jaws of an animal's mouth. This refers to the number of incisors, canines, and molars in each of the four quadrants. Starting from the center and moving outward, our formula, and that of most anthropoids, is 2/1/5. The dental formula for carnivores is 3/1/5-to-8. |
| **Teeth** | The molars of a carnivore are pointed and sharp. Ours are primarily flat, for mashing food. Our "canine" teeth bear no resemblance to true fangs. Nor do we have a mouth full of them, as a true carnivore does. I am reminded of one of Abraham Lincoln's favorite retorts: "If you counted a sheep's tail as a leg, how many legs would it have?" Invariably, people would answer, "five." To which Lincoln would respond: "Only four. Counting the tail as a leg doesn't make it one." |
| **Tolerance for fat** | We do not handle more than small quantities of fat well. Meat eaters thrive on a high-fat diet. |
| **Saliva and urine pH** | All of the plant-eating creatures (including healthy humans) maintain alkaline saliva and urine most of the time. The saliva and urine of the meat eating animals, however, is acidic. |
| **Diet pH** | Carnivores thrive on a diet of acid-forming foods, whereas such a diet is deadly to humans, setting the stage for a wide variety of disease states. Our preferred foods are all alkaline-forming. |
| **Stomach acid pH** | The pH level of the hydrochloric acid that humans produce in their stomachs generally ranges about 3 to 4 or higher but can go as low as 2.0. (0 = most acidic, 7 = neutral, 14 = most alkaline). The stomach acid of cats and other meat eaters can be in the 1+ range and usually runs in the 2s. Because the pH scale is logarithmic, this means the stomach acid of a carnivore is at least 10 times stronger than that of a human and can be 100 or even 1,000 times stronger. |

| | |
|---|---|
| **Uricase** | True carnivores secrete an enzyme called uricase to metabolize the uric acid in flesh. We secrete none and so must neutralize this strong acid with our alkaline minerals, primarily calcium. The resulting calcium urate crystals are one of the many pathogens of meat eating, in this case giving rise to or contributing to gout, arthritis, rheumatism, and bursitis. |
| **Digestive enzymes** | Our digestive enzymes are geared to make for easy fruit digestion. We produce ptyalin—also known as salivary amylase—to initiate the digestion of fruit. Meat-eating animals do not produce any ptyalin and have completely different digestive enzyme ratios. |
| **Sugar metabolism** | The glucose and fructose in fruits fuel our cells without straining our pancreas (unless we eat a high-fat diet). Meat eaters do not handle sugars well. They are prone to diabetes if they eat a diet that is predominated by fruit. |
| **Intestinal flora** | Humans have different bacterial colonies (flora) living in their intestines than those found in carnivorous animals. The ones that are similar, such as lactobacillus and e. coli are found in different ratios in the plant eaters' intestines as compared to those of the carnivores. |
| **Liver size** | Carnivores have proportionately larger livers in comparison to their body size than humans. |
| **Cleanliness** | We are the most particular of all creatures about the cleanliness of our food. Carnivores are the least picky, and will eat dirt, bugs, organic debris, and other items along with their food. |
| **Natural appetite** | Our mouths water at the sights and smells of the produce market. These are living foods, the source of our sustenance. But the smell of animals usually puts us off. Meat eaters' mouths water at the sight of prey, and they react to the smell of animals as though they sense food. |

## So ... What Kind of "Vores" Are We?

Despite the gross perversion of our instincts, they are still alive and well in most people and would reassert themselves should we be relegated back to nature. Therefore, this quest is to ascertain what we would eat in nature.

Our instinctive foods, the foods that helped to develop us to our magnificence, contain all that we need to thrive on. In this section, we inquire about the various types of foods we humans presently eat.

We will evaluate whether each type is an appropriate food for us based on how that food occurs in nature without benefit of cooking equipment, tools, and containers. Remember, your instincts will reject or embrace each food on its merits—that is, its appeals to your senses and palate—the only criteria that guided our food selection in ages past.

Our premise is that Nature served us correctly to start with. We recognize that we thrived and attained our high station, and that what was right for us then is still right for us now, as we are structurally and physiologically the same as we were during most of our sojourn as humans in nature. It is logical that, within our modern context, we can supply ourselves with natural foods.

### *Are We Herbivores?*

Herbivores, or vegetarians, are natural consumers of greenery such as grass, weeds, leaves, stalks, and stems. A broader definition of "vegetarian" includes anyone who eats only plant-derived foods. Typical vegetarian foods may include a preponderance of fruits and greens but, in practice the designation vegetarian means that one eats anything and everything besides animal flesh.

Does foraging in nature for grass, weeds, and leaves appeal to you? Do these items attract your eye, tantalize your sense of smell, and excite your palate? Of course not, for the simple reason that they cannot satisfy your needs. You do not secrete cellulase or other enzymes that break down these plants as herbivores do. Therefore you cannot derive your foremost need from them—namely, simple sugars—which are your body's primary fuel. Rather, the processing and problems caused by their ingestion occasion a net loss of energy.

***What would we eat in nature, without the use of fire, containers, tools, or refrigeration?***

Humans do consume green leafy plants such as lettuce, celery, spinach and the like, as well as the tougher cruciferous vegetables (beets, broccoli, cauliflower, cabbage, collards, kale, and others). Eaten plain, as they occur in nature, these tough vegetables are high in insoluble fiber and therefore difficult for us to digest. Although we can cultivate a taste for them, they really hold only a moderate appeal to us.

All vegetables yield (to the extent digested) proteins, some essential fatty acids, mineral matter, vitamins, and some simple sugars. But if we get enough of these nutrients from our natural foods, then these are not needed from plants that we do not eat raw with keen relish.

So, the answer is yes—humans are biologically equipped to supplement their diets with a wide variety of plant-based "vegetarian" substances. Though we include vegetables in our diets, we're not primarily vegetable eaters by nature. And the divergent array of foods we commonly classify as such are not by any stretch of the imagination our primary ideal, natural source of fuel or other nutrients. Obviously, we're not herbivores.

### Are We Starch Eaters?

Starches can be divided into three general categories: grains (grass seeds), roots and tubers, and legumes.

**Grains.** Creatures that naturally eat grains, which are the seeds of grasses, are called "granivores." A similar term, "graminivore," refers to species whose primary diet consists of grasses. Many birds in nature live on the seeds of grasses and weeds. Included among the thousands of grass seeds that exist throughout nature are wheat, rice, oats, rye, and barley—all of which humans developed as a result of their mastery of nature only within the last 10,000 years.

Of course, in nature we would all reject grass seeds as foods. First, they grow in a form we can neither chew nor digest. Grain-eating birds possess a "crop," a pouch in their throats or gullets, where the grains they swallow whole are allowed to germinate, thereby becoming digestible. Grains are indigestible raw, but even cooked, the complex carbohydrates in them require great digestive effort to break down.

Heavy on starches, grass seeds such as wheat berries would gag us if we attempted to eat the equivalent of a spoonful or two (assuming we could gather them, and remembering that they would have their husks intact, as we would have to eat them in nature) Further, eating a tablespoon of raw flour made from the seeds of any cereal grain would also produce a gag response because it is so dry.

Thus, even though most of the human race presently consumes grains and starches, we can reject them as natural human fare. The fact that grass seeds neither attract, tantalize, nor arouse us in their raw natural state should amply indicate to you that we were not granivores in nature before we mastered fire. Instead of being a palate-tingling delight, these complex-carbohydrate foods in their natural state are a torturesome affair.

***Grass seeds (grains) consumed in their natural form would gag, not tantalize us***

**Starchy roots and tubers.** Animals that grub for roots and tubers are anatomically designed for the task: they have snouts; humans do not. Without tools, humans are very poor diggers. Further, they have no motivation to dig, for there are no foods below ground that, in their natural state, please the palate, and very few exist that our digestive systems can even handle. Some roots, notably turnips, rutabagas, sweet potatoes, yams, beets, carrots, parsnips, and salsify can be eaten raw, though in practice today, next to none are eaten this way.

Humans generally abhor dirt, are quite fastidious, and refuse to eat anything covered in or even tinged with dirt. Hogs and other grubbers pass lots of dirt through their bodies.

In nature, with only handmade tools and without cooking apparatus, we would have to eat roots raw or not at all. In our natural habitat, abundant in our preferred foods, we can be sure that the roots that man could handle without tools received precious little attention as food. In view of these considerations, you can write off humans as natural root grubbers.

**Legumes.** Very few creatures other than birds and pigs readily consume legumes, as legumes in their mature state are indigestible and/or toxic to most mammals. For humans, raw mature legumes are not just unpalatable, they are quite toxic. We simply have no capacity for consuming them in their natural state. Many creatures eat young legumes quite greedily. Pigeons and other birds actually eat the entire legume plant, long before it has a chance to flower. While young legumes are edible and nontoxic, one must question their nutritional makeup.

Legumes are touted as excellent sources of protein, and their protein content is generally quite high. High protein levels are not necessarily a good thing, however, especially for humans, who seem to thrive best on a diet composed of less than 10% of calories from protein. As it is in flesh, dairy, and eggs, the protein in legumes is rich in the amino acid methionine, which contains high amounts of the acidic mineral sulfur.

The carbohydrate levels of legumes are also high enough to make them difficult to digest due to the high protein levels. Invariably when eating legumes, humans get gassy, an indication that their digestive processes have been compromised. The lack of vitamin C, an essential nutrient for humans, also makes legumes a very poor food choice.

From standpoints of taste, nutrition, digestion, and toxicity, legumes simply do not make a viable food option for humans.

To fully digest starchy foods—grains, roots and tubers, and legumes—an animal must produce large quantities of starch-digesting enzymes (amylases). Granivores, root grubbers, and legume eaters all secrete sufficient amylase to digest large quantities of starch. If you view a cow chewing on hay, salivary amylase is dripping into the field. In contrast, the human body produces salivary amylase (also called ptyalin) of extremely limited strength and in relatively low amounts, sufficient only to break down small amounts of starch, such as would be found in fruit that is not fully ripened. The body also produces small quantities of pancreatic amylase for somewhat limited starch digestion in the intestines.

When humans can freely eat starchy grains, roots, tubers, and legumes such as wheat, potatoes, and lentils in their raw state to satiation and proclaim the experience a gourmet treat, then both you and I might accede that we are starch eaters.

### *Are We Consumers of Fermented Foods?*

Substantially all Americans eat fermented and otherwise decomposed substances that are called foods. Most are derived from milk. Some are made from grains (especially the alcohols), fruits (wines and certain vinegars), legumes (especially the soy bean and its suite of putrefactive products), and decomposed meats.

**Carbohydrates** ferment when fungi and bacteria decompose them. Fermented carbohydrates produce alcohol, acetic acid (vinegar), and lactic acid, as well as methane and carbon dioxide.

**Proteins** putrefy (rot) when they decompose. Decomposed primarily by anaerobic bacteria but also by fungi (yeast) and aerobic bacteria, proteins produce as end products ptomaines (cadaverine, muscarine, neurine, ptomatropine, putrescine, and others), indoles, leukomaines, skatoles, mercaptans, ammonia, methane, hydrogen sulfide, and yet other toxic compounds.

**Fats** become rancid and repulsive when they oxidize and decompose.

Oddly, we discard fermented grapes, yet we drink their fermentation end product (wine). Odder still, most Americans consume with abandon something that never occurred in nature—a pathogenic putrefactive product called cheese. We make cheese by taking the casein portion of milk and rotting it with types of bacteria that yield by-products that many palates have come to appreciate. Cheese represents about all the decomposition products in a single package: putrefactive proteins, fermented carbohydrates, and rancid fats.

You need only to refer to a good dictionary to learn just how poisonous these substances are. Yet, Americans eat billions upon billions of pounds of cheese annually. To assert that all these poisons going into the system cause anything less than sickness, disease, and debility is misrepresentation. Tumors and cancer are often the result.

Given that humans could not consume these types of decomposed products in nature without tools and containers, we may safely categorize them as unnatural, and certainly not among the foods we would primarily use for sustenance.

### *Are We Sucklings of Animals?*

I doubt that humans ever directly suckled cattle, goats, mares, camels, sheep, and other animals. And, of course, the idea of doing this is obnoxious to our disposition.

The practice of drinking animal milk as a regular part of our adult diet is only a few hundred years old. Before the advent of the combustion engine, it was not possible to plow, sow, and harvest sufficient grain for most families to support more than just a cow or two. Giving cow's milk to children in lieu of mother's milk is also a relatively new practice that dates back only about two hundred years.

Certain Arabic and African peoples have used animal milk for millennia, but the amount used was extremely small. True, certain peoples, like the Masai, live substantially on milk and blood, but these are by no means our natural foods. They do so primarily for lack of other easily obtainable foods.

No other animals in nature drink the milk of another species; they know instinctively that the milk from their mothers is the perfect food to support their rapid growth and to provide the precise nutrient mix their developing bodies require. We are no more designed for cow's milk than for pig's milk or rat's milk or giraffe's milk . . . or vice versa.

***Cheese contains about all of the decomposition products in a single package***

Milk-drinking is pathogenic. If milk and milk products were discontinued today, millions of people would cease to suffer sicknesses and pathologies within a short period.[13] In fact, if this one dietary practice alone were discontinued, the hospitals would virtually empty out and physicians' waiting rooms would be mostly vacated.

Humans are most certainly designed by nature as sucklings—but only for their early years of life, and only of their own mother's milk. We would do ourselves an astronomical favor if we had the good sense to stop consuming milk after weaning age, as does every other milk-drinking creature on Earth.

## Are We Eaters of Nuts, Seeds, and Other High-Fat Plants?

There is no doubt but that early humans in nature did consume some nuts and seeds, though certainly plants create them for reproduction, not for consumption. The various types of seeds, most prominently grains, weeds, fruit seeds, and nuts (all nuts are seeds) have protective outer coatings that range in texture from fibrous to hard and woody. We do not have razor-sharp teeth and massive jaw power that squirrels use to extract nuts from their shells.

Both seeds and nuts are endowed with nutrients sufficient to initiate and sustain a certain minimum growth of their plants. As with all foods, we derive the greatest nutritional benefit from nuts and seeds when we eat them in their raw state. Heated fats and proteins are quite pathogenic—even carcinogenic. We should eat nuts raw or not at all.

Most people in modern society, however, have never tasted truly raw nuts and seeds. High in water content, genuinely raw nuts have a texture more like apples (in the case of almonds) or nut butters (in the case of macadamias). Virtually all commercially available nuts and seeds have been oven-dehydrated at "low" temperatures, (perhaps 160 F) often for days, to prevent them from going moldy, thus extending their shelf life.

***Truly raw nuts taste nothing like the "raw" nuts we buy in stores***

Unfortunately, our ability to digest nuts and seeds—whether raw, dehydrated, or heated—is rather poor. Ranging from about 55 to 85% fat, nuts and seeds are best eaten infrequently and in very small amounts. Even then, their breakdown into fatty acids, amino acids, and glucose requires a drawn-out process that takes hours. Fats may lie in the small intestine for several hours before the gallbladder secretes bile with which to emulsify (break down and liquefy) them.

In contrast, high-fat fruits like avocados, durians, akees, breadfruit, and olives are rich in easily digestible fats (when ripe). These fruits range in fat content from 30% of calories (durian) to 77% (avocado). Coconut meat, also high in fat (ranging perhaps 20 to 80%, depending on maturity), is easily digested in the jelly-like state but almost impossible to digest when matured and hardened.

Leafy greens and other vegetables, when eaten raw and fresh, contain a small amount of fatty acids in an easily usable state. However, some (primarily the cruciferous vegetables) contain unwanted toxic sulfur compounds. We derive our best predigested fats adequate to meet our fatty-acid needs from fruits and tender leaves.

Biologically we are not a species of fat eaters, but merely incidental eaters of fats. Although an occasional avocado or small handful of nuts and seeds is quite satisfying and complements our natural diet, we are primarily carbohydrate eaters.

### *Are We Omnivores—That Is, All of the Above?*

Of course, humans are omnivores in practice, with the aid of cook stoves, condiments, taste excitants, camouflaging seasonings, spices and so on. But, in nature, we could not do more than eat foods in season, and we would have to eat them in the raw state on the basis of their effect on our taste buds. Without tools, technology, packaging and containerization, and taste-masking agents, we would soon lose our omnivorous tendencies out in the wild … and wet, sweet fruit would look better and better every day.

## We're Frugivores!

In nature, humans would be frugivores only. A frugivore is a creature that lives primarily on fruits, with the addition of tender greens. (This includes the nonsweet seeded fruits we generally eat with vegetables, such as tomatoes, cucumbers, peppers, okra, zucchini and other squashes, and eggplant.) Like all animals, we can indeed survive (albeit less successfully) on a wide variety of foods. Nonetheless, our bodies are designed to thrive on a diet of mainly fruit.

Some people adopt a totally fruitarian diet, meaning they attempt to live exclusively on fruits, but I do not recommend this practice. Dark-green leafy vegetables provide minerals and other nutrients essential for optimum nutrition and health.

Nutritionally, fruit comes closer to satisfying all of our needs (including, of course, our desire for delicious soul-exalting fare) than any other food, as meat does for a carnivore. Fruits are replete with the nutrients our bodies require—in the proportions that we need them. Yes, some vegetables and other foods may have "more" of a particular nutrient or class of nutrients, but fruits tend to contain the types and quantities of nutrients our bodies require. More does not mean better.

Humans are sweet seekers by nature, designed to eat sweet fruits. Taste buds on the very tips of our tongues recognize sweet tastes. Most of us are attracted to sweet fruits in their raw state, regardless of what else our culture and circumstances dispose us to eat.

When ripened, fruits accommodatingly convert their carbohydrate components into glucose and fructose, simple sugars we can use without further digestion. Enzymes in the fruit convert proteins into amino acids and fats into fatty acids and glycerols. Thus, when we eat fruits, all we need do is savor their goodness.

### *Fruits and Tender Greens?*

You may have noticed that I described the frugivorous diet as one consisting primarily of fruits, with the addition of tender greens. Where do the rest of the vegetables fit into this picture?

This may shock you, but by every indication, our digestive physiology was designed to process the soft, water-soluble fibers in fruits and tender leaves, almost exclusively.

It is true that cruciferous vegetables like broccoli, cauliflower, kale, collards, Brussels sprouts, and cabbage are loaded with nutrients, including soluble fiber. But they also contain cellulose and other tough, difficult-to-digest fibers. These vegetables are best digested when eaten in their youngest and most tender state. For best results, they must be thoroughly chewed or mechanically predigested via the use of a blender or shredding device.

***Eat your vegetables— but make them the tender leafy kind.***

To assimilate completely, we need to digest completely, and every time we eat foods that are more difficult to digest, we compromise our nutrition and, over time, our health. To be sure, we are capable of swallowing vegetation that contains cellulose and other rough, insoluble fibers, but such foods put a great load on our organs of digestion and elimination.

Where health is concerned, we want to derive the greatest benefits while minimizing the detriments or outright harm. When we apply this idea to nutrition, we are looking for "enough" of the nutrients we need, not necessarily the most we can get. The indigestible fibers in the harder-textured vegetables are very difficult for our bodies to digest, relative to the soft, soluble fibers in fruits and tender leafy greens. Thus, they are not among our ideal foods.

## Our Senses Confirm

Imagine for a moment that you are about to eat some delicious piece of fruit—perhaps a grape, peach, melon, banana, apple, plum, orange, mango, fig, or berry … you choose the variety. Picture holding the fruit in your hand, admiring its beauty. You hold it to your nose and smell its sweet and distinctive fragrance. It tempts you to take a bite, but first you appreciate the fruit in your mind just a little more, increasing the pleasure. At this point, your mouth should be watering. The fruit requires no preparation; it is a finished product, ready to be consumed exactly as Nature prepared it. For humans, fruits attract the eye, tantalize the sense of smell, and taste divine in their raw, natural, ripe state.

Now, try the same thing again, this time imagining a field of wheat, or a herd of cattle, or a flock of birds in flight. Does your mouth water? When pressed to imagine themselves foraging for food in nature, even those who vehemently question the frugivorous disposition of man have to admit that they would choose little other than fruits. This does not mean we should eat fruits totally and exclusively in our present circumstances, but it does mean that, in nature, they would comprise the overwhelming majority of our food choices.

Allowing fruit to predominate in your diet makes succeeding on the 80/10/10 plan easier than any other approach to eating, raw or cooked. To develop the healthiest and sanest relationship with food, and in order to stick with a dietary plan that will work for you for the rest of your life, have all the fruit you care for to take you through your breakfast and lunch meals. Even your vegetable meals should begin with fruit, as much as you like, until you are certain that you will not crave sweets at the end of the meal.

# Chapter 2
# Meeting Fruit Concerns Head-On

*Do you know anybody whose candida was caused by eating fruit?*
*Do you know anybody whose diabetes was caused by eating fruit?*
*Do you know anybody whose cancer was caused by eating fruit?*
If eating fruit didn't cause these maladies,
why would you believe that avoiding fruit would correct them?

In spite of the fact that fruit has been treated as health food throughout history, condemning fruit has come into vogue in many circles of late. Invariably, when people hear me espousing a diet that is exceptionally high in fruit, they respond with a well-rehearsed litany of questions—the supposed "facts" about the many hazards of fruit eating.

Is there any truth to the allegations about the supposed evils of fruit? Let us take some time to look at a few of them.

## Fruit and Blood Sugar

The mistaken notion that eating fruit causes blood-sugar problems underlies most admonitions to steer clear of fruit, especially sweet fruit. Granted, high blood sugar does lead to candida outbreaks, chronic fatigue, hyper- and hypoglycemia, diabetes, and a host of other conditions and diseases, even cancer. "Too much" sugar is indeed bad for you, though it is almost impossible to get too much sugar from the consumption of fresh fruit. Eating fruit is not the cause of blood sugar problems … it's just not that simple.

I know what I am saying sounds counterintuitive. It is something like telling people that osteoporosis is not a calcium problem (see "The Dangers of Eating More Than 10% Protein" on page 110). Nevertheless, both are true: taking in more calcium cannot alone shore up brittle, osteoporotic bones … and fruit sugar alone does not cause high blood sugar. Stick with me, if you will, while I explain the real cause.

***It is almost impossible to get too much sugar from eating whole, fresh fruit.***

Eating a diet of mostly fruit, including generous amounts of fresh sweet fruit, does not create high blood sugar … not when you are eating a low-fat diet, that is. When the system is not gummed up with excess fat, the sugar from even "high-glycemic" fruit moves easily in and then out of the blood. Blood-sugar levels in a healthy individual do not vary much in spite of changes in the diet.

## Glycemic Index and Glycemic Load

The glycemic index ranks carbohydrate foods based on how quickly they break down during digestion and thus how quickly their sugars enter the blood. Essentially, the glycemic index tells you how quickly carbohydrates turn into blood sugar. However, it doesn't tell you how much of that carbohydrate is in a serving of any food. Both items of information are essential in order to understand a food's effect on blood sugar.

That is where the concept of "glycemic load" comes in. Used in conjunction with the glycemic index, glycemic load information more accurately predicts the extent to which a food elevates blood glucose than does the glycemic index by itself. This is because by definition, the glycemic index measures carbohydrate *quality* but not *quantity.*

The glycemic load is calculated by multiplying a food's glycemic index value by the amount of available carbohydrate per serving (grams of carbohydrates less fiber), then dividing by 100.[14] Thus, fruits, which are mostly water, have a low glycemic load even though they rate high on the glycemic index. For example, bananas rate 52 on the glycemic index (where glucose = 100). But because water accounts for 75% of the weight of a banana, its glycemic load is only 12 (52 x 24 grams of carbs, divided by 100 = 12; based on a 118-gram medium-sized banana). *All fruits fall into the low or medium categories on glycemic load/glycemic index charts (with the exception of watermelon, whose GI ranks barely high).*

It is best to eat fruit fresh, as drying and dehydrating both concentrate fruit sugars to an unnatural level that the body is not designed to handle. It is also important to eat fruit whole, not juiced, as the fiber in fruit slows sugar absorption to its natural speed. In all cases and with all foods, whole, fresh, ripe, raw, and unprocessed is the way to go.

As you will see in the upcoming pages, the speed at which sugar enters the blood is not really the most important factor. When fruits are eaten whole, with their fiber intact, as part of a low-fat diet, their sugars do indeed enter the bloodstream relatively quickly. But then they also exit just as quickly, making them the ideal food, one that provides the perfect fuel for human consumption.

The American Diabetes Association says, *"The use of added fructose as a sweetening agent is not recommended; however, there is no reason to recommend that people with diabetes avoid naturally occurring fructose in fruits, vegetables, and other foods."* [15]

**Glycemic Index/Glycemic Load**[16]

A comparison of common foods (listed in order of glycemic load)

| Food | Glycemic Index (GI)<br>Low 1-55 · Med 56-69 · Hi 70+ | Glycemic Load (GL)<br>Low 1-10 · Med 11-19 · Hi 20+ |
|---|---|---|
| **Fruits (120 grams)** | | |
| Strawberries | 40 | 1 |
| Watermelon | 72 | 4 |
| Cantaloupe | 65 | 4 |
| Peaches | 42 | 5 |
| Apples | 38 | 6 |
| Pineapples | 59 | 7 |
| Grapes | 46 | 8 |
| Bananas | 52 | 12 |
| **Starchy vegetables, grains, and other complex carbohydrates (serving sizes vary)** | | |
| Carrots | 47 | 3 |
| Beets | 64 | 5 |
| Bran cereal | 42 | 8 |
| Popcorn | 72 | 8 |
| Corn, sweet | 54 | 9 |
| Whole wheat bread | 71 | 9 |
| Wild rice | 57 | 18 |
| Spaghetti | 42 | 20 |
| White rice | 64 | 23 |
| Cous cous | 65 | 23 |
| Baked potatoes | 85 | 26 |
| Sweet potatoes | 61 | 27 |

## Fat, Not Fruit, Causes Blood-Sugar Problems

The raw food movement is renowned for its use of great quantities of nuts, seeds, avocados, olives, flax and olive oil, coconuts, and other high-fat foods. On a high-fat diet, whether cooked or raw, people experience nutritional deficiencies, plummeting energy, hormone imbalances, intense cravings, and mood swings … everything goes haywire, not the least of which is blood sugar.

The mechanism that causes blood sugar to rise out of control is actually very easy to understand. Let's begin with a highly simplified description of how our bodies process sugar.

### Sugar's Three-Stage Journey Through the Body

To be used as fuel for our cells, the sugars we eat travel a three-stage journey through our bodies:

**Stage 1:** Sugars start out in the digestive tract when we eat them.

**Stage 2:** They pass through the intestinal wall, into the bloodstream.

**Stage 3:** They then move smoothly and easily out of the bloodstream and into our cells. This occurs rapidly, often in minutes.

When we eat a high-fat diet, the sugar gets trapped in stage 2, and the body works overtime, sometimes to the point of exhaustion and disease, in an effort to move the sugar out of the bloodstream.[17] Meanwhile, the sugar backs up in the blood, creating sustained, elevated blood sugar that wreaks havoc on the body in the form of candida, fatigue, diabetes, etc.

### *The Role of Insulin*

What happens in the presence of fat that causes sugar to pile up in our bloodstream? It has to do with the pancreas. Under the direction of the brain, the pancreas is responsible for producing a hormone known as insulin. One of insulin's roles is to function as a doorman, allowing sugar molecules in the blood to find an insulin receptor in the blood vessel wall. The insulin can then transport the sugar molecule through the blood vessel membrane to the interstitial fluid (the fluid between the cells) and continue to escort sugar across another barrier—the cell membrane—and into the cell itself.

In the body, fat provides many needed insulating functions, including conserving body heat, absorbing shock, preventing too much water from escaping through the skin, and protecting nerve fibers. But excess dietary fat in the bloodstream creates some negative insulating effects. When we eat too much fatty food, a thin coating of fat lines the blood vessel walls, the cells' insulin-receptor sites, the sugar molecules, as well as the insulin itself. These fats can take a full day or more to "clear" from the blood, all the while inhibiting normal metabolic activity, and preventing these various structures from communicating with each other.

Thus, too much fat in the blood impedes the movement of sugar out of the bloodstream. This results in an overall rise in blood sugar, as sugars continue to travel from the digestive tract (stage 1) into the blood (stage 2) but cannot escape from the blood so they can be delivered to the cells (stage 3), which await their fuel.

## High-Fat, Low-Carb Diets Raise Insulin Levels[18]

The entire theoretical framework of low-carb diets, like Atkins and The Zone, hang upon the notion that insulin is the root of all evil. In the view of their promoters, one needs to limit carbohydrate intake in order to limit insulin release. What they overlook is that protein- and fat-rich foods may induce substantial insulin secretion as well. For example:

- A quarter pound of beef raises insulin levels in diabetics as much as a quarter pound of straight sugar. (Diabetes Care 7 (1984):465)
- Cheese and beef elevate insulin levels higher than "dreaded" high-carbohydrate foods like pasta. (American Journal of Clinical Nutrition 50 (1997):1264)
- A single burger's worth of beef, or three slices of cheddar, boost insulin levels more than almost two cups of cooked pasta. (American Journal of Clinical Nutrition 50 (1997):1264)

In fact, the American Journal of Clinical Nutrition article referred to above reports that meat, compared to the amount of blood sugar it releases, seems to cause the most insulin secretion of any food tested.

A study done at Tufts University, for example, presented at the 2003 American Heart Association convention, compared four popular diets for a year. Out of the four (Weight Watchers, The Zone Diet, the Atkins Diet, and the Ornish Diet), Ornish's vegetarian diet (almost all carbohydrates) was the only one to significantly lower insulin (27%), even though that's supposedly what The Zone and Atkins (very little carbohydrates) diets were designed to do.[19]

Eating a high-fat diet, cooked or raw, contributes not peripherally, but directly and causally to all of the misleadingly named "blood-sugar metabolic disorders." Given this new perspective, one might more accurately classify these diseases as "lipid metabolic disorders."

### But What About Those Live Blood Analyses?

It is true. Raw food experts give lectures, write books, and travel with convincing stories, slide shows, and videos that support their stance against fruit. How can it be denied? Right there before our eyes, they show us pictures from their dark-field microscopes. We can see for ourselves the misshapen, cloudy, fungus- and yeast-infected blood cells of real patients who were so misguided as to eat a diet high in fruit!

Their "scientific" information seems conclusive: Fruit is clearly the culprit in blood-sugar problems for raw fooders. But let's step back for a minute: Take a look at the high-fat recipes in the books, newsletters, and websites of those so quick to tell you to avoid fruit. Note the fat-laden foods they serve guests at their institutes, retreats, and rejuvenation centers. Pay attention to the rich tasty morsels they serve up at food demos and festival booths.

Nuts, seeds, and avocados all run 75% fat or more, as a percentage of their calories. Oils are 100% fat. It takes very little of these foods to push us way over the edge in terms of blood fat. And raw fooders, as I will demonstrate, do not eat "very little" of these foods.

*Are you starting to see your raw diet and your intolerance for fruit in a new light?*

### Timing Is Not Everything

Unfortunately, taking care to avoid sugar/fat combinations at the same meal is not sufficient to alleviate blood-sugar problems. Eating a high-fat diet creates elevated blood sugar whenever fruit and other sweets are eaten, regardless of timing. Here's why:

Sugars require little time in the stomach. Immediately upon putting a simple sweet fruit into your mouth, some of the sugars are absorbed into the bloodstream from under the tongue. Fruit eaten alone or in simple, well-chosen combination on an empty stomach requires only a few minutes in the stomach before passing to the small intestines, where the sugars can be quickly absorbed. Most of the sugar from fruit travels from the intestines, to the bloodstream, and then to the cells where they are needed within minutes of its consumption.

Fats, however, require a much longer period of time, often twelve to twenty-four hours or more, before they reach their destination, the cells. In the stomach, fats are subjected to a digestive process that usually takes several hours. When they finally do proceed to the small intestine, they are absorbed into the lymphatic system, where they often spend twelve hours or more before passing to the bloodstream. Most important, fats linger in the bloodstream for many hours longer than do sugars.

On a high-fat diet, therefore, the bloodstream always contains an excessive quantity of fat, and more is coming in at almost every meal. Essentially, even when you eat a fruit meal alone and wait hours before eating fat, those sugars are likely to mix in your bloodstream with the fats you ate the day before.

This is the primary reason raw fooders experience digestive difficulties, malaise, "spaciness," and blood-sugar disorders whenever they eat fruit. When your diet is predominated by nut pâtés, seed cheeses, and flax crackers, it's no wonder you're told not to eat fruit. Whether or not we eat fruit in the presence of such tremendously high levels of fat, we set ourselves up for health problems and inability to remain raw.

### Sugar + Fat = High Blood Sugar

Too much sugar in the blood is as life threatening as too little, and both are dangerous for human health. Unfortunately, the fruit-phobic "experts" focus on the wrong portion of the equation, keeping raw fooders so busy avoiding fruit that they somehow miss the fact that they are eating *more* fat than our friends who eat standard American fare. In Chapter 8, I outline just how much more.

## Fruit and Chronic Fatigue

"How could the consumption of fruit be connected to chronic fatigue," I wondered years ago, after hearing about the millionth person tell me that is what they had heard. After all, fruit is considered "energy food," isn't it? I researched the physiology of chronic fatigue a little more deeply and was intrigued by what I found.

When pancreatic function is sluggish, as happens when the pancreas is fatigued or overused, the adrenal glands serve as a backup mechanism. The adrenals produce the hormone epinephrine (adrenaline), which stimulates pancreatic function and effectively increases insulin production.

As I described in the previous section, abnormally high fat exists in the blood for several hours every time we eat a high-fat meal. As blood-fat levels rise, the "normal" level of pancreatic function is simply insufficient to clear sugars from the bloodstream. Eventually, if we eat a high-fat diet for a long enough period of time, the pancreas begins to fail at producing sufficient insulin to maintain healthy blood-sugar levels. Rather than the typical gentle rise-and-fall fluctuations in blood sugar, we begin to experience increasingly higher peaks and deeper valleys. Blood-sugar levels become unstable due to the overconsumption of fat in the diet.

This sets up a situation where most of us rely upon adrenal-assisted pancreatic function virtually every time we eat, placing constant excessive demands upon both our pancreas and adrenals. This adrenal/pancreas relationship was designed for what is known as the "fight-or-flight" response, an appropriate reaction to potentially life-threatening conditions. This response would rarely be called upon if we lived in a natural setting, where, for example, we might occasionally reach the top of a hill at the same time as a bear with cubs, but from opposite sides.

In today's world, however, we experience more adrenal-triggering responses than we did in yesteryear. They seem to come hourly instead of weekly. Almost every time we drive a car in the city, we experience at least one close call worthy of some degree of adrenal response.

### *We're a Society of Adrenaline Junkies*

As a society, we have very much become adrenaline junkies. We are addicted to stimulation, and rely upon our next "fix" constantly. From the shock of the alarm clock and our morning coffee, to the newspaper headlines and the extreme behavior on daytime talk shows, to movies, spectator sports, and "reality" television shows designed to evoke intense emotions, to restaurant meals that are promoted more for their excitement value than for their nutrition, straight through the day till the eleven o'clock news that is filled with stories of death and destruction, we just keep calling for more adrenaline. Should there be a gap in the "action" we feel sleepy, a sure sign of exhaustion. We are literally living in a state of constant adrenal fatigue.

This excessive adrenal demand, coupled with the high stress of our American lifestyle, result in such extreme overuse of the adrenals that they eventually begin to fail.

The symptoms of severe adrenal failure are referred to collectively as "chronic fatigue" in the United States, or ME (myalgic encephalomyelitis) in Europe. Of course, many signs and symptoms usually lead up to chronic fatigue; it rarely comes as a complete surprise. Lack of motivation, malaise, reliance upon stimulants, excessive need for sleep, and bouts of mononucleosis are all indications of varying degrees of adrenal fatigue.

### *The Sugar Highs of Children*

The adrenal response also plays a key role in what commonly happens to children at birthday parties. They eat generous portions of extremely sugary foods, and shortly thereafter they are running about wildly, literally out of control and almost out of their minds. What happens, and why doesn't it happen to adults?

The answer is rather simple. Young children do not drink coffee, smoke cigarettes, use alarm clocks, or watch the eleven o'clock news. Life for them is interesting, full, and never dull. They have a higher level of vitality than most adults, meaning that their adrenal glands still function well. They are, however, on the same high-fat diet as adults.

Thus, when children eat great quantities of sugar on birthdays, Halloween, and other occasions, they set off a particularly vigorous version of the chain reaction I have described in this chapter. The fats remaining in their bloodstreams from their previous day's meals block insulin function just as effectively as they do in adults. Then their young and not-yet-exhausted adrenal glands "kick in" with a jolt, releasing a good amount of epinephrine. The next thing you know, the children are running wild.

Adults do not show such a response because they simply no longer have the vitality to do so. Their adrenal glands are so fatigued that they require a true and serious emergency in order to function at all. Do not blame the children for running wild. Epinephrine is not to blame either, nor is the sugar.

Children on a low-fat diet do not show this same out-of-control response when permitted to eat great quantities of sugar. It is the fat, more than the sugar, that is the culprit for their hyperactivity. In the same way, fat—not sugar—is responsible for the ever-increasing incidence of chronic fatigue syndrome (by whatever name) that we see in the U.S. and the world today.

## Fruit and Candida

The candida issue is riddled with more misinformation than perhaps any other area in health care. It requires a bit of unraveling to make sense of the true candida picture, as there is so much that needs to be unlearned.

Candida is a form of yeast, an organism that naturally occurs in human blood. It is supposed to be there. This microbe consumes sugar for its food. As there is always sugar in the blood (when diabetics check their sugar levels, they are actually monitoring the amount of sugar in the blood), there is always food for the candida organism.

### *Candida Eats Excess Blood Sugar*

The size or "population" of the candida colony in the blood is directly determined by its food supply. If blood-sugar levels are always at a normal level, so is the size of the candida colony that lives in the blood. When the sugar we eat leaves the blood to be distributed and used by the cells of the body, any excess yeast quickly dies off, as it is supposed to.

Should blood-sugar levels rise, however, the candida organisms multiply rapidly ("bloom") as they consume the excess sugar. Once they have done so and blood-sugar levels come back down to normal, so does the number of candida microbes. This ebb and flow happens as a normal part of human physiology and causes no health problems or uncomfortable symptoms.

If fat levels stay chronically elevated due to a fat-rich diet, sugar remains in the bloodstream and feeds the large candida colonies instead of feeding the 18 trillion cells of the body. Starved for fuel, these cells can no longer metabolize energy. You become tired, and feel rundown.

It is important to understand the implications of a rise in the blood-sugar level. If the body is not able to reestablish normal blood-sugar levels, a dangerous situation exists. The only mechanism that remains for bringing the blood sugar back down is the candida.

The candida microbe in our blood is actually a life-saving organism, one that we do not ever want to eradicate. It functions as another backup system—a safety valve that helps to bring the blood-sugar level back down to normal in the event that the pancreas and the adrenals fail at doing so.

### Causing Our Own Candida

As I have described, most people create the conditions that cause pancreatic and adrenal fatigue constantly, throughout the day and at every meal. It is therefore no surprise that candida issues plague people until they actually change their lifestyle habits. Outbreaks of candida are your wakeup call—a warning that your system is rapidly approaching diabetes, and that you would do well to drastically curtail your fat consumption or face dire health consequences.

Once again, the standard advice from the health community, traditional or alternative, tends to be seriously off base. Comprehending only symptomology and not the underlying fat-based cause, they tell us to avoid all sugar, including fruit. But fruit consumption did not cause the candida problem, and avoiding it will not address the real issue.

***Candida is a life-saving microbe, one that we do not ever want to eradicate.***

Granted, once you have gotten yourself into the candida quandary by overconsuming fat, eating sweet-tasting fruits may seem to exacerbate your problem. But eliminating fruit will not remove the cause of your problem, just the symptoms. In the presence of too much fat in the blood, even a small amount of sugar, from any source, can result in abnormally high blood-sugar levels. Furthermore, to the extent that conscious attempts to lower blood sugar succeed, you feel tired. Trying to eliminate candida by controlling a blood sugar problem inevitably fails, which is why we see thousands of people battling candida for years without lasting success.

Because all carbohydrate, fat, and protein that we eat is converted to simple sugar (glucose) if it is to be used by the cells for fuel, the way out of this cycle is not to eat less sugar, but to consume less fat. When fat levels drop, the sugar starts to get processed and distributed again, and the yeast levels drop because there is no longer excess sugar available for it to eat.

The candida microbe is extremely short lived. If folks suffering from candida would simply follow a low-fat diet, most of them would find that their candida issues were completely gone in a matter of just a few days. Of course, they may still have the underlying pancreatic and adrenal fatigue issues to resolve. Health comes only from healthful living.

## Fruit and Diabetes

As I mentioned in the introduction to this book, the U.S. Centers for Disease Control predicts that our incidence of diabetes will more than double by 2050. And here is another recent statistic, perhaps the most startling of all: From 1990 to 1998 alone, the incidence of diabetes in individuals between 30 and 39 years old increased by 70%![20] Before we discuss how these staggering numbers can be true, and how the underconsumption of fruit contributes to them, let me outline in briefest detail this disease called diabetes.

Five percent of diagnosed diabetics are designated "Type 1," (formerly "juvenile") diabetics. From birth, the pancreas of these individuals is unable to produce adequate amounts of insulin for the metabolism of glucose. Although glucose is present, it remains trapped in the bloodstream. The cells receive no fuel from carbohydrates to perform their necessary functions, because glucose requires insulin for entry. Thus, first among the symptoms of diabetes is malaise. You may have noticed that most diabetics complain of being extremely tired most of the time.

***Most Type 2 diabetics produce plenty of insulin. Dietary fat hinders its function.***

The remaining 95% of diabetics are classified as "Type 2" (formerly adult-onset) diabetics. In the vast majority of these cases, the pancreas produces adequate to excessive levels of insulin, but glucose is nonetheless unable to enter the cells. This is in large part a result of the high-fat American diet, which hinders the functioning of both natural and injected insulin.

Diabetics of both types endure an array of increasingly debilitating symptoms, ranging from frequent urination to unquenchable thirst, excessive hunger, sudden weight loss, weakness and fatigue, reduced concentration and coordination, blurred vision, irritability, recurrent infections, numbness in the extremities, and slow healing of cuts and bruises.

Unfortunately, the ravages of diabetes are by no means the end point on this slippery slope toward total health failure. Diabetics also face higher risks for heart disease, stroke, hypertension, kidney disease, gangrene, limb amputations, and blindness, among others.

All cellular function requires action to be followed by recovery, or inaction. Overtrain (or underrecover) a muscle group and it will degenerate rather than grow. The same is true for any organ. The pancreas cannot continue to overwork without showing signs of partial, and eventually, total failure.

## The Fat/Diabetes Connection

Given the horrors of this road to ruin, one would expect the masses to cry out for a solution to the growing epidemic of diabetes. Instead, we seem determined to seal the fate that the Centers for Disease Control has so ominously predicted. How do we ensure the outcome they foretell? We simply need to continue doing what we have done for over sixty years: eating a diet that is predominated by fat.

In this chapter, I have attempted to present a clear, if vastly oversimplified picture of the natural progression of events that we set in motion when we eat insufficiently of simple carbohydrates. Diabetes is but a natural stepping stone on the low-carb, high-fat path to health devastation. Although not all diabetics experience chronic fatigue and candidiasis, these conditions are manifestations of the same underlying condition—high blood fat.

This fat/diabetes connection is not something I fabricated, and it is not unrecognized in conventional medical circles. But its simple truth points to a condition far too easily and naturally remedied for the medicopharmaceutical cartel to want any part of it.

The correlation was documented as early as the 1920s:

**In 1927** Dr. E. P. Joslin of the famous Joslin Diabetic Center in Boston suspected a high-fat, high-cholesterol diet might contribute to the development of diabetes.[21]

**In 1936**, Dr. I.M. Rabinowitch of Canada presented 1,000 case studies demonstrating it to the Diabetic Association in Boston. In his presentation, he proved that the main factor inhibiting the metabolism of blood sugar in the presence of normal insulin was too much fat in the blood.[22]

**In 1959**, the Journal of the American Medical Association also documented this causal relationship between fat consumption and diabetes.[23]

**A 1979** article in the American Journal of Clinical Nutrition states, "Medical research confirms that up to 50% of people with Type 2 diabetes can eliminate diabetes risks and discontinue medication within three weeks by adopting a low-fat, plant food diet and regular daily exercise."[24]

**In 1998**, Duke University Medical Center researchers reported the findings of a study demonstrating that Type 2 diabetes can be completely reversed in mice by lowering dietary fat. The study showed that foods high in fat were responsible for the onset of diabetes in the mice, whereas sugar had no effect at all on diabetes symptoms. The press release states, "Without the fat, the diabetes does not occur, even in diabetes-prone mice. When the high-fat diet is stopped in mice that have been raised on it, the diabetes disappears."[25]

Many other researchers have corroborated this evidence, not the least of whom was Nathan Pritikin, whose work in the 1960s demonstrated that eighty percent of long-term diabetics put on a low-fat diet could be taken off their medication entirely in less than four weeks.

### Fruit Is Not the Culprit

As I have stated repeatedly, consuming fruit does not cause blood-sugar problems, but overeating fat does. If you remove the fat from the diet, in most cases blood-sugar levels return to normal, as does pancreatic functioning. Restricting fruit from the diet is not the cure. In fact, the opposite is true.

***When we eat low fat, the sugar in fruits passes easily into, and then out of the blood.***

Doctors tell us, "You have diabetes. You will have it for the rest of your life. And oh, by the way—you can no longer eat fruit." This certainly does not sound like a "healing profession" to me.

I have worked with many diabetics over the past twenty-five years. Of course, I guided each person individually, according to his or her unique history. Though I use no generic treatment plans, I do follow some general guidelines as I design each individual's program. In every instance, however, without exception, the use of a low-fat raw vegan diet predominated by sweet fruit has resulted in stabilization of blood-sugar metabolism. Most of my clients were able to completely eliminate their need for insulin and other related drugs within a few weeks or less. No one was ever harmed, and I have never seen any negative consequences resulting from these dietary changes.

### You Mean I Really Can Eat Fruit?

Sure, eating fruit raises our blood sugar, but so does eating other foods. Complex carbohydrates (cooked or raw) top the list of foods with the highest glycemic loads, meaning that they cause the largest and most rapid spiking of blood-sugar levels.

A healthy person who eats whole fruits (as a single-ingredient "monomeal" or in simple combination, as is recommended for all meals) will find that the sugar in fruits passes easily into, and out off the bloodstream in minutes, and causes no abnormalities in blood-sugar levels.

It is odd that we expect that fruit will give us problems but that complex carbohydrates and sugary desserts will not. It is reminiscent of the person ordering a hot fudge sundae with nuts, nougats, and whipped cream, who then says, "but hold the cherry, I am on a diet."

### Fruit and Triglycerides

Some people think that triglycerides (a type of blood fat) increase as a result of the elevated levels of blood sugar that occur when we eat fruit. This mistaken belief is what led Nathan Pritikin to shun fruit (and therefore forced him to sanction the consumption of complex carbohydrates, the only other substantial source of low-fat calories on a vegan diet).

However, by now you should understand that eating whole, raw fruit only results in sustained high blood sugar if you are also eating high fat. That is, elevated triglycerides cannot arise from a blood-sugar condition that does not exist. A high-fruit, low-fat diet has only a positive effect on triglycerides. Unfortunately, until Western scientists conduct studies of low-fat, high-fruit vegans, we remain without "proof" of this simple fact, other than that demonstrated by the health and elevated physical performance of the people following such a diet.

## Fruit and Cancer

More than a trillion dollars has been spent on cancer research during the past three decades. Our longstanding "War on Cancer" has brought us no closer to a cure for cancer today than we thought we were thirty years ago. Cancer is proving to be a disease of lifestyle, environment, and culture, and not a condition caused by a microbe, germ, or genetic factor. The "multifaceted causation theory" is gaining more popular acceptance, yet researchers continue to look for one specific cause.

Almost every cancer research organization worldwide is supportive of the consumption of fruit. It borders on amazing to think that a few relatively untrained individuals would come out suggesting that fruit is detrimental to cancer patients. What is more amazing is that people would pay attention to such individuals and even follow their suggestions by eliminating fruit from their diet. Yet somehow a popular notion among the mainstream warns that fruit is bad for anyone with cancer.

Worse yet, many misinformed raw food "experts"—theoretically the champions of fruit and vegetable consumption—parrot the mainstream directive to avoid fruit ... a travesty that produces emaciated, unbalanced, binge-prone raw fooders who give the movement a poor reputation.

Some allegedly scientific studies have concluded that uncontrollable and often unhealthy weight loss is associated with the raw food diet and with the consumption of fruit. The findings of these small-scale studies have strengthened the mainstream notion that fruit is bad for anyone with cancer concerns. Unfortunately, the researchers who designed many of the studies possessed extremely limited understanding of raw food nutrition, and they reached their conclusions after studying subjects who were also essentially inexperienced with the raw food diet. Few if any of these studies have examined successful or long-term raw fooders.

The standard American diet tends to result in unwanted weight gain. Fruit consumption helps to bring weight toward a healthy normal level (one that can appear unhealthfully low to those accustomed to living among a population of mostly overweight and obese individuals). Later in this book, I devote an entire chapter to the topic of body weight, including a detailed discussion of the relationship between a high-fruit diet and body weight.

### Does Fruit Counteract Cancer Treatment Procedures?

The "success" of both chemotherapy and radiation treatments depends upon a lowering of immune function in the body. Medical professionals know that people with suppressed immunity can tolerate treatments that are otherwise completely unthinkable.

In pursuit of this goal, Western medicine sees fit to assault the beleaguered patient with immunosuppressive drugs. Healthy immune function works against the doctors' efforts. Without the suppression of immune function (essentially the lowering of vitality), patients would have such acutely severe negative reactions to these "treatments" as to make them intolerable.

Recognizing the immunity-strengthening qualities of fruit, I have heard of instances where doctors recommend against its consumption for the very people who need it most. Naturally, the real solution is to work with patients to build vigorous health so they never find themselves in the intractable predicament of choosing between their vitality and their life.

This is merely another example of the fragmented view of health. When medical professionals have their blinders on, seeking only to eradicate disease with no mind toward creating overall health in their patients, they produce bizarre and deadly short-sighted solutions.

The use of immunosuppressant drugs has been cited by some scientists as an actual cause of our current epidemic of immunodeficiency diseases. Unfortunately, the pharmaceutical industry today wields more power over public opinion than perhaps ever before in history.

## *Does Fruit Acidify the Cancer Patient's Body?*

Cancer has been associated with an acidic condition in the body. No one has established whether this acidity is a cause of the cancer, a body-generated defensive "effect," or simply an unrelated condition that accompanies the true cause(s) of cancer.

***Predominance of alkaline minerals are the primary factor in an alkaline system.***

Many people mistakenly assume that the sugar in fruits, and especially the acid in "acid fruits," will acidify the body. The chemistry of digestion demonstrates that this is not so. The mineral content of a food is the primary determining factor as to whether the food produces an alkaline or an acid reaction in the body. Once the food has been digested, if acid minerals predominate, as they do in meats and most nuts and seeds, for instance, the food will be said to have an acid reaction in the body, or to be "acid-forming."

Since alkaline minerals predominate in almost all fruits, including the acid fruits, it is safe to say that fruit has an alkalizing effect upon the body. Fruits may not be as alkalizing as greens, but their reputation as acidifying foods is unfounded.

Cancer researchers have demonstrated that when cells in a petri dish are bathed in an appropriate nutritive environment and the toxic waste products of their metabolism are efficiently removed, healthy cells result. To date, it has not been possible to cause cancer in these healthy cells no matter which carcinogens they are briefly exposed to.

We can translate this good news to humans, for whom the high-fruit 80/10/10 diet represents, in my opinion, the ideal "appropriate nutritive environment" in which to bathe the cells of our bodies. We cannot, however, expect to eat acid-forming foods like cooked proteins, heated oils, and fried chips and remain cancer-free just because we also eat large quantities of fruit and greens.

## Acid-Alkaline Balance

Most of our body fluids and cells require a neutral to slightly alkaline environment (a pH reading in the high-six to low-seven range) in order to be healthy. By design, even if we live and eat very healthfully, our cells tend to acidify due to normal daily activities and stresses. Nature in her infinite wisdom set it up so that our natural diet of alkalizing raw fruits and vegetables would neutralize those acids.

If the vast majority of our foods are alkaline forming, we can easily live in a state of balance, or homeostasis. (Meditation, yoga, biofeedback, and gentle exercise may reduce acidity somewhat, but have not been shown to actually alkalize the body). However, if we overwhelm our bodies with unnatural sources of acidity, there is no amount of raw fruit and vegetables that can compensate. What kinds of activities and practices acidify us in this way?

- Consuming cooked foods, heated fats, animal-derived foods, grains (cooked or raw), or more than a very small amount of nuts and seeds.
- Eating poorly combined foods, cooked or raw.
- Smoking or taking any drugs or stimulants, including caffeine.
- Drinking alcohol, carbonated drinks, coffee or tea.
- Lack of exercise, insufficient rest and sleep.
- Sustained stress, anger, fear, or other negative emotions.

Rather than eliminating the unhealthful foods and practices from their lives, some people fall prey to salesmen who claim that juicing greens or grasses or consuming highly concentrated "superfood" powders can provide enough concentrated alkalinity to counteract an acidic condition in the body. Juices and superfoods, none of them whole foods of our biological adaptation (despite marketing to the contrary), serve only to create further imbalances, however. Only healthful living results in health … there is no shortcut.

### *Does Fruit Feed Cancer Cells?*

Cancer cells, like all other cells, use glucose as their primary fuel. But it is not possible to starve cancer cells of their fuel without also starving all other cells, including vital brain, heart, liver, and kidney cells. Of course, to do so would be counterproductive and in fact, deadly.

Cancer cells thrive in an anaerobic environment, meaning one where the oxygen content is very low. Eating a high-fat diet decreases the oxygen content of the blood and tissues and creates an ideal environment for cancer cells to flourish. When we consume a diet such as 80/10/10, which is high in simple carbohydrates and water, we effectively raise the oxygen-carrying capacity of the blood, thus vastly reducing the likelihood that we will create cancer.

The point is not to try to starve the cancer cells of their fuel, as that would effectively kill the patient as well, but to create a well-oxygenated environment that is inhospitable to the creation and subsequent survival of cancer cells.

## Fruit and Acid Indigestion

The popular belief that fruit causes acid indigestion is another case in which a nutritional misconception has mushroomed out of proportion and acquired mainstream momentum. When a person eats a healthy, simple meal, it generally leaves the stomach rapidly, usually in less than an hour. Difficult-to-digest foods can be held in the stomach for twenty-four hours and longer.

***Our breakfast fruit does not cause acid indigestion. Last night's dinner does.***

When a person eats such foods for dinner, they are generally still sitting in his or her stomach the next morning. Should he then have fruit for breakfast, an extremely volatile and incompatible combination is formed, and acid stomach is often the result. Not surprisingly, most people then blame the fruit they ate for the acid condition they experience.

I call this the "kick the dog" reaction. Picture a man having a bad day at work, getting a speeding ticket on the way home, and then running over his child's bicycle as he pulls in to the garage. The dog rushes to greet him and puts his paws on the man's pant leg. The man then kicks the dog as if the dog had been the cause of his entire bad day. The dog was simply the last straw, but not the cause of the man's troubles. Similarly, fruit is not the cause of the indigestion problem but simply sheds light on the fact that a poor food choice was made the night before.

## Fruit and Tooth Decay

Funny thing about teeth—everybody's got them and almost everybody has problems with them. Ask a dentist what percentage of his or her patients have problems with their teeth because they ate too much fruit. The percentage will be so low as to approach zero.

People have problems with their teeth for a wide variety of reasons, including these three:

**Exposure to intense acids**, such as the phosphoric acid in soft drinks, tannic acid in tea, and the various acids in coffee erodes tooth enamel.

**Fluoride in the water supply** often results in eventual tooth decay (as well as other serious health problems). The late Dr. John Yiamouyiannis wrote and spoke with great courage and conviction about the significant dangers of fluoridation.[26]

**Excess acidity in the bloodstream** causes the body to seek stored alkaline minerals (primarily calcium) to neutralize the acids. Eating highly acid-forming foods like meats, dairy products, and grains elicits this intelligent bodily response. The acid minerals in these foods can eventually cause erosion of tooth and bone structure, as the body draws out calcium to neutralize them. (See "The Dangers of Eating More Than 10% Protein" on page 110).

Eating fruit, at least according to the old adage, "an apple a day keeps the doctor away," is actually good for your teeth. So what is it about dentists, teeth, and fruit that scares people? I think it is the fact that dentists don't really understand the relationship between nutrition and tooth decay all that well, yet they are asked to expound upon it daily.

One dentist told a friend of mine that the reason she was having such severe dental problems was that she ate too much fat. Another dentist told another friend that the reason for her severe dental problems was that she ate too little fat. I have heard dentists tell clients that they need to eat more carbohydrates, while others tell their clients to eat fewer carbohydrates. One dentist told me that I was going to have tooth worries if I ate any carbohydrate at all.

It appears that going to the dentist for nutritional information is not much different than asking your local auto mechanic for financial advice. Dentists eat and mechanics make money, but in neither case does that qualify them as experts in the field. Dentists are experts at repairing decayed teeth. Essentially they are construction workers who work on tiny job sites—filling potholes, building bridges, and the like. They are not specialists in nutrition or the biochemistry of the mouth.

### *Dental Hygiene Itself Is a Culprit*

So what exactly is it that results in tooth decay? Good evidence is emerging that much of today's tooth and gum disease is actually caused by the "preventative" procedures we have been taught to give our teeth. Aggressive brushing of the gums can wear them away, resulting in receding gums. Gums are soft and can decay quickly when treated roughly. Receded gums expose the roots of the teeth, which have no enamel and hence no protection from the acids in foods or those produced by bacteria.

Flossing the gums, rather than gently flossing only the spaces between the teeth, can also be detrimental. Improper flossing can irritate the gums and result in unnatural enlargement of the pockets between the teeth and gums. Food and microbes can then be caught in these pockets and wreak havoc on teeth.

***Everybody has teeth, and it seems everybody has issues with them. Is it the fruit?***

Even toothpaste can have a damaging effect upon the teeth. The particulate matter in toothpaste that is designed to scrub the teeth can eventually wear through tooth enamel. The particles in the toothpaste can lodge between tooth and gums, causing irritation and resultant inflammation. Conservative dentists today recommend using only a soft brush that has been wet with water to thoroughly clean teeth without damaging them.

### *Dehydrated Foods, Nuts, Complex Carbs, and Refined Sugars*

It appears that dehydrated foods have the most profound negative effect on teeth, in several different ways. Dried fruit qualifies as a refined carbohydrate, as the water has been removed from what was once a whole food. In this fractional form, fruit is extremely dry and sticky. It sticks aggressively to the first wet surface it contacts—your teeth. Stuck in the crevices, crannies, and corners of teeth, dried fruit will eventually be broken down by bacteria designed to do exactly that job.

***Dehydrated food, including "raw" nuts, produce tooth-damaging acids.***

The bacteria, unfortunately for your teeth, produce an extremely acidic metabolic waste product, and they excrete that waste directly onto your teeth. The acid in the bacterial "excrement" essentially dissolves your tooth enamel. This acid is extremely damaging to the roots of teeth, should any be exposed. Continued exposure to this acid will result in the development of tooth decay.

Nuts and seeds are rarely eaten fresh from the tree. In that state they have an extremely short shelf life at room temperature. To make raw nuts and seeds last longer, food packers dehydrate them so that they will not grow moldy on the shelf. Roasted nuts are even further dehydrated. When we eat nuts and seeds, small particles of them remain on and between our teeth.

The brain controls the pH (level of acidity) of the mouth by directing the type and amount of digestive enzymes secreted by the salivary glands. The pH of the mouth is usually in the alkaline range when we are in a healthy condition. After testing the saliva of hundreds of clients after they ate nuts or seeds, I have found that the mouth often becomes slightly acidic. This acid works to chemically break down the proteins in the nut and seed particles while it also adversely affects the roots and the enamel of our teeth. Once again, cavities eventually form.

Complex carbohydrates, as well as refined simple carbohydrates, stick to the teeth in a similar fashion to dehydrated fruit. The bacteria that digest the carbohydrates also produce acid waste products that corrode tooth enamel. Most complex carbohydrate foods are acid-forming foods.

### Fruits and Vegetables for Healthy Teeth

The solution to healthy teeth and gums is the solution to health overall. Healthful living has no contraindications. Whole, fresh, ripe, raw fruits and vegetables are excellent foods for teeth and gums. Our dental structure, as well as the rest of our anatomy and physiology, are all designed for fruits and vegetables.

Granted, someone could argue, "But what if you sucked lemons all day, wouldn't that be bad for your teeth?" Yes, sucking lemons all day long is likely to harm your teeth, but who would want to do that? Just use some common sense, and by all means—enjoy your fruit!

# Chapter 3
# Raw Food for Ultimate Health

Unheated or raw foods are the natural and optimal choice for the cellular health of all creatures. One of the major differences between people and the other animals on planet Earth is that we cook our food and they do not. Where our health is concerned, this is not a good thing.

Raw foods make a lot of common sense, and the sciences completely support the raw food concept. Unfortunately, the doctors and scientists who study nutrition, for the most part, are cooked food eaters, and they see the world through a cooked food perspective. They cannot see beyond their accustomed view to envision another approach. The very idea of a diet of all raw foods is unthinkable to most of them. Rarely do they even consider it.

These professional men and women spend a good deal of their time coming up with scientific arguments to support the way of life to which they are accustomed. Common sense does not support cooking, however, as not a single creature other than man cooks its food. In general, the animals that suffer from degenerative "human" diseases are domesticated or caged ones that are routinely fed cooked food by their human caretakers.

If we observe nature, we will find that all creatures are born with or develop everything they need to secure their natural food. No human has yet been born with a stove on his back or the keys to a tractor in her hand.

## The Folly of Cooking Food to Kill Microbes

Prior to and throughout most of the 19th century, fresh fruit was a very popular food item, and people did not eat the high percentage of cooked food that they currently do. In fact, the raw food movement was almost as big 120 years ago as it is today, if not more so. But the whole concept was essentially shot down with a single word: germs.

***The "germ theory of disease" is just that...a theory.***

After scientist Louis Pasteur (1822–1895) published his "germ theory of disease" in 1878, fear of microbes developed into a full-blown phobia for many people (one that lives on—and continues to grow—to this day). This fear led the medical fraternity to suggest that all foods be cooked, for the safety of the consumer. People began cooking their apples, their tomatoes …

essentially everything they ate. Due to the overwhelming power of doctors to influence society, cooking fruit became the norm.

Pasteur's untenable theory lives on as the foundation that underlies the medical model of disease and healing. Society accepts it as truth, despite the fact that it is fraught with inconsistencies. In more than one hundred years, the germ theory of disease has yet to be proved as fact … while having been disproved repeatedly by Koch's postulates.

## Koch's Postulates

The famous nineteenth-century bacteriologist Robert Koch set forth the following set of four logical rules, all of which must be satisfied to prove that a particular microbe or germ is the cause of a particular disease.[27]

1. The germ must be present in every case of the disease, but not in healthy subjects.
2. It must be isolated from the patient and grown in vitro (culture).
3. It must be introduced to a susceptible new host and in that host produce the original disease.
4. The same agent must be isolated once again from the experimentally infected host.

This line of logic, long held as the gold standard for identifying infectious diseases, is the minimal evidence necessary to have confidence in the existence of a pathogen and its causal link to a disease.

The germ theory of disease is destined to remain a theory forever, for it takes very little effort to find evidence refuting Koch's postulates. Here are two of the more obvious examples:

Healthy people often harbor the germs that are said to cause one disease or another, while remaining totally symptom free. This fact stands in opposition to postulate #1.

Conversely, many people with a given disease have been shown not to be hosting the alleged "causative agent," also refuting postulate #1.

The story of Pasteur's life and illustrious career is fascinating. After years of debate with colleagues, he is said to have capitulated from his deathbed, admitting that microbes are not the primary and sufficient cause of disease. Rather, he acquiesced, a toxic "milieu interieur"—the inner environment of the body in which the microbes live—provides a breeding ground for disease. In other words, regardless of the germ's origin or type, it presents far less threat than commonly believed, unless the body is in a run-down state resulting from a disturbed and deteriorated interior environment.

Maintaining our inner terrain in a healthy (undisturbed and undeteriorated) state of homeostasis is one of the key benefits we derive from eating a low-fat diet of whole, raw plant foods in their freshest, least processed form. Just as mosquitoes do not cause stagnant ponds and flies do not cause piles of manure, the "germs" (bacteria, viruses, and other microorganisms) around and inside of us do not cause the toxins in our bodies. Yet like mosquitoes and flies, microbes are more than happy to set up shop in toxic locations that provide them with plenty to eat.

***Germs do not cause disease ... at least not in the way we have been taught.***

If we drain the stagnant pond or clean up the manure pile, the mosquitoes and flies migrate elsewhere. Likewise, the viruses and bacteria that feed upon the toxic wastes inside of us simply move on and cease to be a problem when we clean up our diets and other sources of inner pollution. At this point, our bodies are no longer capable of acting as hosts for such pathogens.

To do justice to Pasteur's story, or to expound upon the fallacies of germ theory, are beyond the scope of this book. But you can find detailed accounts of both of these topics in many publications. One excellent source is a book by Ross Horne, entitled *Health & Survival in the 21st Century.*[28]

## What's the Big Deal About Cooking?

It is true ... people have been setting fire to their food for millennia, and we seem to be doing fine. So what's the big deal about cooking?

Experiments have shown that people can survive on diets as restricted as flour and water, at least for a period of time, but they cannot thrive on such a regimen. This is a testament to the nutritional reserves, resilience, and vitality of the body, not to the nutritional value of the food. The difference between "normal health" and actually thriving is vast.

### *Humans Have Not Been Cooking Long*

Historically, as pre-human hominids moved away from the tropics, they started eating the (cooked) flesh of animals and experimenting with foods such as (cooked) tubers and other complex carbohydrates to substitute for unavailable fruits and vegetables. Evidence tells us this practice has been going on for at least 200,000 years. However, it was only with the advent of grain agriculture, in the past 10,000 years, that we began deriving the vast majority of our calories from cooked carbohydrates.[29] Even if we have biologically adapted to this practice, it would be hard to argue that our basic digestive physiology, like that of every other creature on the planet, was designed for the raw foods found in nature. Any adaptations to the nutritional losses and toxins created by cooking foods could only be considered "devolution," rather than evolution.

In terms of human evolutionary history, 10,000 years is an extremely short period of time, not nearly enough for our digestive physiology to have adapted to the kind of wholesale degradation that cooking causes to our food. Physiologists suggest that it generally takes 50,000 to 500,000 years or longer for evolutionary change to occur. Even then, however, we could not adapt in a healthful fashion to the nutritional losses or the toxins created by cooking food.

***10,000 years of cooking is not nearly long enough to have adapted to it.***

Many foods that are cooked, such as meats and grains, would otherwise be unappetizing or inedible to humans. Cooking allows foods to bypass sensory safeguards that would normally protect us from ingesting unnatural and unhealthful substances. Essentially, cooking makes it possible for us to eat (and to call "good") food we would otherwise consider to have gone "bad." On certain rare occasions, cooking might enable us to sustain ourselves on the only foods available to us. To be sure, however, we pay with our health when we cook foods as a regular practice.

### High Fat

High fat content is another common problem with cooked foods. In particular, meats, grains, and other starchy foods often contain far more fat than is healthful.

The fat is not always visible, however. It is absorbed into starchy foods in the cooking process. Fried potatoes don't look fatty; we like to think of them as a carbohydrate food. Yet the average serving of french fries provides about half of its calories from fat. Apple pie, you would think, is all carbohydrate, right? It is made of sugar and apples and a grain-based crust, all high-carbohydrate foods. Think again, as this delicacy tips the scale at 50% of calories from fat. Not even a baked potato qualifies as a low-fat food, once we add butter or sour cream.

Fat is hidden in the structure of animal foods. The fat content of meat varies by cut, but the majority of meats are very high in fat.

### Toxicity and Disease

To varying degrees, the different methods of cooking introduce toxic substances that the body must eliminate. The repeated consumption of cooked food results in a detrimental enlargement of the pancreas, as well as damage to the liver, heart, thyroid gland, adrenals, and most other organs, as a result of toxic exposure combined with reduced oxygen availability.

Eating cooked food has also been shown to provoke degenerative changes in almost all aspects of blood chemistry. These changes usually reverse rapidly when exposure to cooked food is eliminated.

Studies have shown that our immunes system often reacts to the introduction of cooked food to the bloodstream the same way it does to foreign pathogens such as bacteria, viruses, and fungi: The body literally attacks the food, sending an army of white blood cells to do the job. This phenomenon, which has been linked with the eventual development of AIDS, does not occur when we eat raw foods.

A direct cause-and-effect correlation exists between the cooked food diet and American culture's two main killers, cancer and heart disease. Many of these relationships have been documented for decades, and the evidence is mounting. Obesity, too, is directly associated with cooking our food. Heated foods are nutritionally inferior, which is one of the reasons people commonly overeat cooked food. Their stomachs feel full, but their cells crave nutrients and remain nutritionally starved.

***Like Humpty Dumpty, a cooked food can never be what it was before.***

To escape the destruction of cooked food, one must be willing to recognize that, as a culture, we have been eating ourselves into poor health, early death, and disease ridden old age. Americans consume ever-increasing amounts of cooked, processed food while worrying about the sharp increase in obesity and juvenile diabetes and the staggering cost of their ever-increasing healthcare needs. Few people seem to be connecting the dots publicly, but as these problems become larger social issues, I predict they will soon hit critical mass.

### Cooking Damages Nutrients

The damage done to food when it is cooked provides enough material for a separate book. Cooking renders food a bit like Humpty Dumpty after he fell off the wall, in that once a food is cooked it can never be, nutritionally, what it was before. Foods can only withstand about as much heat as your hand—or the roof of your mouth—can take before their nutrients are irrevocably damaged. Let's take a look at some examples.

### *Protein*

It makes sense that we would want to derive the full nutritional benefit from the protein foods we eat. But few people realize that high-temperature cooking denatures the proteins in foods, fusing the amino acids together with enzyme-resistant bonds that preclude them from being fully broken down, thus rendering the proteins substantially useless—and in fact toxic—to us. All proteins that we consume must be broken down into single, individual amino acids before they can be of any use to us; our bodies cannot use "protein" for any purpose whatsoever.

#### Definition of "Denature"

Merriam-Webster's Collegiate Dictionary, Tenth Edition defines "denature" as follows (emphasis added):

de•na•ture verb transitive: to modify the molecular structure of (as a protein or DNA) esp. by heat, acid, alkali, or ultraviolet radiation so as to destroy or diminish some of the original properties and esp. the specific biological activity. 

Hair is primarily protein. A strand of hair can be rolled into a ball and then pulled back into a strand. However, if a strand of hair is rolled into a ball and then held over a candle flame, even for just a moment, chemistry happens. The hair literally attaches to itself in new places. It can never be returned to its original form as a strand. When an egg hits a frying pan, a similar irreversible chemical change takes place. Our digestive enzymes cannot easily break down coagulated protein molecules once they fuse together. The best they can accomplish is partial breakdown, into polypeptides.

The body recognizes clumps of partially broken down proteins, known as polypeptides, as foreign invaders to be attacked, contained, and eliminated through the kidneys. The cell walls of the kidneys do not allow for easy transport of these substances, and their buildup causes the distress that leads to kidney stones and eventually to kidney failure. Undigested proteins also produce allergies, arthritis, leaky gut syndrome, and other autoimmune disorders.

### Carbohydrates

We must heat starchy carbohydrates to "dextrinize" them, thus facilitating their breakdown into glucose. Unfortunately, heating caramelizes these complex carbohydrate foods, fusing their molecules into a sticky, molasses-like goo. (Dextrin and starch are the two principal vegetable-based adhesives, commonly used as glue for corrugated packaging and wallpaper.) The body can realize only perhaps 70% of the energy potential of cooked starchy foods.

This melting of sugar molecules occurs in carbohydrate-based foods subjected to cooking temperatures whether or not we witness it, and it causes them to produce an extremely high glycemic response in the body. Blood-sugar levels predictably spike after we eat cooked carbohydrate foods, especially grains that have had their fiber refined out of them. Heat the carbohydrates further and they will char, or blacken, as happens to burnt toast. This blackened carbohydrate is toxic, a known carcinogen.

***Heating fuses foods into molecules our digestive system cannot easily process.***

The digestion of cooked complex carbohydrates is typically impaired by the fatty and sugary foods with which they are consumed, leading to fermentation. The byproducts of fermentation are gas, alcohol, and acetic acid. Alcohol is a protoplasmic poison that kills every cell with which it comes into contact. Acetic acid in its pure form is a known poison. When diluted with 19 parts water, it is called vinegar. The acetic acid in vinegar is still toxic, regardless of dilution.

Of great concern, mainstream science is tying itself in knots over a lethal poison, called Of great concern is "acrylamide," recently discovered to be produced in high-carbohydrate foods by the chemistry of cooking. This potent chemical killer was found in high concentrations in the food supply in 2002 by a Swedish researcher. High levels of acrylamide are found most prominently in bread, chips, crackers, french fries, and other dry-cooked carbohydrates. See the FAQ entitled, "How important is it to eat organically grown food?" on page 257 for information about this grave toxin in the food supply.

### Fats

All manner of nutritional and health problems occur when fats are heated. Heated fats interfere with cell respiration, leading to cancer and heart disease. Heating fats also reduces the functional value of their antioxidant properties.

Once fats have been cooked, they quickly go rancid, at which point they become carcinogenic. Thus, it's important to understand that while even freshly roasted nuts are harmful for us, they become more so the longer they sit out. The longer fatty foods are exposed to oxygen, the more their nutrients become deranged. Keeping raw dehydrated fat-based crackers unrefrigerated for days or weeks (not to mention months or years!) is not such a good idea, either.

Many high-temperature methods of cooking (deep frying, broiling, roasting, barbecuing to a char, etc.) cause fats to produce carcinogenic substances including acrolein, hydrocarbons, nitrosamines, and benzopyrene, which is one of the most virulent carcinogens known to man. Frying temperatures range from about 400° to 1,000° F. When unsaturated vegetable fats and oils are heated to such temperatures (and especially when polyunsaturated oils are repeatedly reheated, as in fast-food deep-fry establishments), their naturally occurring "cis" bonds are converted to "trans" bonds, creating trans fatty acids. Trans fats are recognized as one of the most dangerous dietary health hazards of our time.

***Keeping dehydrated raw crackers unrefrigerated for days is not such a good idea.***

Food manufacturers "hydrogenate" unsaturated fats to extend shelf life and improve food texture by heating them and exposing them to hydrogen while they are under pressure. Ingested saturated fats are of no use to us, and they seriously clog arteries and capillaries, reducing oxygen delivery to every part of the body.

If you must eat heated fats, I implore you to begin reading food labels and steer clear of foods where saturated fat is more than 20% of the total fat. Also avoid foods that list any hydrogenated oils (partially or otherwise) among their ingredients.

### Water

In terms of volume, water is our greatest nutrient need—second only to oxygen. Cooking drives water out of food and alters it drastically. Dehydration oxidizes the nutrients in food, and their nutrient value is duly degraded. We cannot eat cooked or dehydrated foods and then make up for the water and nutrients lost by drinking water, juices, or any other "supplement." Doing so simply does not compare to eating a daily diet predominated by whole, water-rich foods. Fruits and vegetables are nature's perfect water filters, and the water within them is the purest available on Earth. All efforts to purify or "structure" our drinking water are merely attempts to replicate the water we were designed to ingest in our raw fruits and vegetables.

Ask yourself: Just how whole is a food that has had its water removed? Soberingly, the water in our foods is vital and definitely not to be considered expendable. We should feel duly concerned if high-water foods do not heavily predominate in our diet. Dehydrated raw foods and powdered "whole-food" supplements are not whole foods, nor are they as nutritious as their whole-food counterparts.

***Dehydrated raw foods and powdered "whole-food" supplements are not whole foods.***

### *Micronutrients*

Most other nutrients—vitamins, enzymes, coenzymes, antioxidants, phytonutrients, and fiber are damaged or devitalized by the heating process, leaving behind "foods" with substantially empty calories.

## The Lycopene Myth

Applying heat to foods provides no nutritional benefit and is detrimental to the person ingesting the cooked food. A few examples exist where, by heating food, certain nutrients are more easily released and more bioavailable to our cells. The lycopene in tomatoes and the iron and beta-carotene in vegetables are often-cited examples.

However, taking this viewpoint ignores the fact that hundreds of thousands of identified and not-yet-identified nutrients in the heated foods are damaged by the heat. For every nutrient that becomes more bioavailable due to the cooking process, countless other nutrients become less so. We don't know for certain, however, that even the ones that become more available are doing us any favors once altered by heat.

More important, this viewpoint assumes that more of a nutrient is better, instead of trusting that Nature has provided the perfect balance of nutrients we need for optimal health in the fresh, raw plant foods we eat.

## Benefits of Eating Raw

If you adopt a natural diet of raw foods, your body can easily cope with cleansing itself of past toxic accumulations and normalize its weight. Here are some of the benefits you can expect:

**Maximum nutrition:** Even those who never question the practice of cooking food have to admit having heard that we discard vitamins when we drain our vegetable cooking water. Sadly, vitamins are not the only nutritional casualty caused by setting fire to our food. To varying degrees, heating food for any appreciable amount of time above a comfortable eating temperature (approximately 105 F) damages most every category of nutrients. Western science is only beginning to recognize the nutritional damage done by the cooking of food.

**Detoxification:** A major benefit of eating unprocessed raw food is that the body's vital energy is freed up for healing and cleansing. When you stop eating cooked foods, you stop abusing your body at each meal with toxic, dehydrating residue that it must work hard to eliminate. When your liver and kidneys do less work detoxifying you, they are free to keep your system cleaner, making for a healthier body.

**Quick digestion:** A proper raw diet eliminates constipation, and the transit time of waste matter shortens to 24 hours or less, eliminating the toxemia that occurs as the colon recycles toxins. Most people on the standard American diet experience transit times of 72 hours or more, during which time their food ferments and putrefies inside them. The resulting foul gas and unpleasant-smelling feces highlight the putrefaction caused by anaerobic bacteria breaking down undigested proteins in the colon. These rotting proteins are said to lead to various forms of colon disease, including polyps, colitis, and cancer.

**Overall improved health and energy:** Many people on a raw diet (even the high-fat way) lose some excess weight and experience clearer sinuses, improved breathing, better sleep, clearer skin, less mucous discharge, increased energy, and heightened mental clarity.

### Additional Benefits of Eating Raw the Low-Fat Way

**Oxygenated cells:** Cleaner blood and healthier red blood cells better transport fresh oxygen to all the cells in the body, resulting in heightened mental clarity and allowing subtle healing to take place within the body that may not be easily noticed.

**Optimal body weight:** If you follow the raw vegan version of the 80/10/10 diet to the letter, including the elimination of all forms of salt and condiments, you will lose any remaining excess fat and water weight, but not healthy lean tissue. It's important to make sure you're eating enough calories, however, as foods with fewer calories per bite require more bites. (See Chapter 10, "Overcoming the Challenges of Going Raw" on page 159) If you need to put on weight, this plan supplies you with the fuel to undertake the weight-bearing exercise that adds muscle—which is something no food can do (see Chapter 9, "Stabilizing Body Weight" on page 147.)

**Ultimate well-being and vitality:** People who take their diets "all the way" to low-fat raw vegan (80/10/10rv) experience markedly fewer colds, flus, and aches than people who eat a high-fat diet, raw or cooked. Acne disappears, and permanent relief from persistent diabetes and candida symptoms finally occurs. More important, people on this program have the opportunity (given proper sleep, exercise, sunshine, and so on) to experience a quantum leap in overall physical, mental, and emotional health that surpasses the mere absence of disease or symptoms. The ultimate benefit is greater longevity and improved quality of life.

## Making the Transition

The switch from cooked to raw is actually a fairly easy one. It is simply a matter of increasing the percentage of raw foods in your diet. Some people find it easiest to begin by simply eating raw for breakfast while leaving everything else the same as always. When they get comfortable with that, they add in raw lunches as well. In time, the raw dinner becomes a realistic challenge. Other folks prefer to start meals raw but finish with cooked, gradually increasing the amount of raw food that is eaten at the beginning of the meal until finally they are eating some meals that are completely raw.

Eventually, you will come to love the raw foods and their effects upon the way you look and feel. Once you start to experience the results, your motivation level will rise dramatically, and it will become ever easier to continue increasing the percentage of raw foods that you eat.

At some point, you may begin to question why you are still eating the cooked foods at all. Sure, you love them; the question is, do they love you back? Cooked foods eventually show themselves for what they truly are: health destroyers. Though you may find that you have many emotional attachments to your cooked food, in due time you will come to no longer look at cooked food as a "treat."

## "Detox" Symptoms: Cause for Celebration

Many people experience temporary symptoms of detoxification when they begin a raw diet, as the body is no longer being overloaded each day with so much toxic residue. The symptoms arise as the body cleanses and heals naturally, releasing toxins into the bloodstream that may have been buried deep within tissues and organs for many years. The body is wise, however, and it always eliminates toxins in a way that requires the least effort and does itself the least harm.

***Detox symptoms are sure to be less severe than the dis-ease they would have become.***

Detoxification symptoms are generally mild but can range from uncomfortable to downright miserable. They are really a cause for celebration, however, as any discomfort in the present is sure to be less severe and of shorter duration than the dis-ease it would have become in the future.

Such symptoms often include tiredness, runny nose, headaches, digestive challenges, weight loss, skin conditions, and drops in blood pressure. Less common but not unusual are diarrhea, vomiting, and all manner of retracing phenomena (reexperiencing past symptoms to complete a healing process that was interrupted by medical intervention or other forms of treatment). All of these and other symptoms are indications that the body is making healthy adjustments.

Initially, intestinal gas problems may arise in people who have damaged digestive tracts. The intestines can hold food in little "outpockets," out of the main flow. There, stagnant foods may ferment or putrefy and cause gas. Over time, the gas will diminish as the intestines heal. Long-term gas problems on the raw vegan diet are generally corrected by being attentive to proper food combining.

Most of what is called "detox" is actually just the reaction of a body that is no longer being irritated or stimulated—effectively "forced" to function. The secondary effect of stimulation is sedation. Thus it is common to feel tired when a person first attempts the raw diet. It is not that the raw diet is making them tired; it is that they are actually "coming down" off of the influence of coffee, refined sugars, meats, and other stimulating foods.

### The Law of Dual Effect

The Law of Dual Effect states that those substances, influences, forces, and conditions to which the body is subjected result in two responses by the body:

- The primary effect is the more acute of the two, and the shorter lasting.
- The secondary effect is less intense, but it lasts longer.

When we drink coffee, for instance, the primary effect is one of stimulation. The secondary effect is only visible after the primary effect has worn off. In this instance, the secondary effect of coffee is to leave us even more tired than we were before drinking the coffee. With our fractured view of health, we tend to look only at the primary effect or acute influence of such a substance while ignoring the secondary effect or chronic influence.

Each person is unique; therefore, the duration and degree of detoxification will vary. Detox can be intense or mild, and can last from a few days to several years, depending on the individual's health, vitality, environment, and the degree to which one follows a healthy lifestyle.

We must also remember that we live in a constant state of retoxifying and detoxifying. In the course of our day, we absorb environmental toxins, and the body works to eliminate them. We ingest foods, even the best sort, and the body creates toxic waste as a result of its cellular metabolism. This toxin production is not cause for worry, however, because we are equipped with kidneys and a liver—eliminative organs designed to rid ourselves of these toxins. Should these organs become overloaded, the skin, lungs, bowels, mucous membranes, and other areas of the body are equipped to help handle the toxic load.

## Which Road Do You Choose to Travel?

Eating raw poses many challenges, of that there is no doubt. But the benefits of this way of eating so far outweigh the negatives that little room exists for argument against eating raw.

If we are honest with ourselves, there is simply no room for cooked food if we desire a vibrantly healthy existence. It is like any other journey. If you are going down the road that is taking you where you want to go, you will likely continue to follow it. If you find yourself going down a road that will not bring you to your desired destination, of course you will switch roads.

At your chosen speed, cooked food can increasingly become a thing of your past. There is no hurry; you can cross that bridge when you come to it. Even then, you are not making an irreversible decision. In any case, I guarantee that after a year of eating low-fat raw vegan food, should you choose to revert to your old style of eating, the high-fat cooked foods will still be available.

But don't be surprised if you discover that the 80/10/10 raw vegan diet is the sweet road to well-rounded health and happiness.

## Our Natural Diet: A Summary

In this age of junk food, manufactured foods, and agrochemicals, the issue of food quality has become increasingly important for those who seek long, productive, vital lives. The relationship of health to diet is becoming ever more profoundly obvious, and more and more people are looking to increase the quality of their food than ever before. The market for organically grown foods is growing rapidly, and farmer's markets are proliferating like never before as more and more of us are waking up to the necessity of a high-produce lifestyle for health and longevity.

Many years ago, the great health educator T. C. Fry, organized his thoughts on how to make the finest food choices and came up with these four excellent guidelines. I have reproduced these timeless words of wisdom here, as a fitting summary to this chapter.

## Criteria for Selecting the Highest-Quality Foods

**By T. C. Fry**

**First Criterion**

*Can the food be eaten in its natural state? Is the food palatable, that is, delectable or delicious? Can it be eaten with keen relish in its natural state?*

If a food cannot be eaten with joy and delight to individuals in normal good health who have an unperverted sense of taste, then the food must be considered to be of low quality. Eating should be a gustatory delight. If a whole, fresh, ripe, raw, organic food is a taste delight, it is perfect. Its quality is reduced commensurate with the reduction in taste.

If the food cannot be ingested in its natural state—that is, uncooked, unprocessed and otherwise untampered with—it does not belong in the human diet. We humans were for millions of years adapted to a diet obtained directly from nature in its fresh raw natural state. There have been no adaptations noted in human physiology to the consumption of cooked, processed, or otherwise devitalized foods. This determines the character of our diet and also the manner in which we were accustomed to ingesting it.

Therefore, cooking and processing foods to make them palatable is unacceptable to the health enthusiast. Cooking destroys enzymes totally. While a healthy individual will synthesize some 1,000 enzymes required for digestion, assimilation, and utilization of foods, the body is, nevertheless, dependent upon the enzymatic action of the foods for the most perfect digestion. Consequently, it is absolutely essential that our foods have their full complement of enzymes intact.

Cooking is the worst "health" practice that humans have ever adopted. It destroys not only the enzymes but deranges and destroys almost all known food factors. Cooking disorganizes, oxidizes and makes nonusable a food's mineral content. It deaminates the food's protein content, thus rendering it worthless in human nutrition. Cooking reduces the value of a food from its wholesome state all the way down to worthless ashes, depending on the degree of cooking to which it has been subjected.

To the extent that a food has been cooked—reduced to inorganic minerals, caramelized sugars and starches, coagulated and deaminated proteins, poisonous acrolein-laden fats, devitalized vitamins, and the like—

it is not only worthless, but the ash becomes toxic debris in the body.

That cooked foods are poisonous in the body is easily demonstrable. White blood cells function as janitors in the blood. A normal white count is around 3 million. If toxic substances enter the bloodstream, the white blood cell count will rise, rapidly and dramatically, in order to clean up the blood. After eating a cooked meal, the white count typically rises as high as 15 or even 18 million, and even higher. After eating a meal of raw fruit, there is usually no discernable rise in the white count. So the rule is this: If we can't eat the food "raw," if it is not delicious and palatable in its natural living state, it is not a food for us.

**Second Criterion**

*Does the food introduce harmful or toxic substances into our digestive system?*

If the food is proper to the human diet it must contain no noxious or unwelcome substances. We do not want poisons in our system, no matter how little or how "mild." Anything that interferes with vital activities or destroys cells and tissue is poisonous to our system.

*[Author's note: Since the time of this writing, science has progressed remarkably. We now know that various toxins exist even in the most preferable of foods. Terry was correct in his concept, however; just the wording was off. I believe that today he would likely replace the thought of "no" toxins with the reality of "the lowest possible amount."]*

**Third Criterion**

*Is the food easy of digestion and assimilation?*

Foods to which we humans are ideally adapted require a minimum of vital energy for their digestion and assimilation. To be of greatest value to us, foods must be efficiently digested and assimilated, granting, of course, that we have unimpaired digestive systems.

Humans have become highly efficient at digesting and assimilating foods to which they, in nature, became adapted. Millions of years of development made certain foods very easy of digestion—we developed constitutions, enzymes, and processes that appropriated, digested and assimilated certain foods with a minimum expenditure of vital resources and time.

The water and sugars of fruit, which make up almost its entire digestible portion, require virtually no digestion whatever. They simply require absorption. Shortly after their absorption, they are very easily and rapidly assimilated.

**Fourth Criterion**

*Does the food contribute a broad range of nutrients? Does the food possess great biological value for us?*

Though many foods are rather complete in their range of nutrients, none is suitable for a "mono diet" such as grass is for cattle. But most of the fruits and vegetables are quite suitable for "monomeals." And, certainly, if properly combined, these foods furnish all the nutrients we humans need.

The objective is not that we should eat a great variety in hopes of getting all the nutrients needed, but rather to eat simply to afford our bodies every opportunity to easily digest and assimilate what the foods offer. What does it matter the range of nutrients we put into our bodies if we ingest them in such manner as to vitiate and tax the digestive process? We can compromise digestion such that we fail to derive the goodness intended. Thus we would penalize our bodies and rob them of nutrients as well.

We should never take more than four or five foods at a single properly prepared and combined meal. Almost no preparation other than cleansing is necessary, but we must make sure to eat in strictly compatible combinations. The ideal is a single food per meal! There is no particular penalty in eating two to four different items at a meal if they are compatible in the digestive process.

To really simplify the digestive process and to assure ourselves of easy digestion on a continuing basis, we may select a rather narrow range of foods according to the season and stick with them. For instance, we may make one meal a day of just bananas with some lettuce and celery and another meal of a salad with citrus and nuts.

This can go on day after day in the winter season. In summer we might have melon rather consistently for just one meal and at a second meal of the day, mangos, peaches, or other summer fruit and a green salad with tomato. The objective is to eat a diet to which we are biologically adapted, that gives the highest potential for wonderful health.

Green leaves possess the highest and most complete range of micronutrients. This is one of the primary reasons we must have them often in our diet for the best health. Of course the body is provident—missing them on occasion is not particularly harmful and would not prove disastrous unless we missed them for some length of time, usually months or more.

While we do not spell out the nutrient contents of various foods—that knowledge not being necessary—we should plan our meals so that we receive the benefit of foods that complement each other in their nutrient contents essential in human nutrition. A variety of fruits and vegetables eaten throughout the year will easily guarantee nutritional sufficiency.

# Chapter 4
# Understanding the Caloronutrient Ratio

We get our calories from three sources: carbohydrates, proteins, and fats. I refer to these as "caloronutrients," a term my wife (who at that time was known as Professor Rozalind Gruben) and I coined. Thus, I refer to the proportion of carbohydrates, proteins, and fats in a person's diet as their "caloronutrient ratio." You will see these terms used throughout this book. For consistency, I list all ratios in my writings in the same order: carbohydrates/proteins/fats (CPF for short), separated by slashes. Thus, "80/10/10" is shorthand for 80% carbohydrates, 10% protein, and 10% fat.

## "Goldilocks" Nutrition

I believe we benefit from fat—and all other nutrients—in appropriate, moderate amounts. In this book, I propose that too much of a good thing (in this case fat) is as harmful, and in many cases much more harmful, than not enough. I call it the "Goldilocks" approach to nutrition: for best results, you don't want too much of any nutrient and you don't want too little; you want the amount to be "ju-u-ust right."

## 80/10/10 for Health, Beauty, Energy

That amount, I assert—at least in terms of caloronutrients—turns out to be 80/10/10: a minimum of 80% of your calories from carbohydrates, primarily from whole, sweet fruit, and a maximum of 10% protein and 10% fat.

***Not too much, not too little… ju-u-ust right.***

On the 80/10/10 plan, a person who eats 2,000 calories a day would shoot for approximately 1,600 of those calories to come from carbohydrates, 200 from protein, and 200 from fat. Naturally, not all sources of these nutrients are the same, and I have devoted much of this book to discussing just what forms those caloronutrients should take for best results.

After two decades of research, coaching amateur and professional athletes, and assisting health seekers worldwide, I have come to believe that 80/10/10 is the overall target for long-term health and dietary success. When we consume our food in this proportion—the one for which our species was designed—we enjoy glowing health, superb energy, and ideal body weight, effortlessly.

Sometimes in my lectures, I simplify this formula even further, referring to it in shorthand form as 811—as in "Dial 811 for the healthiest, trimmest you!" This short form is commonly used in conversation, e-mail, and my online discussion group, as you will notice in the testimonials in Appendix C.

## 80/10/10 for Longevity

Eating foods of low caloric density, such as fruits and vegetables, has been cited as a probable method of extending longevity. Experts in the field of human longevity have long held that refraining from overeating is the surest method of extending the lifespan, as it most effectively reduces the likelihood of obesity. Obese people live shorter lives, on average.

One very healthful method of not overeating is to increase caloric demand by raising activity levels while eating primarily fruits and vegetables, foods that are relatively low in calories per bite.

### Long-Lived Cultures Eat High Carbs, Low Fat

In John Robbins' book, *Healthy at 100: The Scientifically Proven Secrets of the World's Healthiest and Longest-Lived Peoples*, he describes the lifestyles and eating patterns of the long-lived cultures of Abkhasia (Russia), Vilcabamba (Ecuador), and Hunza (Pakistan). This table is taken from Robbins' book:

| | Abkhasia | Vilcabamba | Hunza |
|---|---|---|---|
| Percent of calories from carbohydrate | 69% | 74% | 73% |
| Percent of calories from fat | 18% | 15% | 17% |
| Percent of calories from protein | 13% | 11% | 10% |
| Overall daily calories | 1,800 | 1,700 | 1,800 |
| Percentage of diet from plant foods | 90% | 99% | 99% |
| Percentage of diet from animal foods | 10% | 1% | 1% |
| Salt consumption | low | low | low |
| Sugar consumption | 0 | 0 | 0 |
| Processed food consumption | 0 | 0 | 0 |
| Incidence of obesity | 0 | 0 | 0 |

The Abkhasians, Vilcabambans, and Hunzakuts have traditionally consumed high carbohydrates and little fat mostly out of necessity, eating strictly from the foods that have been available to them. They have done so naturally, without any science to guide them and without options for choosing or adjusting their caloronutrient ratio.

## The Ratio for Humans ... By Design

People ask me how the 80/10/10 diet can apply equally well to people of all ages, sizes, activity levels, etc. "Aren't we all individuals, with different nutritional requirements and different bodily makeups?" they ask.

Despite all the hype about metabolic typing, I do not believe this ratio varies to any appreciable degree on the basis of our individual needs. (See the FAQ entitled "What about individual differences?" on page 241)

Like high-performance race cars, the human body is designed to get its best results from a very specific fuel mixture. Think about it: Can you find any example in nature of a mammalian species whose individual members eat foods from completely different categories, based upon their blood type, their geographical location, their metabolic type, or any other factor? Can you imagine a "kapha" bear eating more fat than a "pitta" bear? Or a "fast-oxidizing" monkey avoiding bananas because they are too high in sugar? This is nonsense.

***Do not let anyone tell you that humans are the one exception in the animal kingdom.***

The fact is, Nature has seen fit to provide the ideal food for every creature on Earth, and all creatures of similar type eat similarly. For example, horses—and all creatures that look like horses (zebras, donkeys, mules)—eat from essentially the same category of foods—those for which their biological systems were designed. Do not let anyone tell you that humans are the one exception to this rule (called the Law of Similars) in all of the animal kingdom, for there are no exceptions: Animals that are anatomically and physiologically similar thrive on similar foods. Cows eat grass, leopards eat meat, and hummingbirds eat nectar. There is simply no need to complicate this simple program, presented in perfection by nature in thousands of examples.

All of the creatures that are anatomically and physiologically like us (known as the anthropoid primates: gorillas, orangutans, chimpanzees, and bonobos) thrive on a low-fat diet that is predominated by fruits and vegetables. Their caloronutrient ratios closely approximate 80/10/10. With the exception of the gorilla, whose great weight makes it almost impossible to climb the skinny branches of trees to procure fruit, they get more than 80%

of their calories from the carbohydrates in fruit. The combined caloronutrient average for chimpanzees, bonobos, and orangutans is about 88/7/5. Add in the gorilla's numbers, which come closer to 70% carbohydrate, and the average decreases, making the ratio almost exactly 80/10/10 for all of our anthropoid relatives.

The actual *foods* humans eat differ according to season, geography, availability, personal preference, etc., but not according to anything pertaining to our physiology. The total number of *calories* each person needs varies according to many factors, including gender, size, age, activity level, fitness goals, health status, and so forth. But the ratio of carbohydrates to protein to fats we need remains relatively the same. This is true regardless of the dietary specifics, food choices, or total volume consumed. As I explain in Chapter 5, no amount of adaptation or relocation has changed the basic digestive physiology with which we have been endowed since the beginning of time.

## Why Percentage of Calories?

In this book, I use "percentage of total calories consumed" as my primary model for discussing carbohydrate, protein, and fat consumption. Although this approach has its drawbacks, it is the best way I have found to help people gain perspective about, discuss, and compare the macronutrients they eat.

The scientifically accepted measure of food and nutrient consumption is mass (weight in grams, ounces, etc.). However, providing dietary guidelines in those terms requires unnecessary complexity that offers no incremental benefit. Many factors combine to determine the amount of food an individual should eat for optimal health and body weight, some of which are gender, age, height, muscle mass, amount and intensity of physical activity, digestive efficiency, food choices and, to a very limited degree, metabolic rate.

***The calorie model allows us to discuss caloronutrient intake for all of us at once.***

Using the percentage of calories model allows us to discuss appropriate carbohydrate, protein, and fat consumption, despite our individual differences. For example, both a sedentary woman who eats 1,600 calories per day and an athletic man who eats 4,000 calories per day will thrive eating in the 80/10/10 proportion. The only difference is that the former would eat far fewer calories than the latter.

I realize that most of my readers have never learned how many calories are in the foods they eat. And I concede that the calorie concept has its limitations. More than one person has aptly pointed out to me that not all of the calories we consume are used for energy. One person insists (and rightly so) that calorie-equivalent quantities of carbohydrate, protein, and fat cannot be considered identical (or even reasonably similar) where our digestive biochemistry is concerned. Technical detractors sometimes suggest to me that because we as humans do not actually burn our foods—as is done in a bomb calorimeter in order to determine a food's calorie content—we should dispense completely with the notion of calories.

I agree with these and other objections to thinking in terms of calories for diet analysis. Yet numerous peer-reviewed nutritional studies in the finest journals have seen fit to use the model, including those from top-caliber nutritional scientists like Dr. T. Colin Campbell of Cornell University. The World Health Organization and governmental nutritional agencies around the world use both percentage of calories and absolute amounts in grams to express their dietary recommendations. Even with its flaws, the calorie concept is the only generally accepted model of energy requirements that relates to everyday activity. With my background in exercise physiology, I have found the calorie concept particularly useful in helping athletes perform at their peak and get enough fuel.

### Pros and Cons of the "Percentage of Calories" Model

I am aware of the concern that people could be dangerously misled if they try to compare the caloronutrient ratios of foods with wildly differing caloric densities. Below is an example that highlights this potential confusion, followed by another example that illustrates why I nonetheless choose to calculate nutrients using the percentage of calories approach.

#### How Percentage of Calories Can Seem Misleading

Let's look at some numbers that could be confusing to those new to the calorie concept:

- Spinach contains 30% protein (30% of its calories come from protein).
- Macadamia nuts contain "only" 4% protein.

Given just this information, one might be led to believe that a pound of spinach provided more protein than a pound of nuts. However, knowledge of total calories, and not just percentages, is required to make sense of this data. A pound of spinach contains 104 calories (31 of which are protein) and a pound of macadamia nuts has more than 3,250 calories (125 of which are protein). In terms total calories, the nuts yield four times as much protein as the spinach.

**How the Calorie Model Is Useful**

Imagine that a person eats 7 pounds of food in a day, and only 3.5% of that weight consists of high-fat food. This sounds like a low-fat day, right?

Not hardly. Let's look at a simple example of a "healthful" day's intake that comprises 7 pounds of food and only 4 ounces of fatty food:

- **4 lbs. fruit (1814g)** — about 900 calories, 60 fat
- **1 lb. lettuce (454 g)** — about 75 calories, 11 fat
- **1.75 lbs. other vegetables (794 g)** — 240 calories, 12 fat
- **1 ounce olive oil (28 g, just over 2 teaspoons)** — 250 calories, 250 fat
- **3 ounces almonds (85 g, about 45)** — 490 calories, 360 fat

**Total: 1,955 calories, 693 fat**

The nuts and oil in this example weigh only ¼ pound but amount to 740 of the 1,955 total calories. Since the nuts are not all fat, and the plants do contain some fat, the total comes to 693 fat calories, or 35% of the day's intake. This is the same percentage of fat found in the standard American diet. This quantity of fat, of any type, is not "low," or healthful, by any standard!

### *Comparing Apples to Apples*

Often, when caloronutrient numbers are being bandied about, things can become extremely misleading. A pint of liquid contains 96 teaspoons. Add just one teaspoon of oil to a pint of water, and you have a fluid that is 100% fat in terms of calories but only 1% fat by weight.

It is important to understand the units of measure used by other diet gurus when comparing their carbohydrate/protein/fat recommendations to those expressed in this book. These teachers sometimes use different units for different foods, or change units over time, or use different units when referring to liquids than they do for solids. Often too, they use numbers in their presentations that sound good when taken at face value. But if you roll up your sleeves and do the math, the figures simply cannot add up.

Recognizing that calculating percentage of calories produces a vastly different caloronutrient ratio than percentage of weight, percentage of dry weight, percentage of volume, etc., making sure you are comparing apples to apples (so to speak) is an important factor when evaluating other programs in relation to the 80/10/10 diet.

For example, one popular author recommends consuming anywhere from 10 to 25% of the diet from fat (depending upon one's body type and level of inner toxicity). But at retreats and other events where his recipes are served, fat routinely accounts for 30 to 60% of the total calorie content of the meals. How can this be? The seeming contradiction stems from the fact that this author's recommended caloronutrient ratio is based on volume of food (cups and spoons), rather than percentage of calories. Further complicating things, he quotes his ratio guidelines in terms of "percentage of high-carbohydrate, high-protein, and high-fat foods." Given that the items raw fooders deem "high protein" (nuts and seeds) average 75% of calories from fat, the problem becomes apparent rather quickly.

When you follow this author's "low-fat" guideline ("50% carbohydrate, 30–35% protein, and 10–15% oils,") you end up eating about 30% fat. The high-fat version of his plan ("50% protein, 30–35% carbohydrate, and 20–25% oils") yields a minimum of 60% fat. Although he acknowledges the necessity to moderate the fat content of "protein foods" by consuming expensive high-protein powdered supplements, my experience is that adherents of his plan slather on the fat with abandon, with little or no awareness of the extent to which their diets are predominated by fat.

The table below provides another example of the misleading results we get when analyzing nutrient content by volume rather than calories. Consider a salad made of just two ingredients: 6 cups of lettuce and ¼ cup of almonds. As this table shows, the almonds account for just 4% of the volume but—surprisingly to many—nearly 80% of the calories.

| Measuring Percentage by Volume vs. Calories | | |
|---|---|---|
| | **Lettuce** | **Almonds** |
| % of salad volume (6.25 cups total) | **96%**<br>(6 of 6.25 cups) | **4%**<br>(0.25 of 6.25 cups) |
| % of salad calories (262 calories total) | **22%**<br>(57 of 262 calories, 7 from fat) | **78%**<br>(205 of 262 calories, 151 from fat ) |

In Appendix A I provide analyses of sample meals that use real recipes and quantities, to help you begin to get a sense of how your daily meals stack up in terms of caloronutrient ratio.

## The Bull's Eye: 80/10/10rv

For those who choose to follow the healthiest version of 80/10/10 in order to achieve off-the-charts results in every aspect of your well-being, we add the suffix rv, standing for "raw vegan," to the 80/10/10designation. Also called the "low-fat raw vegan diet," 80/10/10rv presents you with the life-changing opportunity to partake exclusively of Nature's bounty—consuming only whole, fresh, unprocessed and undressed plant foods in the form Mother Earth presents them to us.

I have eaten substantially this way and used the 80/10/10rv program, as it has evolved, with clients for more than twenty years, —with astonishing results. This approach to diet and nutrition has proven over that time to be the healthiest dietary regimen known to man. By the time you finish this book, you will have the specifics you need to implement this program in your life.

## How Close to 80/10/10 Am I?

How does 80/10/10 compare to *your* caloronutrient ratio? Well, naturally, each of us is unique, but the generalizations are telling. Various sources suggest that Americans consume 40 to 50% of calories from carbohydrates, about 16% protein, and about 35 to 45% fat.[30] After twenty years of doing dietary analysis for my clients, I have observed that 42/16/42 is typical for most people.

As this book explains, most of us in the U.S.—even vegetarians and vegans—tend to gravitate toward this 42/16/42 average, a proportion that provides far less fuel (carbohydrate) than our bodies need in order to thrive … and a seriously dangerous level of fat.

You will also step through some calculations so that you can assess the caloronutrient ratio of commonly consumed raw food plans. You will see for yourself, through simple examples, something that became apparent to me years ago: Raw fooders, for the most part, are consuming astonishing levels of fat—sometimes twice that of the fast-food-eating mainstream! Naturally, cooked fat carries with it a host of problems not present in raw fats, but high levels of either can wreak tremendous havoc with our health.

***80/10/10rv—whole, fresh, unprocessed plant foods as Mother Earth presents them.***

If you are new to the high-produce way of eating, consider yourself lucky to have encountered this information early in your quest. With this book, you can steer clear of the pitfalls that leave so many vegetarians and raw food enthusiasts disheartened and unsure of where to turn next. If you are a raw fooderfooders, this book may catapult you into a whole new reality, as answers to long-standing nagging questions begin to emerge. You may find light bulbs going on as you begin to understand why you or your friends may not have quite thrived as promised on this "healthiest of all diets."

## Tracking Your Own Numbers

In Appendix D. "Resources for Diet Analysis", I describe online tools and other resources that you can use to get a sense of what you are eating. I encourage you to take the time to learn to use a nutrient-analysis tool, at least for a short while. Perhaps the most important use of these automated calculators is to make sure you get enough calories for your size and activity level. This is of critical importance, as undereating in terms of calories is one of the main reasons that people fail to thrive on a high-produce diet.

To keep it simple, a week or so of tracking your meals online can give you sufficient information to begin seeing the true composition of your diet. From there, you will be able to recognize pitfalls and start adjusting your caloronutrient ratio. After that, you may want to log on and catalog a day's consumption here and there, or as new foods come into season, just to make sure you are still on track … but soon 80/10/10 will become second nature, and no such effort will be necessary.

## Relax ... We'll Get There Together

Most folks find dietary changes more challenging than almost anything else in life. Many patients have come to me desperate to solve some serious health issue, saying "Doc, I will do anything you say, follow any program you suggest. Just don't mess with my diet."

Rare indeed (and gratifying) are the few who are so motivated to feel better that they change directions on a dime. But I acknowledge that dietary shifts are daunting for nearly everybody. With this in mind, I created the 80/10/10 diet to allow everyone to transition at a comfortable speed.

By focusing on the caloronutrient ratio (the percentage of carbohydrates, proteins and fats), rather than on the specific foods, this plan allows you to set your own pace. Succeeding on 80/10/10 is simply a matter of adjusting the volume of the foods you eat, in relation to each other, to move yourself in the direction of your target. Gradually increasing healthful carbs from whole fruit and decreasing fat will work just fine and is far better than making no change at all. The results, especially when tracked with colorful graphs on Nutridiary.com (See Appendix D. "Resources for Diet Analysis" on page 335), will provide you with motivation to continue making improvements.

***Dial 811, for the healthiest, trimmest you!***

Though food diaries and numerical analyses can be helpful, you do not need to buy a food scale or log meals each day to receive value from this book. On the pages that follow, I provide the information, meal plans, and sample calculations to give you a clear idea of how to incorporate the 80/10/10 formula into your life, with or without the high-tech tools.

Just giving conscious thought to what you eat with the caloronutrient ratio in mind is a first step in the right direction. You can spend as much or as little effort as you want becoming familiar with your current diet and how it compares with the 80/10/10 plan.

Please, look to this book for inspiration and guidance toward the body and the health you desire, but do not be discouraged. Some people tell me that they feel overwhelmed as they become painfully aware of how much fat they have been eating and how far they have strayed from their goals. To those I say take heart ... and relax. The confusion will clear as we step through these pages together.

By the time you finish reading this book, I venture to say that the road to success will seem nearer and easier for you to follow. If what you read makes sense and you are ready to take your health and your body to new levels, simply start steering toward 80/10/10 … the results will come quickly. If you need support and more information, visit my online discussion forum, at http://foodnsport.com, visit the raw natural hygiene forum at www.RawNaturalHygiene.ning.com.

Even when you have the 80/10/10 concept down to a science, you will never eat in that ratio at every meal, nor even every day (nor should you). In reality, you will you eat a bit more fat on some days and less on others. The goal is to eat 80/10/10 as an average, for an entire year or more. Once you have done that, I'd wager you will never look back.

# Chapter 5
# Carbohydrate: 80% Minimum

Nutritionists and health-minded diet professionals generally agree that 60 to 80% of our calories need to come from carbohydrates. Having established so far in this book that the percentage of total calories in our diet to be provided by both fat and protein should run in the single digits (not more than 10% each), we can see that the high end of this range is just about right. For most people, I recommend 80% carbohydrates, or even higher. In fact, if we consume much less than 80% of our calories as carbohydrates, we are destined to consume too much protein, fat, or both—but more likely it will be fat.

Insufficient carbohydrate in the diet leads to an array of health concerns, primary among which are eating disorders, severe food cravings, lethargy, weakness, and all of the conditions associated with the overconsumption of fats. As we increase protein intake above ten percent of daily calories from protein results in, we start seeing low energy and increased acid toxemia, a precursor for osteoporosis, kidney disease, arthritis, immune dysfunction, and cancer. Eating substantially more than ten percent of daily calories from fat can lead to diabetes, cardiovascular disease, stroke, cancer, and many other maladies. Any way you slice it—too few carbohydrates, too much fat, or too much protein—you will suffer serious health consequences.

## Sugar: The Fuel We Are Designed For

Before our cells can utilize any food for fuel, whether it contains primarily carbohydrate, protein, or fat, it must first be converted into simple sugars. Carbohydrates are by far the easiest to convert to useful sugars. Glucose (a simple sugar) is the primary, preferred source of fuel for every tissue and cell of our bodies. In fact, some of our cells (the brain, red blood cells, and some nervous tissue, for example) depend almost exclusively on glucose as their fuel source.

***Any way you slice it—too few carbohydrates, too much fat, or too much protein—you will suffer serious health consequences.***

### Fuel vs. Energy

A major misconception people have about food is that it is a source of energy. This fallacy is partly supported by the fact that in the nutritional sciences, the words "fuel" and "energy" are used synonymously. The lethargy that follows a holiday meal easily demonstrates the fault in this line of thinking.

In health sciences however, the term "energy" is defined as a low-voltage electrical current produced by your brain during sleep, which runs through your body via your nervous system (also known as vital nerve energy). When you are awake, you use nerve energy more rapidly than the brain can produce it. Hence, you eventually run out of energy. After an appropriate period of hours procuring sleep, you awaken, fully recharged and full of nerve energy again.

On the other hand, food is referred to as "fuel." We need to consume fuel for three primary reasons— nutrition, hydration, and pleasure. Through the process of digestion, we "burn" our fuel (food) to release its own energy potential and utilize it for ourselves. During this complicated process, we receive a net gain in energy by using our own nerve energy to release the potential in food.

To help explain the difference, we can apply the analogy of a car. We have no difficulty understanding that the fuel in our gas tank (food) is completely different than the energy supplied from the battery of our car (vital nerve energy). Either without the other is completely useless, but in combination they work to create motion and activity.

Humans have little or no capacity for storing excess protein or excess carbohydrate, but we can convert both to fat stores for later use as fuel. When we do not eat sufficient carbohydrates to meet our fuel needs, our bodies break down stored fats into glucose through a complex chemical process called gluconeogenesis (literally, "the creation of new sugar"). While this can be a lifesaving process in times of hardship, in the absence of sufficient carbohydrates, gluconeogenesis results in the production of by-products known as ketones.

Circulating in the bloodstream, ketones adversely affect our decision-making abilities, because they exert an influence upon brain chemistry similar to that of alcohol. Effectively, a heavy ketotic state renders us "under the influence." In such a state, we should not make decisions important to our life and health, such as those made when driving a car, doing sports, or performing any work that requires precision of body or mind.

## Types of Carbohydrates

The definitions of carbohydrate and its constituents are evolving. Among lay people, carbohydrates are thought to fall into two broad categories, complex and simple. Science recognizes intricate differences between the various carbohydrate compounds, and considerable confusion exists in the literature that describes them. Here is a simplified summary of terms, which is by no means definitive; you will find many variations on this list:

**Simple sugars** (mainly monosaccharides consisting of one sugar molecule and disaccharides made of two monosaccharides). Primary among these are glucose, fructose, galactose, and dextrose (monosaccharides), as well as lactose, maltose and sucrose. They are found in most foods, including fruits, vegetables, milk, and honey.

**Oligosaccharides** (short-chain sugars consisting of three to nine sugar molecules): Oligosaccharides include raffinose, stachyose, verbascose, fructo-oliogosaccharides, and maltodextrins. Most renowned for causing the flatulence associated with beans, some oligosaccharides are entirely indigestible, while others are partially digestible.

**Polysaccharides** ("complex carbohydrates" that contain 10 or more—as many as several thousand—sugar molecules): These include starches (amylose and amylopectin) and dextrins found in grains, rice, and legumes, as well as nonstarch polysaccharides, also known as fiber (cellulose, pectin, gums, beta-glucans, and fructans), found in grains, fruits, and vegetables.

Together, monosaccharides and disaccharides comprise the "sugars" found on the Nutrition Facts portion of food labels. Monosaccharides are the only carbohydrates that can be absorbed directly into the bloodstream, through the intestinal lining. Our digestive system easily breaks down disaccharides into their monosaccharide constituents.

Simple carbohydrates come in two forms: refined sugars (extracted from fruits, grains, tubers, and sugar cane) and whole-food sugars (the sugars found in whole, fresh plant foods, primarily sweet fruits). Both refined and whole-food simple sugars taste sweet to the tip of the tongue. Unfortunately, widespread misinformation and general ignorance about nutrition causes the great majority of the population to equate simple carbohydrates with the nutritionally bankrupt refined sugars. Unaware that whole-fruit sugar is profoundly different in nature than extracted sugar, these misguided dieters lump all simple carbohydrates together and then shun them as a category. Government guidelines and short-sighted nutritionists perpetuate this misconception, admonishing us to avoid simple sugars like the plague.

Complex carbohydrates, found in grains and other starchy foods, do not taste sweet, even though they are made from chains of sugars. Complex carbohydrates are more difficult to digest than simple carbohydrates. They require substantial amounts of energy in the conversion to sugar, and eating them cooked generates toxic byproducts.

Later in this chapter, I discuss each of these broad categories—complex carbohydrates, whole-food simple carbohydrates, and refined simple carbohydrates—in some detail.

## Two Carbohydrate Camps

Although there are a tremendous number of variations on the theme, two basic schools of thought exist regarding what to eat. There are the low-carbohydrate/high-fat proponents, and then there are the supporters of the high-carbohydrate/low-fat approach to food.

### *The Low-Carb/High-Fat Faction*

In recent decades, high-fat (disguised as low-carb) diets have taken the country by storm. In response, grocery stores, restaurants, fast-food chains, airlines, and even doughnut shops have begun marketing their "low-carbohydrate" options with pride. If the trend continues, I predict that fat consumption will show a concerted rise by the next time national statistics are released.

Why? It's a simple proposition: If your daily caloric "pie" is made of only three slices (carbohydrate, protein, and fat), and you decrease one of them, one or both of the other two must increase.

People generally believe that the decrease in carbohydrates in their "low-carb" meals is offset by an increase in protein. This is incorrect.

As I describe in the protein chapter, only exceedingly rarely does anyone eat even a quarter of daily calories as protein. The vast majority of

Americans eat about 16% protein each day, and only a very small fraction of the population consumes 20% protein or more.

The balance of our daily calories, at least 80%, must come from some combination of carbohydrates and fat. Essentially, any decrease in carbohydrates must be accompanied by an increase in fat, assuming we continue to consume the same number of calories.

Unfortunately, each gram of fat contains more than twice the calories of a gram of carbohydrate. So if you eat the same general quantity of food on a "low-carb" program, you will increase not only your percentage of calories from fat but also your total calories for the day.

So how do people lose weight on low carbohydrate diets? In brief, research shows that these people invariably consume fewer total calories. Dr. Michael Greger's superbly comprehensive and condemning eBook, Atkins Facts, sums it up well:

In 2001, the medical journal Obesity Research published "Popular Diets: A Scientific Review." Claiming to have reviewed every study ever done on low carb diets, they concluded, "In all cases, individuals on high-fat, low carbohydrate diets lose weight because they consume fewer calories." (Obesity Research 9(2001):1S.)

I urge anyone who is considering destroying their health with any low-carbohydrate diet to read this riveting 47-page document in its entirety.[31] The following sidebar is excerpted with Dr. Greger's permission from that publication.

### The Deadly Low-Carb Craze

When one is eating enough carbohydrates, fat can be completely broken down as well. But when one's body runs out of carb fuel to burn, its only choice is to burn fat inefficiently using a pathway that produces toxic byproducts like acetone and other so-called "ketones."

The kidney uses minerals such as potassium and calcium to help rid one's body of toxins like ketones. People on the Atkins Diet are urinating these minerals away. And critically low levels in the blood of these electrolytes can lead to fatal cardiac arrhythmias—lethal heart rhythms.

The current director of nutrition at Harvard advises that all physicians should produce a handout warning about all of the adverse effects of the Atkins Diet. The symptoms of ketosis [a metabolic state where the body "switches" from primarily using glucose for energy to primarily using fat for energy] include general tiredness, abrupt or gradually increasing weakness, dizziness, headaches, confusion, abdominal pain, irritability, nausea and vomiting, sleep problems, and bad breath.

After running through the adverse effects associated with ketosis, the American institute for Cancer Research wrote, "Those are the short-term effects. The long-term effects are even more dire."

Dr. Greger's full document details literally dozens of additional diseases and problems brought on by this deadly diet, including:

- Malnutrition (compromised vitamin and mineral intake).
- Cancer, stroke, gout, osteoporosis, and diabetes.
- Potential kidney, bone, liver, and cholesterol abnormalities.
- Cardiac disease, arrhythmias, contractile function impairment.
- Impairment of physical activity.
- A rise in blood pressure with age.
- Rapid falling blood pressure upon standing (orthostatic hypotension).
- Sudden death.

Dr. James W. Anderson, professor of medicine and clinical nutrition at the University of Kentucky School of Medicine, said of the Atkins plan, "This is absolutely the worst diet you could imagine for long-term obesity, heart disease, and some forms of cancer. If you wanted to ruin your health, you couldn't find one worse than Atkins'."

Having bought into the health-destroying mythology of low-carbohydrate plans, some dieters avoid all forms of carbohydrate, including grains, starchy vegetables, and fruit, attempting to derive their fuel instead from dangerously high proportions of fat and protein. Although we were designed with survival/backup mechanisms that allow us to transform noncarbohydrate foods into sugar in case of starvation or other extreme conditions, this capability was intended to be invoked only on rare occasion.

We pay a huge price in terms of health and optimum functioning whenever we force our bodies to resort to fat (or worse, to protein) to fuel our cells, as these conversions are chemically inefficient compared with using carbohydrate for fuel. The body can only do so by expending substantial amounts of vital energy and producing toxic waste products along the way.

Proper body weight is an effortless, natural outcome of optimum health, but optimum health is unlikely to result from a diet designed solely for weight loss. The followers of low-carbohydrate diets may achieve their weight-loss goals, but they imperil their long-term health in doing so. The admonition to consume tremendous amounts of animal fat and protein is creating millions of cases of deadly disease that will become ever more apparent in the years to come.

### Starch-Based Diets: The Other Camp

The vast majority of diet/nutrition experts whose patients and clients consistently experience reversal of degenerative disease, however—including renowned medical doctors like Dean Ornish, John McDougall, Michael Klaper, Caldwell Esselstyn, Neal Barnard, Joel Fuhrman, Matthew Lederman and his wife Alona Pulde, and Michael Greger, as well as professionals at the world-renowned Pritikin Longevity center—recommend that we base our diets instead around starchy complex carbohydrates. These experts emphasize the importance of consuming starches (beans, legumes, tubers, roots, starchy vegetables, whole grains, and whole-grain products).

***Diets high in complex carbohydrates miss the mark where optimum nutrition is concerned.***

This advice could be seen as a step in the right direction, because, as I discussed in the introduction to this book, whole foods are always more nutritious than fractional foods. Yet due to the nutrient losses incurred during the cooking process, no cooked food can be viewed as a true whole food. In fact, the cooking process itself actually removes the water from food (with the exception of certain dehydrated foods that are actually rehydrated as they are cooked in water). No food whose water has been removed can realistically be viewed as a whole food.

Agreeing that we are designed to run on simple sugars from carbohydrate, these highly respected professionals perceive that there is no other substantial whole-food source than complex carbohydrates. Coming from a cooked food perspective, although they often acknowledge the nutritional superiority of raw fruits and vegetables, they do not consider basing the human diet on the sugars in fruit to be a feasible option, primarily for three reasons.

**First,** when most people talk about eating fruits and vegetables, they tend to think of the vegetables being predominant. Yet nutritionists are very familiar with the studies that have concluded that a diet predominated by vegetables simply cannot supply sufficient caloric density to support human health. On a diet of just vegetables, I agree, it is highly unlikely that any human beings could maintain their health. They would lose weight at a steady rate that would eventually become unsustainable, and they would suffer unyielding health decline.

**Second,** in all likelihood, they simply don't conceive of consuming fruit in sufficient quantity to meet our caloric needs, even though doing so is quite pleasant and not difficult. They dismiss this possibility wholesale, as it is entirely outside of their framework of reference. After all, who knows anyone who lives primarily (but *not* entirely) on fruit? I must admit that in today's world, it is a rare individual who lives this way. Yet almost every person I have ever met who eats great quantities of fruit has written a book extolling its virtues. There must be a reason these fruit eaters are so excited about the excellent health benefits that result from such a foodstyle.

**Finally,** their misguided notions about the glycemic index and their unnecessary worries about elevated triglyceride levels literally prevent them from considering fruit as a primary source of calories. And so, in spite of the fact that fruit is universally promoted as the ultimate health food, and in spite of their own conclusions that carbohydrates must predominate the diet in order for health to be possible, the majority of the world's health professionals fail to see the obvious: A fruit-based diet is the finest possibility we have for developing optimum health.

No one can deny that the low-fat vegetarian diets recommended by Pritikin, McDougall, and their colleagues produce phenomenal results in terms of health, vitality, and body weight. When they substitute cooked starches for meat in their diets, program adherents show a marked reduction in cardiovascular disease and an initial improvement in overall health and well-being.

Yet starch-and-grain-based diet proponents still broadly miss the mark where optimum nutrition and health are concerned. These complex carbohydrate foods lack in areas such as vitamin C, soluble fiber, and several hundred thousand phytonutrients. The experience of eating them can't compare to the ease, simplicity, cleanliness, and natural satiation of eating sweet fruit.

### Grains: Pritikin's Downfall

*In 1988, a gentleman named Ross Horne wrote a book entitled Improving on Pritikin*—You Can Do Better.[32] *His story is fascinating. In the 1970s, Horne was the "best disciple and staunchest supporter" of Nathan Pritikin and his renowned grain-based diet. But after experiencing himself and observing in others some serious deleterious effects of the Pritikin plan (including arthritis and cancer), Horne wrote this book. In more than 150 pages, Horne details the health perils that accompany a grain-based diet and precisely where Pritikin's logic fails. With utmost respect for the superb results of Pritikin's low-fat plan in reversing heart disease, Horne points out the following:*

*Although Pritikin's low-fat regimen is nothing short of miraculous in terms of reversing heart disease, a healthy heart does not ensure a healthy person. Pritikin's emphasis on grain (and, interestingly, its excess protein, which averages "only" 12% of calories) creates other health issues, ranging from arthritis to cancer.*

*Horne's book presents a compelling and spellbinding argument against the consumption of grains. Here is an excerpt from Chapter 10, "Grains Are for the Birds".*[33]

Pritikin's mission, first and foremost, was the reversal of coronary heart disease. This was uppermost in his mind and so his reasoning followed:

- We must lower fat, cholesterol and protein, the causes of atherosclerosis and heart disease. To do this we must cut out foods of animal origin. We must become vegetarian.
- As most of the food we eat goes into the production of energy, if we cut out animal foods which provide most of the energy in the American diet, as well as the protein, where then will we get our energy and sufficient protein?
- The only other suitable foods available are cereals, root vegetables, and fruits, because green vegetables are so low in food value that you

would have to eat them constantly all day long like cattle do to get enough. We must therefore choose between starch foods (cereals and potatoes) and fruit, and consider green vegetables mainly as a source of vitamins and minerals.

So far Pritikin's reasoning was correct, but at this point his preoccupation with eliminating atherosclerosis became an impediment. He knew that cholesterol and triglycerides (blood fats) were the two factors most implicated in atherosclerosis and he was determined that his diet should diminish these in the blood to as low levels as possible. Cutting out animal derived foods completely eliminated cholesterol and the harmful animal fats from the diet, but what about triglycerides from vegetable sources? Pritikin knew that concentrated sugar of any kind—refined sugar or even extracted natural raw sugar—entered the bloodstream too quickly, upsetting the normal blood sugar levels and resulting in the production of triglycerides, his number-two enemy. His reasoning logically continued:

- If out of our two remaining sources of energy and protein, one of them contains sugar, a substance which elevates triglycerides, we cannot entertain it as a principal source of nourishment.
- We must therefore severely ration fruit because of its sugar content and rely almost entirely on cereals to provide our energy and protein.

What was the outcome of this reasoning? It was a great outcome; Pritikin first of all eliminated his own atherosclerosis and then proceeded to eliminate the atherosclerosis in the bodies of thousands of people who followed his teachings.

This is how the current rage on complex carbohydrate started and why companies who make whole-grain bread, pasta, cookies and crackers are doing so well.

But the reversal of heart disease and its associated problems is not the be-all and end-all of health and longevity. There are other things to consider besides restoring good circulation. Unsticking the blood is only the first step in optimizing health, the second step is to get the blood's chemistry right. Pritikin had taken the lipo from lipotoxemia but much toxemia still remained. ***When he grouped the natural sugars contained in fruit in with other sugars, Pritkin had made a fatal mistake.***

Because cooked grains create a condition known as acid toxemia, people who adhere to starch/grain-based diets eventually fall victim to cancer, arthritis, chronic fatigue, hypothyroidism, and a host of other health challenges. A diet of grains and cooked vegetables provides most of the vitamins; however, vitamin C—the most important vitamin of all for the maintenance of tissue integrity and immune system function, and the most easily destroyed by heat—is seriously lacking unless the diet also includes a great deal of fresh fruit.

I maintain that whole, fresh fruits—"the other carbohydrate"—contain precisely the fuel upon which we were designed to thrive.

Let's step back for a moment and examine in more detail the three types of carbohydrates—complex carbohydrates, refined simple sugars, and whole-food simple carbohydrate from fruits.

## Complex Carbohydrates

We find complex carbohydrates in rice, corn, and other grains; roots and tubers (potatoes, sweet potatoes, yams, carrots, beets, turnips, parsnips, and the like); and legumes (beans, peas, and lentils). We make breads, cakes, pastas, cereals, pancakes, and pastries from these complex carbohydrate sources.

Across the board, complex carbohydrate foods are nutritionally inferior to fruits and vegetables, which are the two highest sources of vitamins, minerals, and phytonutrients. Grains, for example, are low in vitamins A, B, C, and E, as well as sodium, calcium, sulfur, and potassium. The phytic acid in grains is an antinutrient that drastically reduces zinc absorption. Legumes are low in vitamins A and C as well. Both grains and legumes contain more protein than I would recommend eating in quantity (their percentages averaging in the teens and twenties, respectively) to be eaten in quantity.

With the exception of corn, peas, and some root vegetables like carrots and beets, we cannot even attempt to eat most complex carbohydrate foods from the garden, unprocessed, in the form Nature gives them to us. Even if we can physically chew and swallow starchy carbohydrates, they are very difficult for our bodies to digest. This is true whether they are eaten raw, soaked, cooked, processed, or refined. We do not have the digestive enzymes to break down the oligosaccharides in beans, nor the polysaccharides (cellulose and other fibers) in grains and starchy vegetables, a sure sign that they are not designed for human consumption. Biochemistry tells us exactly which foods we can and cannot digest, and therefore what foods we should eat.

In the raw food world, creative chefs have devised recipes that utilize soaked lentils, wild rice, oats and other grains. The dishes they create from these easier-to-swallow yet still substantially indigestible "staples" allow them to replicate many of the tastes and textures we once enjoyed with cooked food. In all cases, however, grains, starchy tubers, and legumes create nutritional, digestive, and health problems for those who eat them. Even when soaked and raw, grains are acid forming in a body that needs to be slightly alkaline.

### Complex Carbohydrates and Disease

Many research studies link diets high in complex carbohydrates to negative health conditions. The gluten-containing grains[34] (primarily wheat, but also rye and barley, and oats) contain at least fifteen opioid sequences, which are strongly addictive, morphine-like substances that have potent psychoactive properties and produce serious neurological disorders, constipation, urinary retention, nausea, vomiting, cough suppression, and other symptoms.[35]

***Biochemistry tells us exactly what we can digest, and therefore what we should eat.***

Gluten intolerance (celiac disease) contributes to or causes a wide range of other diseases, including asthma, arthritis, chronic fatigue, Crohn's disease, Type 2 diabetes, depression, eczema, fibromyalgia, irritable bowel syndrome, migraines, lymphoma, and gastrointestinal cancers. Gluten intolerance may also be linked to autism, schizophrenia, and several autoimmune disorders.

### Masking the Bland Taste of Complex Carbs

Most people who attempt to thrive on a high-carbohydrate diet devoid of fruit run into health problems. Primarily, this is because most starchy carbohydrates are completely unappealing if served as is. Society has proven repeatedly for more than forty years that people will not, in fact cannot gravitate toward a diet dominated by plain, undressed complex carbohydrates.

Brain-destroying, neurotoxic, and profoundly addictive flavor enhancers, called "excitotoxins," are added to almost all processed foods, especially frozen and diet foods.[36]

## Excitotoxins Enhance Flavor While Poisoning Our Foods

In his book, *Excitotoxins: The Taste That Kills,* Russell L. Blaylock, MD suggests that the prolific use of excitotoxic flavor enhancers in almost all processed foods is a major cause of obesity and disease in our country.

The most common and dangerous excitotoxins include Nutrasweet, (aspartame) and MSG and its derivatives, which show up on food labels as innocuous-sounding ingredients like hydrolyzed vegetable protein, autolysis yeast, yeast extract, textured protein, soy protein extract, sodium caseinate, natural flavoring, and spices.[37]

Excitotoxins are substances that react with specialized receptors in the brain in such a way as to lead to destruction of certain types of brain cells. These highly addictive, neurotoxic substances accelerate aging and stimulate the nervous system, causing neurodegenerative diseases, neurological disorders, endocrine disorders, heart attacks, strokes, tumors, vision loss, migraines, seizures, and many other diseases. They also worsen or mimic the symptoms of such diseases and conditions as fibromyalgia, MS, lupus, ADD, diabetes, Alzheimer's, chronic fatigue, and depression.

Excitotoxins are used heavily in both sweet and salty snack foods, and no laws restrict the use of these substances. Fast-food chains hire food chemists to load our pizzas, tacos, fried chicken, bento boxes, and the like with as much of these deadly additives as possible, which keep us feeling "high" and coming back for more. All of the salty soy products, as well, (whether or not they purport to contain MSG) are laden with highly excitotoxic free glutamates. This is of special concern for the raw food community, which tends to consume a tremendous amount of soy sauce, shoyu, liquid aminos, miso, and tamari.

***Excitotoxins give the phrase, "Nobody can eat just one" a whole new meaning.***

In his personal film documentary, "Supersize Me," Morgan Spurlock created a vivid description of his experience living exclusively on McDonalds' food for 30 consecutive days. Although he did not specifically use the term "excitotoxins," he clearly described the symptoms of addiction and withdrawal he experienced during that month. News of the widespread use of excitotoxic additives in junk foods is getting enough press that soon people are coming to perceive a whole new level of reality in the 1960s Lay's potato chip jingle "nobody can eat just one." Can you forget the taste of Planter's dry-roasted peanuts? ("Monosodium glutamate" sits unabashedly on the label). Other junk foods, like Frito Lay's "playfully mischievous" Cheetos snacks, boast multiple sources of excitotoxic free glutamate. (Flamin' Hot Cheese Flavored snacks, for example, list monosodium glutamate, autolyzed yeast extract, hydrolyzed soy protein, and sodium caseinate on the ingredient label.)

### *Fiber*

Our commonly consumed cooked foods—meats and refined grain products—are extremely low in fiber. In fact, animal foods contain no fiber.

Many health-minded people, thinking they are doing their bodies a favor, endeavor to eat whole-grain complex carbohydrates to get fiber in their diets. They are on the right track, as fiber is what we remove from whole grains in order to make refined grains—and dietary fiber is absolutely essential for digestive and overall health.

Unfortunately, these health seekers have been misled to believe that the fiber in grains is good for us. This is not true. There are two broad categories of fiber, referred to as soluble and insoluble. Soluble fiber is an essential nutrient (one we cannot make within our bodies and must therefore eat), found primarily in fruits and to some degree in vegetables. It absorbs water and helps to keep the stool bulky and soft. It functions as a sticky gel-like absorptive medium to keep all substances moving through the intestines. Insoluble fiber is found primarily in grains.

Pectin and guar are the two most common soluble fibers. They are used in recipes as thickeners because of their ability to hold water. They also slow sugar absorption from the intestines, functioning as built-in protection that prevent the sugars in fruits from being absorbed into the bloodstream too rapidly. Ironically, in their isolated form, pectin and guar are being used by the medical establishment in the treatment of diabetics, while doctors insist that diabetics should not consume fruit.

***The fibers in grains irritate and scrape our intestinal walls.***

Before doctors truly understood the function of fiber, it used to be described as a "scrub brush" for the intestines. The insoluble fibers in grains (raw, sprouted, or cooked), however, are harsh on our delicate digestive tracts. Since they do not absorb water, their edges and points remain sharp. These fibers literally scrape at the delicate walls of our intestines, irritating them and causing a thickening of the intestinal wall. This makes the fiber less irritating but also reduces the body's ability to absorb nutrients.

This irritation of the intestines and colon is what gives bran its reputation for encouraging bowel function. The body senses an irritant and attempts to expel it as rapidly as possible, along with whatever else is in the colon at the time. Anyone who uses bran fiber for this purpose has noticed that after a short time they must increase the quantity of bran that they use in order to get the same effect. The more the body increases the thickness of its mucous membrane to protect itself from irritation, the more bran must be ingested. It is an endless cycle, similar to that of all substance abuse.

Reduced absorption, impeded assimilation, adhesion development, scar-tissue formation, leaky gut syndrome, irritable bowel syndrome, spastic colon, colon blockages, diverticulitis, ulcerative colitis, Crohn's disease, and other digestive maladies are often the outcome of consuming insufficient fiber or fiber that is too harsh. The soft, soluble fibers found in fruits and vegetables are necessary for optimum digestive and colon function.

## Refined Simple Carbohydrates: Junk Food

The second category of carbohydrates is the refined simple carbohydrates found in cookies, cakes, candies, and other confections. Refined sugars are also added to drinks, cereals, complex carbohydrate foods of all types, and anywhere else that you see the word "sweetener" or "sweetened." If the ingredient list includes corn syrup, fructose, galactose, sucrose, dextrose, maltodextrin, dextrin, maltose, levulose, lactose, or almost any word ending in "ose," refined sugars have been added.

If people don't eat lots of fruit, they typically eat something sweet at almost every meal anyway. Orange juice, sweetened cereals, jellies, jams, sweet rolls, and sugar in coffee ensure that the day starts off with sweets. Lunches and dinners usually are not complete unless some type of sweet dessert follows. Be it coffee and cake, milk and cookies, or any of dozens of other typical combinations, we have found a way to replace the healthy "sweet and juicy" provided by fruit with unhealthy, refined sweet and (well ... wet, or at least gooey) choices.

***Refined simple sugars are classic examples of "empty calories."***

Refined simple sugars, a category that includes table sugar, are the classic all-time-best examples of "empty calories," that is, calories without their full complement of original nutrients intact. In all forms of refined foods, some part or parts of the original nutrient package have been removed. Regardless of method, the refining of a food reduces its nutritional value and creates nutrient imbalances. In my opinion, refined foods have no place in the diet of anyone wishing to improve their nutrition or any aspect of their health.

Foods can contain partially empty or completely empty calories, depending upon the amount of refinement the food has undergone. When people add such empty calories to other ingredients to create a dish, I refer to the finished product as "junk food."

Consumers have come to mentally lump all sugars—in fact all carbohydrates—into one group, to which they attribute mostly negative connotations. Along with complex carbohydrates, refined sweets and fruits are commonly considered nothing but "another source of sugar."

The meat and dairy industries like to point fingers at sugars, declaring them synonymous with empty calories. They have done such a good job of marketing that to this day most people do not understand the differences between refined simple sugars (empty-calorie junk foods) and the simple sugars in fruit (health food), thinking that "sugar is sugar."

The empty calories in refined simple carbohydrates are so devoid of food value as to bankrupt you nutritionally while they also function as stimulants. Both the stimulation and the nutritional deficit accelerate aging.

## Fruits: Whole-Food Simple Carbohydrates

Whole, fresh fruit is the third and most overlooked source of carbohydrates. Fruit comes in an intricate, highly nutritious package that matches our nutritional needs better than any other category of food. I recommend that virtually our entire carbohydrate intake—80% of calories or more—come from the simple sugars in whole, fresh fruit. These sugars are the optimal fuel source for humans. The soft, water-soluble fiber in whole fruits allows their sugars to absorb slowly and gradually, so high blood sugar is not an issue (as long as your diet is low in fat … see Chapter 2 "Meeting Fruit Concerns Head-On" on page 31.)

***Whole, fresh fruits: "The Other Carbohydrate"***

Fruits are the obvious choice for obtaining our carbohydrates, as they provide the only substantial and healthful whole-food source of simple sugar. Many classically trained nutritionists, and most doctors, still erroneously refer to fruits as complex carbohydrates, because some of their fiber (such as the skins, pith, etc.) is composed of complex carbohydrates. Though these indigestible fibers are complex carbohydrate in nature, virtually all of the carbohydrate calories in ripe fruit are simple mono- and disaccharides. This misunderstanding has long been pointed out by sports physiologists, who rely on the fact that the sugars in fruit are simple in design and hence work extremely well before, during, and after all physical exertions.

Fruits never require cooking in order to be delicious and nutritious, and our bodies digest them quickly and easily. (Some vegetables with a slightly sweet taste—like some lettuces, garden-fresh baby peas and corn, and young roots—also contain simple carbohydrates, but they are so low in calories that chewing them may utilize more fuel than they provide.)

### *Think Fruit Meals for Health*

Fruit is considered "health food" by almost everyone in the health field. A director of nutrition for the U.S. Olympic teams once called fruit "magic food." All the major organizations of health and disease, from the government to private businesses, from the National Heart Foundation to the American Cancer Society, agree that we should increase our consumption of fruit.

As a category, fruits are our least toxic food choice. They digest cleanly, leaving only water as residue, which is easily expelled from the body. I see no healthful reason to look anywhere else for the vast majority of our calories. The health, nutrition, energy, and human performance results available on a high-fruit, low-fat, raw vegan program eclipse even the proven, consistent benefits of low-fat, starch-based diets.

### Fruit As a Staple: An Idea Whose Time Has Come

The practice of eating enough fruit to make complete meals of it is alien to most of us. Yet it is an idea whose time has come. Fruits are designed to be our staple; they contain everything required to be the source and mainstay of our nutritional sustenance.

We have been trained to think of fruit as a treat, something to eat at the end of a meal, or perhaps as a snack between meals when nothing else looks good. But I invite you to begin thinking of fruit as real food, and even as a meal unto itself.

If fruit is to become a primary food source for us, we must be willing to explore new avenues, think new thoughts, and ask new questions like the ones below. The consumer has a lot to learn—as we literally have no frame of reference for such a concept—and now is the time to get started. In this book, I answer some of these questions and many others:

- How do we know when fruit is fresh?
- How many blueberries (or oranges, or mangos, or bananas) does it take to make a meal?
- How can I tell if I ate enough fruit?
- Is there such a thing as eating too much fruit?
- Which fruits provide us with the most carbohydrates per bite?
- Which fruits provide the least?
- Which fruits are best at the different seasons of the year?
- Where does each fruit come from?

Eating 80% of our calories in the form of uncooked simple carbohydrates can become easy and natural once we learn to eat a moderate amount of nuts and seeds, all the green leafy vegetables we care for, and great quantities of whole, fresh, ripe, in-season fruit.

## We Are Designed for Tropical Fruit

As a species, humans originated in a warm climate and eventually spread throughout the "tropical belt," the warm zone that extends through most of the thousand-mile range above and below the equator. This is the environment where tropical fruits abound.

Some folks suggest that wherever they live, they should eat food that is locally grown, as "logically" that must be the best for them, at least, that is what they have heard. In the U.S. and Europe, people often argue that since they live in a northern climate, it is only appropriate that they should eat foods of northern origin.

Think about this: If you have a goldfish, cat, or dog, do you change the very nature of their diet every time you move? Do zoo animals get entirely different classes of food, depending on the latitude of the zoo that houses them? Viewed in this way, it becomes obvious that we must honor the unique dietary requirements of each species, based on its particular digestive physiology.

Further, many people live in climates that only produce food for a few months of the year. What should they eat the rest of the year? Humans are anatomically and physiologically adapted to the food of the tropics, predominantly fruit, as are almost all of the tropical creatures. In Central America, for example, all mammals with the exception of the river otter and the jaguar are known to eat fruit, as are most of the birds, many of the amphibians, and quite a few of the reptiles.

No logical or scientific reason exists to conclude that simply because we have moved away from the tropics, we should therefore change what has been our natural food for the great majority of our time on Earth. Regardless of where we go on this planet (or even whether we ever venture off of the planet to other worlds), tropical fruits remain our natural foods, the only cuisine for which we are perfectly designed.

### *Our Own Private Tropics*

Historically, it was only the population explosion caused by the advent of tools and hunting, and exacerbated by the introduction of farming, that resulted in humans being forced to move into what would otherwise have been considered inhospitable and even uninhabitable areas. We effectively took the tropics with us, though, as we had no other choice.

Every one of us lives almost every minute of our lives in a miniature tropical environment, keeping ourselves in the tropics by the judicious use of clothing, bedding, and heat. Even the Eskimos surround themselves with enough clothing and keep their homes warm enough so that they can spend almost all of their time "in the tropics."

We have been trained from early childhood, and have learned through repeated experience, that it is extremely uncomfortable and can be potentially dangerous, even lethal, for us to leave the safety of our own private tropics, and early in life accepted the wisdom and seriousness of this warning. We go through the rest of our lives without ever questioning that we must maintain ourselves in the warmth of a tropical environment.

### *Fruit Is a Natural*

Fortunately, most people love fruit. Children are naturally inclined to eat it. Our ever-present sweet tooth is a signal from nature that drives us to eat enough fruit to provide the simple carbohydrates that fuel every cell of our bodies. Whenever I introduce someone to a delicious tropical fruit that they have never tried, it is met with delight. It doesn't seem to make any difference what the fruit is, people almost always "connect" with it immediately. Almost invariably, I hear something like:

- "Wow, this is the best thing I have ever tasted!"
- "I just found my new favorite food!"
- "I could live on this!"
- "Where can I get this at home?"
- "Do you know of any mail-order catalogs that can ship some to me?"
- "Is this expensive? I want to buy lots of it!"
- "How do I learn more about other fruits like this?"

The entire conversation points to the fact that people not only love fruit, they are designed for fruit. Wherever humans have chosen to venture on planet Earth, they have carried this physiological predilection for tropical fruit with them. People who live in temperate areas still require the foods for which they were designed, just as zoo animals that are geographically relocated still retain their physical requirements.

In fact, it may be even more important for people who live in a cool climate to obtain tropical fruits, as these people often must do without other essential healthful-living conditions that are common to the tropics (warm temperatures, clean air, rural living, year-round sunshine, sounds of nature, pure water, etc.). If you live in an area where tropical fruits are scarce, it may be well worth your while to consider which other environmentally essential factors you are also doing without, and to supply them to the best of your ability.

Training ourselves to once again eat fruit, a practice that held us in good stead for thousands of generations, is as rewarding for our health as it is delicious.

# Chapter 6
# Protein: 10% Maximum

Of the three caloronutrients, protein is certainly the most discussed, and the most misunderstood. I begin with a discussion of protein in order to clear the air about this vital nutrient, with the intention of not discussing it again in the remainder of this book.

The need for protein has been greatly exaggerated by market forces, and protein's functions have been misrepresented. This chapter discusses why we need protein and where we obtain protein on a low-fat 80/10/10 diet. We put the protein issues to rest and then get to the heart of the 80/10/10 diet, carbohydrates and fats.

## How Much Protein Do We Need?

I often respond to the question, "where do you get your protein?" with several questions of my own: "How much protein do you think we need?" "How much protein do you think you currently eat?" "What exactly is the function of protein?" "Have you ever met anyone with a protein deficiency?"

Although I have met many people who have begun to or are considering vectoring their diets away from animal foods, I rarely meet anyone who has a reasonable response to these queries. Usually they tell me that we need large quantities of protein for energy, or to stay strong, or to keep us from getting sick. Nothing could be further from the truth. Protein's primary function is growth, which is negligible in adults, as well as repair from injury and replacement of worn-out cells.

***Compared to a rapidly growing infant, adults need minimal protein.***

## Official Guidelines Recommend 10% Protein

Sometimes I wonder whether the official nutritional guidelines for caloronutrient consumption are intentionally vague and confusing in order to better serve influential market forces. I mean, after 100+ years of testing we have a fairly good idea of which foods are most nutritious for us. Still, the U.S. government officially recommends that our protein intake should be somewhere between 10 and 35% of total calories consumed. It is extremely difficult to consume more than a quarter of your % of total calories from protein, however, unless you are following a strict regimen of refined protein powder and egg whites. Currently fewer than 5% of Americans eat more than 21% of their calories from protein, with the bell curve ranging from 11 to 21%.[38]

Despite the advertising hype of the meat and dairy industries, humans require an extraordinarily low amount of protein in their diets. Many official groups, including the World Health Organization,[39] the U.S. National Academies' Institute of Medicine,[40] and the National Research Council[41] suggest that eating a mere 10% of our total calories as protein is sufficient.

Mother's milk provides on average approximately 6% of calories from protein for growing infants.[42] This should be ample proof that adults do not need more protein per calorie than this, as infants, with their extremely rapid rate of growth, have the highest need for protein per calorie of all humans.

Proteins (or more accurately, amino acids) are the building blocks of living cells. Once we have done our growing, we have very little requirement for the raw materials of which we are made. Think of the analogy of building a brick house: you need truckloads of bricks during the construction stage. Once the house is built, however, if trucks continue to deliver bricks, you have a problem on your hands. The same is true of protein in the human diet: too much creates emergency conditions and keeps the body in a constant state of toxicity.

***Once our house (body) is built, we have very little need for more bricks (protein).***

For those accustomed to seeing your protein recommendation in terms of grams or calories per unit of body weight, the 2003 U.S. RDA for protein is 0.36 grams per pound of body weight, or 0.8 grams per kilogram (1 kilogram = 2.2 lbs). The RDA calculates these numbers for a "typical" (sedentary) female and male who eat 1,600 and 2,200 calories per day, respectively, arriving at a suggested 44 grams of protein for a female and 55 grams for a male. See the sidebar entitled "Calculating Your Protein Intake" on page 111 later in this chapter for sample calculations.

## 10% Protein Includes a Wide Safety Margin

The national and international organizations that set nutrient guidelines build into their numbers a margin of safety that increases the recommendations substantially, often near double. The 1989 U.S. RDA for protein of 0.8 g/kg/day, for example, was designed to meet the needs of 97.5% of a normally distributed population. It was calculated as follows:[43]

- Conduct nitrogen balance studies to determine the mean amount of protein required to replace daily "obligatory losses" through sweat, urine, feces, and sloughed skin, hair, and nails.
- Add two standard deviations (25%) to this mean value.
- Add margins for digestibility and protein quality.

In his book The China Study, renowned Cornell University professor emeritus of nutritional biochemistry T. Colin Campbell states that we require only 5–6% of our total calories to come from protein in order to replace the protein we routinely lose, and that "About 9–10% protein has been recommended for the past fifty years to be assured that most people at least get their 5–6% 'requirement.' [44]

In addition to the safety margin, this recommendation assumes that people eat their protein cooked. Given that cooking substantially deranges protein and other nutrients, we can safely consume far less raw plant protein and still be assured of sufficient nourishment. Thus, you can see that 10% protein (maximum) is both sufficient and reasonable.

The additional protein afforded by the built-in safety factor is not a problem, per se, except that overconsumption of protein can lead to health problems, which will be discussed later in this chapter. The more important concern is relative overconsumption of protein. In other words, if we overconsume one of the three caloronutrients, we are likely to underconsume one or both of the others.

The fact that our protein needs actually run in the single digits (under 10%) often surprises people. Most all of us have unwittingly fallen prey to meat-industry propaganda that would lead us to believe otherwise. Truly, advertising has influenced our perception of reality so widely that the concept of "getting enough protein" is embedded in the culture.

## Athletes and Bodybuilders: 10% Still Plenty

Bodybuilders have long consumed extra protein and lowered carbohydrate intake in the mistaken belief that dietary protein builds muscle. In reality, only weight-bearing exercise builds muscle. When insufficient carbohydrates are supplied, it is true that protein requirements go up, as the body transforms the protein into carbohydrate (an energy-expensive process) and utilizes it for fuel. This does not, however, bring about the result they desire.

### No Extra Protein Required for Physical Activity

Bodybuilders may be interested to note that in its extensive study of protein requirements, the Institute of Medicine/Food and Nutrition Board determined that no additional protein needed to be added to the RDA to account for physical activity:

"There is little evidence that muscular activity increases the need for protein, *except for the small amount required for the development of muscles during physical conditioning* (Torun Et al., 1977). Vigorous activity that leads to profuse sweating, such as in heavy work and sports, and exposure to heat increases nitrogen loss from the skin, but with acclimatization to a warm environment, the excessive skin loss [loss by perspiration through the skin—DG] is reduced and may be partially compensated by decreased renal excretion (WHO, 1985). *In view of the margin of safety in the RDA, no increment is added for work or training.*"[45]

Bodybuilders following the 80/10/10 program have found that if they supply sufficient calories from carbohydrate, their protein needs go down dramatically, and their energy to train and their muscular growth both increase.

Lisa O'Borne (see page 301), a professional bodybuilder in Canada for many years, says that she got the best results of her career when switching to the 80/10/10 diet, gleaning a growth spurt the likes of which none of her trainers had ever seen.

## All Plant Foods Contain Protein

Consuming approximately 5% of calories from protein is difficult to avoid if you are eating enough food to meet your daily calorie needs. All plant foods contain protein, and even if you ate a diet of only white rice, (not recommended) you would still end up with 8% protein for the day! But would it be the "right kind" of protein?

Proteins are complicated molecules made by assembling simple building blocks (amino acids) together in a "polypeptide" chain. Some 20 different amino acids are used to synthesize proteins, eight or nine of which are designated essential (depending upon whose information you read). The term "essential" in nutrition means that the nutrient in question must be eaten or otherwise consumed, as the body cannot synthesize it.

### The Complete Protein Myth

In the 1970s, people often concerned themselves with combining proteins so that all of the essential amino acids were available at each meal. Later research has determined that this is not necessary, and in fact the author of the "incomplete protein theory," Frances Moore Lappe, recanted 20 years later, saying that she was utterly mistaken. We do need all of the essential amino acids, but we do not have to eat them together, or even each day.

### Sources of Protein

Dietary protein is not the only source for building the proteins we need. Instead, our bodies efficiently recycle between 100 and 300 grams of our own protein every day. We have an amino acid pool from which to build new proteins. We add amino acids to the pool by breaking down the proteins we eat and the proteins in our bodies.

We can easily meet our protein requirements on a vegan diet, with no particular attention focused on combining proteins or selecting certain foods for each meal.

The table below shows the percentage of calories from protein in twenty-one common fruits and vegetables and in five animal foods, for comparison.

**Protein Content of Common Foods[46]**
**(percentage of calories)**

| Food | Protein | Food | Protein |
|---|---|---|---|
| Apricots | 10% | Asparagus | 27% |
| Bananas | 4% | Broccoli | 20% |
| Cherries | 6% | Cabbage | 15% |
| Cucumbers | 11% | Carrots | 6% |
| Grapes, red | 4% | Corn | 10% |
| Oranges, Valencia | 7% | Kale | 16% |
| Peaches | 8% | Lettuce, green leaf | 22% |

| Strawberries | 7% | Spinach | 30% |
|---|---|---|---|
| Tomatoes, red | 12% | Cheese, cheddar | 26% |
| Watermelon | 7% | Milk, whole | 23% |
| Potatoes, baked | 7% | Egg, poached | 37% |
| Rice, white | 8% | Ice cream, chocolate | 8% |
| Spaghetti noodles | 14% | Beef, ground (avg) | 50% |

Another chart more specific to the 80/10/10 diet can be found in the back of this book on page 340. This chart shows values not only for protein but also for calories, carbohydrates, fat, water, and fiber for selected whole plant foods. In them, you will see that fruits generally contain 4 to 8% protein, and a few contain more. Surprisingly, the vegetables we commonly eat raw range from about 10 to 30% protein. (Vegetables are so low in calories, however, that even huge quantities add very little overall to one's daily protein percentage.) Nonetheless, when we calculate the caloronutrient ratio of a week's worth of food consisting strictly of a variety of raw fruits and vegetables without the addition of concentrated proteins, it generally weighs in just shy of 5% of calories as top-quality protein. A few ounces of nuts or seeds puts us at around 8% protein, well into the —an adequate and healthful amount range.

Mainstream nutritional science defines protein quality in terms of how efficiently the protein promotes body growth, rather than whether it produces health. Thus, milk and egg protein are considered the highest quality. However, in the words of T. Colin Campbell, "There is a mountain of compelling research showing that 'low-quality' plant protein … is the healthiest type of protein." [47]

Although many people are surprised to hear it, they understand the logic of this line of thought when they stop to consider what anthropoid primates in the wild eat: a diet that is made up primarily of fruits and vegetables. We have never heard that chimpanzees or orangutans—which are typically five times stronger than humans, pound for pound—need more protein than the amount they get from their plant-based diet.

## Americans Eat 16% Protein

As a percentage of calories consumed, the standard American diet, replete with meat, dairy, and eggs, runs in the teens. As stated above, the bell curve that describes protein consumption for the vast majority of the population ranges from 11 to 21% of calories from protein. Outliers on the low end include the small population of people who eat low-fat vegan fare, who can easily and healthfully reduce that number to single digits. At the high end, people who intentionally consume high-protein diets can approach 30%, but only bodybuilders and athletes who eat massive quantities of egg whites and isolated protein powders are likely to reach 40 or 50+ percent protein.

People are generally doubtful that protein could comprise such a small percentage of their diets, but I am not making these numbers up. According to the Centers for Disease Control and Prevention, average U.S. protein consumption was 15.5% for men and 15.1% for women in 2000. These numbers have been consistent for decades; in 1970 they were 16.5% and 16.9%.[48]

The U.S. Recommended Dietary Allowances, 10th Edition (1989) says, "Food consumption data from the U.S. USDA's 1977–1978 and 1985 surveys indicate that 14 to 18% of the total food energy intake is derived from protein. Despite wide variations in food energy intake, this proportion remains similar for both sexes and all age groups except infants. There is also little change as a function of household income, urbanization, or race. Food items likely to be underreported in surveys (e.g., alcoholic beverages, confections) would provide energy but little protein; hence, the percentage of energy from protein may be overestimated.[49]

***The standard American diet averages only 16% protein... 10% is a not a stretch.***

How can it be that as a nation we gorge on "high-protein" foods, yet we end up with less than 20% of our calories from protein? The answer is that the vast majority of our commonly consumed "protein" foods—meat, egg, and dairy products, as well as all nuts and seeds, contain such an overwhelming amount of fat that the protein numbers go way down as a percentage of total calories consumed. For example:

***In truth, there really is no such thing as a "high-protein" diet.***

- Eggs contain more than 60% fat.
- "70% lean" ground beef also weighs in at 60% fat.
- Cheddar cheese contains 72% fat; cream cheese 88%.
- Almonds and sunflower seeds each contain 73% fat.

In truth, there really is no such thing as a "high-protein" diet—at least not one in which protein comprises the majority of a person's calories. Typical quantities of high-protein "superfoods" increase protein consumption as a percentage of daily calories very little. For example, 10 grams of spirulina provides about 7 grams of protein, which might increase one's protein percentage from 16 to 17.2%. In other words, without serious powdered protein supplementation, most people would find it extremely difficult to consume even a third of their total calories from protein on a sustained basis.

This is good news, indeed, for even the 10% of calories from protein that I recommend is in truth the maximum that can reasonably be considered healthful, in my opinion.

## The Dangers of Eating More Than 10% Protein

To listen to the proponents of the meat industry, one would think we are in imminent danger of disease and death if we fail to eat meat three times a day. The truth is that eating meat this often causes the very conditions we're taught to fear. This is a surprise to most people, who have been taught, incorrectly, that they need large amounts of protein to be healthy. Actually, the reverse is true: Most people suffer from an overdose of protein each day, and this accounts for a great deal of our ill health.

Too much protein in our diets is associated with all manner of health impairments, including such symptoms as constipation and other digestive disorders that often lead to toxemia (toxic blood and tissues) and, eventually, cancer. Autoimmune dysfunction, arthritis, and all other autoimmune conditions, premature aging, impaired liver function, kidney failure, osteoporosis, and many other degenerative and pathogenic conditions result from eating more protein than we need.

In general, protein-based foods are highly acid forming in the human body (even the high-protein plants, such as legumes). This is because their predominant minerals are the acidic minerals—chlorine, phosphorus, and sulfur. To maintain homeostasis, the body must counterbalance the acidity caused by excess protein consumption. Unfortunately, it does so in part by taking a precious alkaline mineral—calcium—from our bloodstream. The body replaces calcium into the bloodstream, where calcium levels must remain relatively constant, by removing it from our bones and teeth, setting the stage for osteoporosis and tooth decay.

It is no coincidence that fruits and vegetables contain just the right amounts of protein to build and maintain the human body. Nor is it a coincidence that the minerals they supply are predominantly the alkaline ones: calcium, sodium, magnesium, and potassium.

## Calculating Your Protein Intake

The following examples show how a to calculate protein intake and how to convert gram measurements to percentage of calories. Calculations are based on the U.S. RDA of 0.36 grams of protein per pound of body weight (the *upper* limit of protein intake on the 80/10/10 diet).

My guidelines vary from these slightly, as I make my recommendations as a percentage of total calories consumed rather than by body weight. I believe this system works far better, because it allows for individual differences in fuel use, which can vary by a factor of ten for extremely sedentary people and extremely active people of the same weight.

125-Pound Woman: 45g

- 0.36 grams of protein 125 pounds = 45 grams of protein per day.
- 45 grams of protein contain approx. 180 calories (45 4 = 180).
- If this woman is sedentary and eats about 1,800 calories per day, this amount of protein would come to 10% of her total calories for the day.
- If this woman is more active and eats perhaps 2,300 calories per day, 180 calories of protein would amount to 8%.

175-Pound Man: 63g

- 0.36 grams of protein 175 pounds = 63 grams of protein per day.
- 63 grams of protein contain approx. 252 calories (63 4 = 252).
- If this man is sedentary and eats about 2,400 calories per day, this amount of protein would be just over 10% of his calories for the day.
- If this man is more active and eats 3,000 calories per day, 252 calories of protein would amount to 8%.

In light of the near-double safety factor of the U.S. RDA, I have no concerns when I see my clients consuming even less protein relative to their size.

In my experience, about 5% of calories from protein, especially when it is high quality and unadulterated by heat, is adequate and healthful.

That last statement, "5% of calories is adequate and healthful," is not a radical concept, not by a long shot. If you have any question whatsoever that this level of protein intake is healthy, or if you want indisputable evidence of the toxicity of higher protein consumption, I highly recommend that you pick up a copy of T. Colin Campbell's outstanding book, *The China Study*.[50] I cannot recommend it highly enough.

A consummate nutritional scientist, Dr. Campbell was at the helm of the most comprehensive study of health and nutrition ever conducted. His blockbuster book will leave you with no doubt that 5% protein, *exclusively from plant foods*, is more than enough.

## Protein from Fruits and Vegetables Only

On a diet of fruits and vegetables only, it is likely that your total protein intake will average about 5% of calories or slightly lower. Adding a small quantity of nuts or seeds results in a slight increase in protein intake percentage. For example:

- A meal of 10 peaches (420 calories) yields 7 grams of protein.
- Another meal of 10 bananas (1,085 calories) supplies 12 grams of protein.
- A bowl of soup made from 3 tomatoes blended with 2 cucumbers (150 calories) supplies more than 7 additional grams of protein.
- A pint of fresh-squeezed orange juice (225 calories) offers nearly 3.5 grams of protein.
- One medium head of lettuce (about 50 calories) provides about 5.5 grams of protein.
- Though we have only eaten 1,930 calories so far, the total protein consumed is 35 grams (over 6% of calories).

My recommendations for total calorie consumption are somewhat higher than most official recommendations. I do this not because I wish to see people gain fat, but because I know that an increased calorie intake— when accompanied by a commensurate increase in fitness activities—results in an overall higher level of fitness and health. It is this rise in calorie consumption, from an increased intake of fruits and vegetables, that assures the consumer of nutritional sufficiency.

In nature, we would have to be fit in order to survive. We would also eat fruits and vegetables, the most nutritious of all foods. In order to be well nourished, we are designed by Nature to consume the significant quantities of fruits and vegetables that would be eaten by a fit, active person.

## Protein Deficiency Does Not Exist

On a whole-food diet that provides sufficient calories, there is no such condition as a protein deficiency. A brochure from the Vegetarian Society of Colorado says, "Studies in which humans have been fed wheat bread alone, or potatoes alone, or corn alone, or rice alone, have all shown that these plant foods contain not only enough protein, but enough of all of the essential amino acids, to support growth and maintenance of healthy adults."[51]

A 1999 journal article entitled "Optimal Intakes of Protein in the Human Diet" confirms this fact, saying "… the true minimal [protein] requirement is likely to be so much lower than the amounts provided by natural diets (which are providing sufficient energy and other nutrients) that its magnitude becomes to some extent an issue of scientific curiosity only."[52]

In developing nations where insufficient food is available and people are literally starving to death, protein/calorie malnutrition conditions known as marasmus and kwashiorkor do exist, but these do not occur in developed countries. The symptoms—extreme emaciation, lassitude, and muscle wasting—resolve equally as well by the introduction of high-carbohydrate or high-fat foods as they do from the consumption of concentrated protein, and usually better. Protein deficiency, it turns out, just is not the cause of these problems. It is simply a shortage of food, a chronic severe deficiency of calories, that causes people to literally digest their own muscle tissues for fuel.

It is much more likely however, that a person would run into a huge host of other social, health, and nutritional problems long before developing the dreaded protein deficiency. Protein deficiency simply is not part of our reality. This is the main reason that this book focuses on just two of the three caloronutrients: only our fat and carbohydrate consumption rates tend to vary appreciably. As one goes up, the other, fairly reliably, goes down.

# Chapter 7
# Fat: 10% Maximum

Nutritionists have told us what to do in order to be healthier: increase our carbohydrate consumption and eat less fat. But knowing what to do does not mean that we will do it, of course. A prime example is quitting smoking. We have known for decades that smoking is killing us, yet according to the World Health Organization, more than a billion people continue to smoke. In order to make successful long-term changes, we must not only anticipate health as an outcome, we must also be happy about it.

Apparently we have not found a way to be happy while eating less fat. We certainly have not implemented this relatively simple change into our diets. Even the recent threats of morbid obesity, epidemic diabetes, bovine leukemia, and mad cow disease have not gotten us to reduce our intake of meat, dairy, poultry, fish, oils, or fats in general.

## How Much Fat Do We Need?

In its 2002 Dietary Reference Intakes (DRIs, which replaced the 1989 Recommended Dietary Allowances, or RDAs) the U.S. Department of Agriculture recommends that 20 to 35% of our calories be consumed as fat.[53] This advice is significantly skewed to the high side by the financial and lobbying influence of the U.S. dairy and meat lobbies.

In his book *The China Study*, Dr. T. Colin Campbell sheds some light on this longstanding problem. In 1982, while serving on a National Academies of Science expert panel, Campbell coauthored a report entitled *Diet, Nutrition and Cancer*. This was the first public scientific panel to openly question the wisdom of certain widely accepted nutritional standards. In particular, the panel recommended a substantial reduction in fat intake.

Campbell writes, "*The first guideline in the report explicitly stated that high fat consumption is linked to cancer, and recommended reducing our fat intake from 40% to 30% of calories.*" The report acknowledged that the 30% goal was an arbitrary cutoff point that represented a "moderate and practical target," but the data could easily have justified a greater reduction in recommended fat intake.

A more healthful "greater reduction," however, was not to be. As Campbell describes, "The director of the USDA Nutrition Laboratory told us that if we went below 30%, consumers would be required to reduce animal food intake and that would be the death of the report."[54]

In spite of such continuous industry pressure, some public agencies have succeeded in publishing lower guidelines. For example, a 2003 report on diet and chronic disease, commissioned by the World Health Organization and the Food and Agriculture Organization recommends a diet consisting of 15 to 30% fat.

Private sources offer an even more conservative perspective on healthful levels of fat consumption:

**Udo Erasmus**, author of *Fats That Heal, Fats That Kill*, has extensively researched the topic of fat consumption and health. What's more, he sells fat for a living. Yet in his book he recommends we eat just 15–20% of our calories as fat.[55]

**The Pritikin Longevity Center**, a facility that holds the finest heart disease reversal record of any such organization in the U.S., recommends a dietary fat consumption of 10%.[56]

**Dr. Dean Ornish**, a renowned cardiologist and author, also guides his heart patients to greater health and disease reversal through his near-vegetarian dietary program that includes not more than 10% fat.[57]

**Dr. Caldwell Esselstyn**, surgeon at the famed Cleveland Clinic and author of *Prevent and Reverse Heart Disease*, also recommends a low-fat cooked vegan diet where approximately 10% of calories come from fat.[58]

**Dr. Neal Barnard**, president of the Physicians Committee for Responsible Medicine and author of several books on vegan nutrition, is another proponent of approximately 10% fat for health.[59]

Many other doctors and PhDs famous for their work in nutrition have written extensively on the health benefits that predictably accompany a drastic reduction in dietary fat consumption. These include John McDougall, Michael Klaper, Alan Goldhamer, William Harris, Ruth Heidrich, Michael

Greger, and Matthew Lederman and Alona Pulde, among others. All of these professionals, as well as many dietitians, nutritionists, sports scientists, and other health experts agree the magic percentage could be as high as the teens, but no not much higher. Only industry-influenced government bodies recommend that we should limit fat consumption to 30% of our total calories. I would steer clear of any health "professional" or diet plan that claims that consuming 20% or more of our calories from fat is healthful (or even acceptable).

Several years ago, I read an interview in an airline magazine with the then-current director of nutrition for the U.S. Olympic Team. In it, she stated that the relative percentages of fat, protein, and carbohydrates in an athlete's diet should not vary, regardless of whether the athlete runs the mile or the marathon, lifts weights or plays table tennis, shoots skeet or puts the shot. She stated that without a doubt, the only nutritional change she would recommend from athlete to athlete would be the number of calories consumed, not the choice of food or caloronutrient ratio. She went on to assert that fruit is like magic food for athletes. The International Olympic Committee, in its book *Food, Nutrition and Sports Performance*, concluded that a diet based on fruits and vegetables was the healthiest for athletes and would result in the best possible performance.[60]

## The Role of Fats

Fats serve a wide variety of functions in our diet and in the human body. It is wrong to think of fats as being all bad. Fats are a concentrated source of fuel, providing more than double the calories per gram of either carbohydrates or proteins. They play an as-yet not totally understood role in satiation, possibly because they are so difficult to digest. The fat in foods serves as the sole carrier/source of our fat-soluble vitamins. Dietary fat is also the source of the widely misunderstood nutrients known as essential fatty acids.

***The roles of fats are many, and all are important. But a little goes a long way.***

Fat plays many important roles in regulation of various bodily functions. It is essential to our production of hormones, although too much fat will exert an adverse influence on our hormones. It also helps to regulate the uptake of nutrients and excretion of waste products by every cell. Fat is the primary insulator within the body. It protects us against cold and heat, keeps the electricity that flows through our nerves on course, and protects our vital organs from jarring and other types of physical shock.

## Types of Fat

Fat is fat, or so a great many people think. Actually, there are many types of fat. Some are considered good; others are considered bad, and still others are a mixed bag. Some fats are solid at room temperature; others are liquid. Many fats are indigestible and unusable by the body, while some are indispensable. There are overt fats and covert fats, short-, medium-, and long-chain fats, saturated, monounsaturated, and polyunsaturated fats. There are cooked fats and raw fats—and yes, there is a difference. There is also a big difference between animal-derived fats and plant-based fats, at least where our health is concerned.

Yet with all the dietary fats available on the planet, a man walking in the jungle with nothing more than his bare hands would have a very difficult time putting his lips to any but a minimal amount of fat, and then only if he hit the season exactly right. Animals that are built similarly to man eat a diet that is very low in fat. They rely upon fruits and vegetables for their calories, not fats. Let's look at fat in a little more detail.

***It's hard to make a meal of in-shell nuts fresh from the tree.***

Fatty acids comprise the basic structural unit of all "lipids" (a term comprising oily, water-insoluble substances that include fats, oils, waxes, sterols, and triglycerides). You can think of fatty acids as the building blocks of fat. They are found, on their own, in all whole foods. When fatty acids are joined to the other more complex lipid structures, the fatty acids are responsible for the properties demonstrated by that lipid.

### *Overt and Covert Fats*

Overt fats are the fats that you can see, or at least tell, are in our foods. Since our taste buds cannot distinguish fat, we only detect it by the greasy feeling on our hands or lips. To us, fat is tasteless. If a food is fatty, oftentimes people have to be told. Many people are surprised to find out the actual fat content of the foods they eat.

### Typical Fat Content of Selected Foods

(percentage of calories)

- Nuts and seeds: 60 to 90% fat
- Wieners and sausages: 70 to 85% fat
- Beef ribs: 65 to 80% fat
- Hamburger patty: 55 to 65% fat
- Chicken with skin, roasted: 36 to 63% fat
- French fries: 45% fat
- Chocolate chip cookies: 45% fat
- Apple pie: 40% fat
- Swordfish, grilled: 30% fat
- Baked potato with ¼ cup of reduced-fat sour cream: 20% fat
- Chicken breast, broiled skinless: 20% fat

Flesh, including fish, fowl, and game, as well as eggs and dairy, nuts and seeds, olives, avocados, and all oils make up the bulk of the overtly fatty foods. Deep-fried foods of all kinds are extremely fatty and also count as overt fats. Many desserts are also overtly fatty, such as cheesecake, ice cream, pastries, and nutty candies. Yet all of these foods account for less than half of the fat consumed in the typical American diet.

The remainder is often referred to as "invisible" fat. We will call it "covert." Covert fats are more hidden. Vegetables, sweet fruits, and nonsweet fruits like tomatoes and cucumbers contain enough fat that should you eat them exclusively (in quantities sufficient to meet your caloric needs) and consume no overt fats whatsoever, you will average between 3 and 5% of your total calories from fat.

Eating primarily low-fat fruits and vegetables—accompanied by a very small amount of nuts, seeds, and fatty fruits such that total fat does not exceed 10% of calories—provides sufficient fat to cover all of our nutritional needs.

### *Solid and Liquid Fats*

We readily identify fat when we see it congealed on the top of soup that has cooled. We have no problem recognizing a stick of butter, or that white stuff around the edges of our steak, as fat. But many people find it difficult to conceive of liquids as fat.

All oils are fats, but all fats are not oils. What is the difference? Oils are fats that tend to be liquid at room temperature. Both solid and liquid fats function nutritionally as fat. Both oils and fats exist within walnuts and avocados. Whereas you can feel the liquid oil in a pine nut, you cannot separate the oil from the lettuce; they are one. The 80/10/10 diet does not recommend the consumption of refined oils, those separated (extracted) from foods; rather, we recommend eating foods with oils in them, especially over foods with solid fats in them.

## How Can 2% Milk Be 35% Fat?

You may have heard someone say that "2% milk" is anything but low fat. Most of us who have not taken the time to learn the nuances of interpreting food labels find this quite paradoxical. How can it be?

The answer lies in the distinction between percentage by weight versus percentage by calories. The following macronutrient calculation example demonstrates this distinction and shows just how misleading food marketing can be.

**100 grams of whole milk contain 60 calories.**

Its weight (100 grams) is distributed as follows:

| | |
|---|---|
| 88.3 | grams of water |
| 0.7 | grams of ash (solid residue) |
| 4.5 | grams of carbohydrates ( 4 calories per gram = 18 carb calories) |
| 3.2 | grams of protein ( 4 calories per gram = 13 protein calories) |
| 3.3 | grams of fat ( 9 calories per gram = 30 fat calories) |

**100 grams total**

As you can see, 88% of the milk's weight (the water) provides no calories. Among the remainder, 3.3 grams out of the 100 grams are fat, which is why the milk label shows "3.25% milk fat."

However, protein, fat, and carbohydrates do not all contain similar energy value; fat packs more than twice the calories of an equivalent amount of carbohydrates or protein. In rough numbers, each of the 3.3 grams of fat contain approximately 9 calories, while the 3.2 grams of protein and 4.5 grams of carbohydrates contain about 4 calories each.

Thus, in terms of calories, 30 of the 60 calories in whole milk come from fat, a fact the dairy industry is very happy to obscure. The table below summarizes the fat content of the common fluid milk products:

| Item (100 grams) | Cals | Fat Cals | % Fat |
|---|---|---|---|
| Whole milk ("3.25% milk fat") | 60 | 30 | 50% |
| Reduced fat milk ("2% milk fat") | 50 | 17 | 35% |
| Low-fat milk ("1% milk fat") | 42 | 9 | 20% |
| Nonfat milk | 35 | 0.7 | 2% |

Interestingly, the "nonfat" milk contains the 2% fat that the dairy industry would like you to think is in its "2%" product!

The idea that all fats derived from animals are solid while all those found in plants are liquid is inaccurate, although this is true in the majority of cases. The primary exceptions are liquid fish oils in the animal kingdom and solid coconut oil in the plant world.

### *Essential and Nonessential Fats*

Essential fatty acids[61] (also referred to as EFAs) are so named because they cannot be synthesized; we must consume them in our foods. They play an integral role in the health of our skin, in growth and development, the stability of our heartbeat, and the clotting and flowing of our blood. Too much, too little, or the wrong ratio of these vital nutrients can wreak havoc on our health.

Currently, two fatty acids are thought to be essential: alpha-linolenic acid (ALA), and linoleic acid (LA), omega-3 and omega-6, respectively. Omega-3 and omega-6 fatty acids are commonly understood as synonyms of the term "EFA," but twelve different fatty acids are actually made from ALA and LA. And all of the fatty acids that stem from these are classified as omega-3 and omega-6. Thus, by definition, not all omega-3 and 6 family fatty acids are essential. Only the polyunsaturated fats ALA and LA must be attained from external sources. The omega-3 fatty acids made from ALA include some notable members such as EPA (eiocosapentaenoic acid) and

DHA (docosahexaenoic acid). In the omega-6 family, the most notable members are arachidonic acid (AA) and gamma-linolenic acid (GLA).

Interestingly, current research in nutritional science is questioning whether ALA is actually essential, since evidence exists that the body may be able to synthesize it, as well. Thankfully, we needn't worry about this, since both linoleic and alpha-linolenic fatty acids are both quite common in the makeup of plant lipids.

There are is no established *minimum* recommendations for EFAs, but we do know that their ratio to one another is as important, if not more important, than the quantity we consume. Scientists generally accept that early man consumed omega-6 and omega-3 fatty acids in roughly a 1:1 ratio. This happens to be the same ratio of essential fatty acids found in the human brain.[62]

Historically, as grain consumption escalated and the use of oils heavily laden with omega-6 became commonplace in our diets, this ratio began to shift. Current recommendations suggest that the ideal ratio is between 1:1 and 4:1 (omega-6 to omega-3). In spite of this "ideal' range, the average American diet shows a ratio ranging from 10 to 30:1, a dietary choice that contributes significantly to the prevalence of inflammatory diseases and other very serious health issues in our nation. This seriously skewed ratio compromises the body's ability to convert ALA into longer-chain fatty acids, such as EPA and DHA.

***Omega-3 and omega-6 are intermediates for a dozen other fatty acids.***

Lacking an agreed-upon minimum EFA requirement, we do have some data to guide us. In November of 2008, the Food and Agriculture Organization of the United Nations and the World Health Organization convened a meeting of experts to review the major developments in the field of fatty acids in human nutrition. Its final report is yet to be published, but a preliminary summary concludes, "the available evidence indicates that 0.5 to 0.6%E [percentage of energy, or calories] alpha-linolenic acid (ALA) per day corresponds to the prevention of deficiency symptoms."[63] Previously in 2002, the Food and Nutrition Board of the U.S. Institute of Medicine (IOM) recommended an "adequate intake" (AI), which is not a minimum, for omega-3 of 1.1 (women) to 1.6 (men) grams per day.[64] If consumed as oil (not recommended), this amount would be extraordinarily small: 1.6 grams equates to approximately a third of a teaspoon, or a couple dozen drops ... and even this low number may be substantially inflated.[65]

The information above can be combined to guide us in determining our nutritional needs. On a 2,000-calorie diet, 0.5% of calories from ALA, or omega-3 represents 10 calories. This is approximately 1.1 grams of ALA, which falls within the IOM's adequate intake levels (albeit at the bottom of the range). This quantity of ALA can be obtained through the consumption of whole fresh fruits and vegetables, with the occasional addition of nuts and seeds. The following table shows ALA and LA content of selected whole foods.

**EFA Content of Various Whole Foods (grams)**

| 1 oz. Fatty Fruits/Nuts | ALA (omega-3) | LA (omega-6) |
|---|---|---|
| Avocado | 0.04 | 0.47 |
| Flaxseed | 6.45 | 1.67 |
| Olive | 0.02 | 0.24 |
| Pine nuts | 0.22 | 7.03 |
| Walnuts | 2.57 | 10.76 |
| **8 oz. Fruits & Vegetables** | **ALA (omega-3)** | **LA (omega-6)** |
| Banana | 0.06 | 0.10 |
| Blueberry | 0.13 | 0.20 |
| Cabbage | 0.08 | 0.06 |
| Fig | 0.00 | 0.33 |
| Kale | 0.41 | 0.31 |
| Kiwi | 0.10 | 0.56 |
| Mango | 0.08 | 0.03 |
| Oranges | 0.02 | 0.04 |
| Papaya | 0.01 | 0.06 |
| Peaches | 0.00 | 0.19 |
| Pineapple | 0.04 | 0.05 |
| Romaine lettuce | 0.26 | 0.11 |
| Strawberries | 0.15 | 0.20 |
| Tomatoes | 0.01 | 0.18 |

Based on the above numbers, on a 2,000-calorie 80/10/10 diet, we could obtain recommended levels of EFAs with the following:

- Breakfast: 1.5 lbs. of mangos (about 3) and 12 oz. blueberries.
- Lunch: 44 oz. of bananas (about 11).
- Dinner: 1 lb. of oranges, 1 lb. of romaine lettuce, and 8 oz. of tomatoes.

According to the USDA nutrient database, this meal plan (totaling 2048 calories) provides 1.3 grams of ALA and 1.4 grams of LA. This maintains the 1:1 ratio and supplies the adequate EFAs without including any overt fats at all. Including healthful (very small) amounts of overt fats on occasion will ensure your needs are met.

Since the average American consumes a higher ratio of omega-6 than omega-3, we are bombarded with nutritional information directing us toward omega-3 supplements. The idea that we need to consume more of some particular nutrient to balance another that is overconsumed is as ineffective as taking vitamin C to minimize the damage from smoking cigarettes. The result of increasing fat consumption, whether from "good" fats or not, is that we end up consuming too much fat. Our need to supplement for nutritional balance would not exist if we were not harming ourselves through our lifestyle and foodstyle choices in the first place. In our natural diet, the foods are automatically balanced to suit our nutritional requirements.

### Cholesterol

Cholesterol, a sterol (combination steroid and alcohol) and lipid, is found in the makeup of every cell membrane and is transported in the blood of every animal. The precursor of the five major classes of steroid hormones (progestagens, glucocorticoids, mineralocorticoids, androgens, and estrogens), cholesterol is not all bad but is vital to human life. Some of its many functions include the production of vitamin D and the formation of the bile salts, the sex hormones testosterone and progesterone, and the myelin sheath that surrounds our nerves.

Discovered during the late 1700s in gallstones, cholesterol is still the subject of much study. We know that cholesterol is not an essential nutrient for humans (we don't need to eat it). Our livers produce all the cholesterol we need. However, when we regularly consume animal foods that contain cholesterol or saturated fat, we ingest quantities that exceed our physiological needs, with deleterious consequences to our health. Excess cholesterol accumulates and forms plaques within artery walls, leading to atherosclerosis (hardening of the arteries), decreasing the oxygen-carrying capacity of the blood, disrupting hormonal balance, and sometimes decreasing cell permeability.

### Saturated and Unsaturated Fats

Saturated fatty acids are so named because their long chain of carbon atoms contains the maximum possible number of hydrogen atoms—in other words, they are *saturated* with hydrogen. These fatty acids have the highest melting point and are solid at room temperature. Saturated fats are stable molecules, and as such are very unlikely to change, making it impossible for the body to do anything constructive with dietary saturated fats.

Yes, our brains are high in saturated fats, but eating saturated fats will not improve brain function or slow its degeneration. In fact, our bodies are simply not capable of utilizing dietary saturated fats. At best, the body stores dietary saturated fats as body fat and at worst, the fats accumulate along arterial walls.

#### Do We Need Lauric Acid from Virgin Coconut Oil?

Lauric acid is the subject of quite a bit of current research. This medium-chain fatty acid is primarily found in mother's milk, coconuts and their oil, cocoa butter, palm oil, and palm kernel oil. The latter three are highly saturated plant fats. While virgin coconut oil may pose less health risk when consumed raw than saturated cooked fats, it is still a fractional, artery-clogging refined saturated fat that our digestive system is not designed to process.[66] Later in this chapter I talk more about why oils in general are unhealthful; please see "Oil Is Not Health Food" on page 130.

The antibacterial and antimicrobial properties of lauric acid are not desirable traits, as slick marketing would have you believe. Antibiotic (literally meaning "anti-life") is not a property that we should seek in food. The internal environment of a healthy adult who eats a low-fat, low-toxin diet does not harbor excess harmful bacteria.[67] When we develop healthful living habits, our body has all the resources it needs to care for itself.

Unsaturated fatty acids make up the bulk of plant fats. *Mono*unsaturated fats contain one double or triple bond; *poly*unsaturated fats have two or more double bonds. Hydrogen atoms are eliminated where double bonds are formed. The body adds hydrogen, a process that saturates the fat. In other words, the unsaturated fat molecule is malleable and is subject to change within the body. The body can work with it and utilize it. It then integrates these self-manufactured saturated fats into our bodily structure as needed.

**Monounsaturated fatty acids** can accommodate a single pair of hydrogen atoms. Monounsaturated oils have a lower melting temperature than saturated fatty acids. Whole-food raw plant sources of monounsaturated fat include avocados, almonds, and other nuts and seeds and their butters.

**Polyunsaturated fatty acids** are the least saturated, with room for two or more pairs of hydrogen atoms. Polyunsaturated oils have even lower melting points, meaning they are all liquid at room temperature. Whole-food raw plant sources of polyunsaturated fat include walnuts and other nuts and seeds and their butters, as well as leafy green vegetables.

Generally, the less saturated the fatty acid, the more easily it can be utilized by the body.

### S/P Ratio

Nutritionists have recommended a healthy ratio of saturated to polyunsaturated fats for the last fifty years. The ratio is called the "S/P ratio." The suggested ratio that is best for health has been placed at 20/80 (20% saturated to 80% polyunsaturated). This is an accepted standard in the world of nutrition.

Note that the S/P ratio of most plants, including nuts and seeds, is ideal: 20/80, or extremely close to it. The proportion of saturated to polyunsaturated fatty acids in most animal foods is 80/20, the exact opposite of the ratio we require.

When we discuss the health values of different types of fat, it is important to remember the S/P ratio. The structure of the fat we consume very profoundly affects bodily function. As this number skews toward saturated fats in the diet, we see increases in atherosclerosis and other forms of heart disease, the number-one killer in the westernized world. It is literally impossible to achieve a healthy S/P ratio while including products of animal origin in our diets.

## How Much Fat Do We Eat?

Americans consume one-third to one-half of their calories as fat. In my experience, the number tends to gravitate around 42% for the average fast-food connoisseur. Government national average statistics weigh in lower, because they include people who eat low-fat diets, people who eat massive amounts of refined sugars, and those on every other conceivable dietary plan.

In 2004, the U. S. Centers for Disease Control and Prevention released a report entitled "Trends in Intake of Energy and Macronutrients—United States, 1971–2000,"[68] which highlights an important distinction: although the average percentage of calories from fat decreased a few percentage points from 1971 to 2000 (4% for men, from 37 to 33% of calories, and 3% for women, from 36 to 33%), the total fat consumed shows a different picture.

On average, total fat intake (in grams) increased among women by 6.5 g and decreased among men by 5.3 g, reflecting a near-zero overall change. This is because a statistically significant increase in average energy (calorie) intake occurred during that period: men's calorie intake increased from 2,450 to 2,618 calories per day, and women's calorie intake increased from 1,542 to 1,877 calories per day. (This data includes numbers for men and women from 20 to 74 years of age; younger people eat more and older people eat less than these averages overall). The bulk of increased calories has come in the form of carbohydrates, as consumption of refined sugary desserts, breads, crackers, pastries, soft drinks, and alcohol have skyrocketed.

People commonly consume more fat than they need in one of the following three ways:

- Some people overeat fat while keeping their total calories at the right level to maintain their weight. To accomplish this, they must, of necessity, undereat carbohydrates. The immediate consequences of eating too few carbohydrates can include lethargy, cravings, bingeing, and emotional instability.

- Other people overeat fat while undereating in terms of total calories. Such a diet produces weight loss, but it falls far short in some nutrients—while providing potentially fatal overdoses of others. If we minimize one of the caloronutrients from our diets (carbohydrates), of course we will lose weight; we will have almost halved our calorie intake. However, we have to learn to ignore our natural sweet tooth, while living with an incessant and ever-growing craving for carbohydrates.

- Finally, there are those who overeat fat while overeating in terms of total calories. The results of this practice are well known. In addition to all the ill effects which result from a high-fat diet, overeating on calories contributes to overweight, obesity, lethargy, digestive illness, a reduced life-span among other illnesses.

Whether they realize it or not, most people tend to gravitate toward 42% fat, regardless of the type of diet that they follow.

### Vegetarians

Many people think of themselves as vegetarians even though they eat at least some flesh food. Their diets are generally skewed toward fish and fowl, under the false assumption that these are more healthful choices. They consider themselves "on the vegetarian path," and they eat flesh "sparingly" compared to the amount they ate in the past.

Lacto-ovo vegetarians, (those who don't eat flesh) tend to make up for the lack of meat in their diets by increasing their consumption of dairy and eggs. Vegetarian options such as cheese sandwiches, fried potatoes, cheese- and oil-drenched pastas, and rich fatty desserts often become the focus of their dietary regimens.

Vegetarians quickly learn to recreate all their old favorite foods in a style that is acceptable to their new ethics. Vegetarian pizza may not have meat, but it often has a double portion of cheese and does not lack at all in fat. Vegetarians are generally happy that they can eat familiar foods while feeling no sense of deprivation. In the final analysis, the vegetarian diet averages around 42% fat.

### Vegans

**_Just because your fats come from plants doesn't mean you should use them liberally._**

In addition to eating no flesh of any kind, including seafood, vegans do not consume dairy, eggs, honey, or any other animal-derived products. Vegan alternatives to most conventional food items are now sold in supermarkets. They are also the stock-in-trade of the larger health-food stores nationwide. Vegan lasagna (using soy cheese) and even vegan milk (from soy, almonds, or rice) are common today. Vegan chefs abound, and big cities like Los Angeles, New York, and Seattle boast vegan restaurants featuring the cuisines of many nations of the world, including India, China, Jamaica, Italy, Thailand, and others.

Margarine, a vegan product, (the health "value" of margarine, even compared with butter, is another story altogether) contains the same percentage of calories from fat as butter: 100%. Oil generally plays a larger role in the vegan diet than in the standard American diet, as it replaces many of the animal fats. Vegans often increase their use of nuts, seeds, avocados, and olives, as well.

Essentially, vegans eat their own version of the standard American diet, with vegan versions of all the same foods that they ate before. It should then come as no surprise that when we analyze the caloronutrient ratio of the vegan diet, we find that it doesn't change much.

If anything, vegans often allow their dietary fat intake to swell even higher than the mainstream. Vegans think that they do not need to limit their fat intake, because they believe that the animal products were the only "offenders" in their old program. Even if their fat intake remains the same, overall calorie intake often drops when vegans replace animal foods with plant foods (which provide fewer calories per bite). Thus, the percentage of the vegan diet that comes from fat rises.

The average, however, remains close to 42%, because a good number of vegans follow "low-fat" programs, as well. Nonetheless, the vegan diet, with its increased use of fruits and vegetables, and its superior S/P ratio, is overall a far healthier diet than the standard American diet or vegetarian options. Still, too much fat is too much fat.

## Eating Fat: Good or Bad for Us?

More fat than we require is not an asset but a detriment to good nutrition. The more fat we eat, the further we stray from meeting our nutritional needs. A steady flow of research comes out regularly relating high-fat diets to almost every type of digestive disturbance, blood disorder, and degenerative disease. Much of this is caused by the body's reduced ability to uptake, transport, and deliver oxygen to our trillions of cells. (We discussed this at length in Chapter 2 . In addition, too much fat reduces the actual number of viable red blood cells. Excessive fat consumption may be commonplace, but it is nothing short of nutritional disaster.

A high-fat diet not only destroys our health, but it ages us, as well. Due to our inability to taste fat, we tend to dress our fatty foods with stimulants and irritating condiments, to give them flavor. These very stimulants and condiments accelerate the aging process. We pay for every "up" with a subsequent down. All isolated substances extracted from whole foods have this effect upon the body, even if they are promoted as supplements, beauty or rejuvenation aids, or other types of health builders. Combine the influence of these food additives with the extra work the body performs to process high-fat meals, as well as the compromises in blood function that plague people in the habit of eating heavy, fatty diets, and you have the perfect recipe for the early onset of aging and health decline.

## Oil Is Not Health Food

While we have learned and repeatedly demonstrated that whole foods are the only source of balanced nutrition, many health advisors tell us that refined, isolated fats and oils should be considered "health foods." They almost all sell some type of "food-grade" oil, which seems like a fairly strong endorsement. Are we just supposed to ignore the obvious contradiction?

Some vendors promote the consumption of oil as part of an internal "cleanse" program. I have even heard oil referred to as "juice," with the suggestion that we drink it as a daily health practice. This is the stuff that draws ridicule from mainstream scientists and nutritionists, and, at least according to many health experts, is why the raw movement is being laughed out of the scientific community.

***A high-fat diet not only destroys our health but it ages us, as well.***

### Oils ... Empty Calories at Best, Carcinogenic Junk Food at Worst

Across the board, refined oils (including coconut, flax, olive, hemp, almond, borage, and the like, which are touted as "pure" or "special" because of their source or careful processing methods) are essentially empty calories, not fit for human consumption. They are stripped of the fiber, protein, and carbohydrates that accompanied the whole foods from which they were derived, leaving an imbalanced fractional product that is 100% fat.

In contrast, whole-food fats eaten sparingly (fresh nuts, seeds, avocados, or young coconut flesh) provide some useful nutrition and are not automatically detrimental to health. Using such intact sources of fat in salad dressings and other dishes with their full complement of macro and micronutrients is by far preferable to using refined oils.

Although oil vendors tout a wide variety of health benefits to be gained from the phytochemicals contained within cold expeller-pressed oils, there can be no doubt that these delicate micronutrients are more potent when left untouched within the whole foods. Maximum nutrition occurs when our teeth are the first thing to break Nature's package ... rather than a machine, an appliance, or even a knife.

Further, the fiber contained in whole plant foods helps keep fats from going rancid. Shortly after extracting any oil from its source and discarding the fiber, early-stage rancidity (and therefore potential carcinogenicity) ensues, even if we cannot detect it. As rancidity begins to set in, micronutrients become deranged.

If calling refined oil "empty calories" doesn't sit well with you, chalk it up to good marketing—because oil (pure fat) fits the description of empty calories perfectly, as do protein powder (pure protein) and table sugar (pure carbohydrate). These include commodities popular among raw fooders such as evaporated cane sugar (Rapadura) and hemp protein. Empty calories invariably provide less nutritional value than their whole-food counterparts.

If we think only in terms of symptoms, we may indeed perceive some benefits from consuming oil. But when we extract the oil from nuts and seeds in a vain attempt to maximize their anticancer properties and concentrate other nutrients, we create (often undetectable) imbalances within the body that inevitably produce unintended health problems. Adding oils into the diet to treat symptoms such as dry skin, eczema, dandruff, candida, joint aches, etc., which were not caused by a lack of oils (no known symptom is actually caused by a lack of oil), is totally nonsensical.

Rather than treat or suppress the symptoms of any condition, it is always a healthier strategy to remove the causes of the condition. True health is created from the inside out, not through lotions, potions, or other aids. Increasing the amount of high-water-content fruits and vegetables while reducing fat consumption to a healthful range is the foundation for creating a healthful life.

Eating for health requires a shift in thinking, from "is this good for me" to "what am I designed for?" No matter how we look at it, oil is simply not necessary in our diet and should never be considered a health food (or even a food, in my opinion).

## 10% Fat for Health

If you are relatively new to the idea of monitoring your caloronutrient ratio, bringing your total fat consumption down to the teens (under 20%) is an excellent initial goal. You can accomplish this by just calculating the fat in your nuts/seeds/avocados/etc., without factoring in the covert fats in your low-fat fruits and vegetables. These foods add only a negligible amount of fat to the daily intake—just a few percentage points total.

As eating a greater volume of fruits and vegetables gets easier, you may decide that it is worth your effort to track the covert as well as the overt fats for a short time, in order to get a more realistic view of your total fat consumption. You may find that you need to be vigilant in monitoring fat intake, at least at first, because fat calories are more concentrated than carbohydrate or protein calories and therefore, are easy to miss.

## The Caloronutrient Seesaw

A truly healthy diet is well balanced in nutrients, but the balance is not the one we have been taught. Eating 80%$^{+}$ of calories from carbohydrates, with fat and protein in the upper single digits, actually balances what I term "the caloronutrient seesaw" quite nicely.

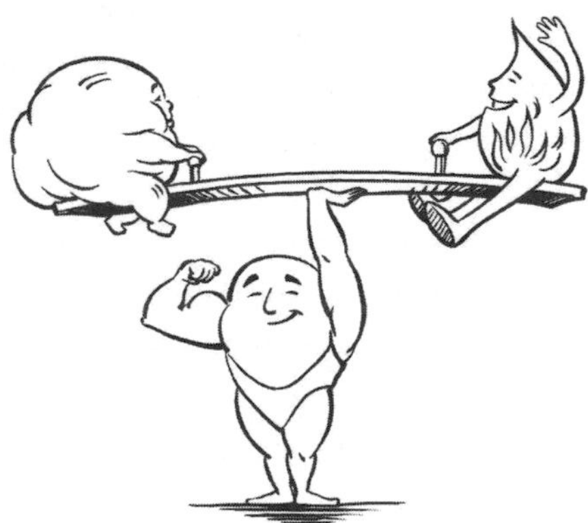

In the graphic above, protein is the fulcrum, and fat weighs so heavy on our system that just a little bit goes a very long way. A balanced caloronutrient seesaw would be 80%$^{+}$ carbs, with single-digit (less than 10%) protein and fats. When this ratio comes from whole, fresh, ripe, raw, organic, plants, all the rest of your food-related nutrients will be consumed in the optimum quantities for human health.

# Chapter 8
# The Big Surprise: Raw Fooders Average 60%+ Fat!

As is true of new vegetarians or vegans, when people initially begin incorporating raw foods into their diets, they almost automatically gravitate toward foods of similar composition to the ones they are used to, in order to feel satisfied. With delight and abandon, they eat their fill of luscious raw concoctions that are tremendously rich and difficult to digest, certain that they have reached "nutrition nirvana." In the back of their minds, they may recall someone having mentioned that these are "transitional" or "celebration" foods, but today they are still celebrating their transition ... and what a party it is!

Can you make raw pizza? Sure, that's easy. You can find hundreds of pizza recipes among the dozens of raw websites and recipe books available today. Virtually any dish from any cuisine can be replicated using only raw ingredients.

In some parts of the U.S. and abroad, it is becoming easier and easier to jump on the raw food bandwagon. The raw-curious can dip their toes into an ever-expanding array of potlucks, food-preparation workshops, chef trainings, and prepared food offerings being presented by local raw chefs, speakers, and food vendors. Prepackaged raw snacks, desserts, and entrées are becoming popular in many health-food stores, sometimes meriting a section of their own with multiple rows of taste sensations. And it seems a new raw restaurant, or at least a deli with a few raw options, opens every week in some area of the country.

***Virtually every raw "gourmet" food you are likely to encounter Is loaded with fat.***

For those with computer access, virtual communities and online discussion boards abound, and it doesn't take much searching to find plenty of helpful support (and confusing information) for your new endeavor. And if you can afford the luxury of travel, you can find raw retreats, festivals, and educational events taking place across the globe year 'round.

Unbeknownst to the new raw food enthusiast, however, virtually every speaker they are likely to hear and every food they are likely to taste will lead them down a garden path to a raw diet that at least equals—and often far surpasses—the fat content of mainstream American fare, in terms of percentage of calories consumed.

Yes, you read that correctly: Almost across the board, raw fooders rank right up there with the burgers-and-fries crowd when it comes to ingesting fat, almost always consuming 50% of their calories as fat, usually far more. I see it all the time: raw fooders who eat a chocolate-coconut-almond shake or a fruit-and-flax-oil smoothie for breakfast, a nut pâté for lunch with an oil-drenched, avocado-laden salad on the side, glorious granola bars or slices of fruit slathered with nut butter as snacks, and tahini-dressed greens and sprouts for dinner with more avocado, plus a plate of seed cheese on flax crackers.

***A high-fat raw diet leaves us dehydrated, deoxygenated, and undernourished.***

Such a regimen can easily top 75% fat and may seem far too heavy for a seasoned raw fooder. Over time, most people who eat a raw diet refine their menus, eventually ending up eating "simple meals," which include more fruits and vegetables and fewer fats. But it takes precious little in the way of nuts and seeds to equal or exceed the percentage of fat consumed by the average American. Even longtime raw fooders who consider their diets massively simplified in comparison to their early days are often astonished to learn that they still consume an average of 40 or 50% fat!

### *"Don't Worry, It's Raw ..."*

Many leaders of the raw food movement endow raw foods with almost supernatural powers, teaching that consuming fat won't harm us "as long as it is raw fat." They tell people that the unstable fats in nuts and seeds can withstand the sustained heat of lengthy dehydration and subsequent room-temperature storage without degrading or going rancid. This is wishful thinking on the part of people wishing to profit from the high-fat raw fad by selling flax crackers, granola bars, and other dehydrated prepared foods. Eating such concoctions within hours of dehydration is safest, but it is still a far cry from eating fresh, unprocessed whole-food fats as they occur in nature. Some even pride themselves on eating 80% of calories from fat and beyond, recommending such a program as perfectly safe, which it categorically is not.

The high-fat raw foods that well-meaning raw chefs, teachers, and authors promote are very likely to cause in raw fooders many of the same health issues that plague cooked food eaters, including candida, chronic and intermittent fatigue, and even heart disease. These maladies result in large part from excess fat in the bloodstream, a correlation explained in "Chapter 2". Sadly, I personally know two raw fooders who have undergone open-heart surgery this decade. Yes ... their high-fat raw diets resulted in the total blockage of their coronary arteries.

Raw fats are without question far better for us than cooked fats—especially when they come from whole plants as opposed to extracted oils or cooked animal products. But do not let anyone mislead you: the habitual consumption of fatty foods is not a healthful practice.

### *Cooked or Raw, Too Much Fat Is Still Too Much Fat*

Whether you eat cooked animal fat, cold-pressed plant oil, or whole-food raw fats, too much fat is too much fat ... and we must recognize its health-destroying potential. Below are a few examples. (See "Cooking Damages Nutrients" on page 57 for more information on the additional health problems we create by cooking our fats.)

- Cooked or raw, higher-than-healthy levels of fat in the bloodstream force fat to "precipitate out" and adhere to arterial walls, a condition known as atherosclerosis. Hypertension, aneurism, atherosclerosis, embolism (thrombus), myocardial infarction, cerebral infarction, and other vascular disorders are all related to excessive consumption of dietary fat.

- Cooked or raw, increased fat in the bloodstream reduces the oxygen-carrying capacity of red blood cells, predisposing us to cancer. A lowered blood-oxygen level also adversely affects all cellular function, including muscle and brain-cell function. Reduced oxygen to the brain results in impaired clarity of thought, poor decision making, and a dull mind. Some researchers have suggested that impaired oxygen delivery sets the stage for senility, memory dysfunction, and learning disabilities.

- Cooked or raw, increased fat in the bloodstream requires an increased epinephrine (adrenaline) response in order to drive the pancreas to produce insulin. Following excess stimulation, adrenal exhaustion sets in, as required by the Law of Dual Effect. Adrenal exhaustion is the precursor for conditions such as mononucleosis, Epstein-Barr virus, chronic fatigue syndrome/myalgic encephalomyelitis (ME), post-viral fatigue syndrome, lupus, and myofascial disease, to name just a few.

- Cooked or raw, increased fat in the bloodstream results in increased demand for insulin, known as insulin resistance. As described in "Chapter 2", the resulting continuous drain on the pancreas eventually leads to pancreatic fatigue and chronically elevated blood-sugar levels. This predisposes us to a group of lipid (fat) metabolic disorders, mistakenly referred to as "blood-sugar metabolic disorders": hyper- and hypoglycemia, hyperinsulinism, candida infections, diabetes, and others.

- Cooked or raw, the excessive consumption of fat has been incontrovertibly linked to the development of cancer, heart disease, and diabetes. Future research is expected to continue to support this statement, as countless thousands of studies have already done, including the Framingham Heart Study and the China Study, respectively the longest and the largest nutrition studies ever undertaken. When other lifestyle factors are equal, the greater the amount of fat that a population consumes, the higher the rates of these dreaded conditions. It has been shown that when we consume more fat than we require, we almost invariably consume less carbohydrate than we require. Insufficient carbohydrate consumption will result in feelings of fatigue, loss of strength, reduced sex drive, and a general lowering of vigor and vitality.

### "Not Me," You Say?

If you have been following a raw diet, you are probably almost certain that it does not contain 60% or more fat. "I love my salads. I eat lots of greens," you say. "I eat tons of fruit, too, compared to most people. There's no way I eat that much fat!" Yet fat has a way of sneaking into the diet, whether it is cooked or raw, and you won't notice it unless you understand where it comes from.

I analyze what people eat on an ongoing basis. While I occasionally meet someone who both claims to consume a low-fat diet and actually does so, far more frequently people are shocked at the analysis they receive. In almost every instance, people discover that the raw food cuisine they consider the ultimate in health has actually become a very high-fat program.

## Low-Fat Cooked vs. High-Fat Raw

People often ask whether it is better to eat a low-fat cooked diet or a high-fat raw one. Some people ask, "which is worse?" It is important to differentiate between eating "just to stay raw" and eating for health. The 80/10/10rv plan represents the ideal—the eating program that is optimal in every way, including your health. If you were asked to choose between shooting yourself in the foot or shooting yourself in the hand, hopefully your choice would be not to shoot yourself at all. Choosing between the lesser of two evils is not the point of The 80/10/10 Diet. Each situation calls for the application of intelligence. You may often have to make decisions regarding the quality of your food. Knowing the ideal will serve you extremely well: whole, fresh, ripe, raw, organic, low-fat plants.

That said, I must emphasize that habitually eating a high-fat raw diet is profoundly damaging to the body, and we do ourselves no favors by rationalizing, "I know all this fat isn't so great for me, but at least it keeps me raw." If I found myself—on rare occasion—with only high-fat raw or low-fat cooked plant-food options, I would make one of two choices: Either I would forgo eating altogether by skipping that meal, or I would indulge in the high-fat meal and then follow it with a day or more where I eat no overt fat whatsoever. The occasional high-fat meal (preferably about six, and an absolute maximum of twelve times per year) is certainly an allowable exception, as the goal is to keep the overall diet as close to the 80/10/10 parameter as possible.

I do realize, however, that for various reasons some people find themselves ongoingly unable to eat enough fruit to make a low-fat raw vegan diet feasible for them. For such people, I must admit that eating in the 80/10/10 proportion, regardless of the food choices, wins hands down over habitually partaking of the high-fat foods popular at raw potlucks, restaurants, festivals, retreats, and workshops. If high-fat raw or low-fat cooked seem your only options, choose the low-fat option, ***every time.***

If you must eat gourmet raw for a handful of "transitional" months, go ahead … but keep your eye on the 80/10/10rv target, if health is your goal. Please, keep in mind that by far the easiest transition to this way of eating is invariably the shortest one, as verified by the many who have gone before you.

## Why Raw Fooders Eat So Much Fat

Just as in the mainstream population, many raw fooders have been taught to fear sugar and, therefore, to fear fruit. Eating lots of low-calorie greens and shunning fruits forces us to consume fats for satiation and caloric sufficiency.

Whereas Americans consume between one-third and one-half of their calories as fat, most raw fooders consume at least 1½ times that amount. They eat a continuous stream of nuts, seeds, oils, coconuts, olives, avocados, and other fatty fruits. Even when the quantities eaten look small, the calories in these foods add up quickly. As a result, many raw fooders attempt to live on a diet where fat accounts for 50, 60, and even 70-plus percent of the mix. Here are some of the reasons why:

### *Nuts and Seeds in Place of Meat and Dairy*

Raw nut and seed loaves, pâtés, and cheeses are staples in every raw gourmet kitchen and sure-fire favorites at raw food restaurants. But nuts and seeds pack a caloric wallop that even the fattiest meats cannot touch.

**Fat in Nut Loaf vs. Ground Beef**

| Item | Cals | Fat Cals | % Fat |
|---|---|---|---|
| Nut loaf: 8 oz. walnuts | 1,480 | 1,240 | 83% |
| Veg-nut loaf: 4 oz. almond/4 oz. carrot | 705 | 520 | 74% |
| Hamburger: 8 oz. ground beef (not lean) | 660 | 410 | 62% |

### *Seeds Instead of Grain*

Flax seeds, sunflower seeds, sesame seeds, hemp seeds, and several others have become popular as the "meal" of dehydrated crackers. Some are more mucilaginous gelatinous than others, but seeds typically are "sticky" enough to hold together when dehydrated, creating a reasonable facsimile of a cracker.

These dehydrates look, feel, and taste pretty much like crackers. They hold dips as well as any cracker. Of course, in contrast to crackers made of grains that offer only a small percentage of their calories from fat, the majority of calories in these crackers (even when "cut" with a huge proportion of vegetables) come from fat, ranging from about 50 to 70%. But they remind us so much of "real" crackers when we eat them that it is difficult to remember they are more than half fat. And what do we eat them with? Why, a nice fatty nut and veggie spread, a seed cheese, or guacamole, of course.

### Fat in Raw vs. Traditional Crackers
**(percentage of calories)**

- 66%: Sunflower flax crackers: (half sunflower seeds, half flaxseeds)
- 58%: Flax crackers (all flaxseeds)
- 49%: Veggie flax crackers (10 C. vegetables, 2 C. flaxseeds)†
- 47% Ritz (9 Ritz = 140 calories)
- 38%: Nabisco Wheat Thins (15 Wheat Thins = 140 calories)
- 34% Triscuit (7 Triscuits = 140 calories)
- 22%: Nabisco Snackwell's Wheat (10 Snackwells = 140 calories)
- 0%: Rice cakes (4 cakes = 140 calories)

†The "Veggie Flax" cracker listed above is an actual recipe from a recently published book by a popular raw food chef. In all likelihood, at 49% fat, it is among the lowest-fat nut/seed-based cracker being consumed in the raw food world today, as flaxseeds contain the least fat (58%) among the nuts and seeds, and the recipe is loaded with vegetables. The regular flax crackers shared at potlucks and sold at festivals are virtually always significantly higher in fat.

This "low-fat" cracker recipe yields approximately a hundred 3 x 3-inch crackers and contains a total of 1,840 calories, or 18.4 calories per cracker. Thus, about 8 of these raw crackers provide the caloric equivalent of 9 Ritz, 15 Wheat Thins, 7 Triscuits, 10 Snackwells, or 4 rice cakes.

### *Nuts As Pastry Substitutes*

Raw food chefs steer clear of bread, because it is a cooked food. But they still like to make pastries, pies, cookies, and other dishes that traditionally call for dough. Hence, they have learned to make pastry dough out of crushed nuts and even fluffy "bread flour" out of leftover nut-milk pulp—both of which work exceptionally well, if your goal is delicious food without regard for health.

Tastewise, raw pastries are definitely a hit. But the caloronutrient ratio is all wrong. As the following table shows, the fat in a raw pie crust makes the Pillsbury Doughboy look lean.

## Fat in Raw vs. Traditional Pie

**Crust Comparison**

Let's examine the high-fat ingredients commonly used in raw desserts. Many raw pie crust or cake recipes call for 2 cups of nuts or shredded coconut, and sometimes a combination of both.

| Item | Cals | Fat Cals | % Fat |
|---|---|---|---|
| Almonds: 2 cups | 1,640 | 1,300 | 79% |
| Pecans: 2 cups | 1,490 | 1,310 | 88% |
| Shredded coconut: 2 cups | 1,320 | 1,085 | 82% |
| Conventional pie crust (for comparison) | 900 | 495 | 55% |

**High-Fat Raw Pie Fillings and Toppings**

Often, the sweet blended fillings in raw fruit pies get their delicious, creamy "mouthfeel" by adding avocado to the mixture. Also, cashew cream is a favorite topping for pies, cakes, and other raw desserts.

| Item | Cals | Fat Cals | % Fat |
|---|---|---|---|
| Avocado: 1 cup | 380, | 290, | 77% |
| Cashews: 1 cup | 720, | 480, | 66% |

True, raw pie crusts usually contain sweet fruits such as dates or raisins, and many fillings also contain fresh fruit. These fruits decrease the overall fat percentage of the recipe, but in even the best case, not likely lower than 40% of total calories. But do not let the percentages fool you. A raw fruit pie with a nut-based crust has a tremendous quantity of fat, even before the filling and topping are added. It is important to understand both calories and caloronutrient ratio in order to fully grasp the caloronutrient picture.

### *Coconuts for All Occasions*

Creative raw food chefs have devised a wide range of culinary applications for coconut meat and dried shredded coconut. Coconut meat shows up in raw items such as icings, sauces, soups, smoothies, cheeses, and creams, whereas the shredded variety adorns granolas, cakes, candies, cookies, pie crusts, tortes, and more.

Many raw fooders plow through a case of young coconuts weekly; some even daily. In addition to the high fat inherent in such a diet, imported coconuts are dipped in fungicide, thus contaminating both the meat and the liquid.

Packaged or bulk shredded coconut, like all other products dehydrated to a crisp, is not really a food in any sense of the word. It is a party item at best. If you include dried coconut at all among your list of acceptable "foods," I urge you to use it sparingly (maybe once or twice per year for very special occasions), and to purchase only the unsweetened, organically grown product. Otherwise, even the shredded coconut found in health-food stores usually contains sulfites to prevent browning, and often other chemical preservatives and additives. Most commercial air-dried coconut is dehydrated at temperatures between 170 and 180 degrees F.

### Coconut Facts

Coconut is a versatile food with a delicious, unique taste. The fruit of the coconut consists of a green or yellow-brown fibrous husk inside which the coconut itself is found. The nut itself has a hard outer shell with a kernel inside.

In the young "green" coconuts, the kernel is soft and jelly-like, and the central cavity is filled with coconut water. As the coconut matures, the kernel becomes harder and the amount of water decreases. The edible parts are the water and meat or jelly.

Below are some of the many ways coconuts are used as food, as well as data on fat content (from the USDA nutrient database).

**Coconut meat:** The solid white flesh inside the mature coconut.

**Coconut jelly:** Young coconut meat still in a semiliquid state.

**Coconut water:** The translucent liquid inside a coconut.

**Coconut milk:** Liquid expressed from grated coconut meat and water.

**Coconut cream:** Liquid expressed from grated coconut meat.

**Coconut oil:** A soft solid at room temperature. Warms easily to liquid.

**Dried coconut:** Air-dried flaked or shredded mature coconut meat.

| Item (100 grams or 3.5 ounces) | Cals | Fat Cals | % Fat |
|---|---|---|---|
| Coconut meat (mature) | 355 | 285 | 80% |
| Coconut jelly ranges from 20% to 85% fat; increases with maturity. | | | |
| Coconut water | 20 | 1.8 | 9% |
| Coconut milk | 230 | 200 | 87% |
| Coconut cream | 330 | 290 | 88% |
| Dried coconut | 660 | 545 | 82% |
| Coconut oil | 862 | 862 | 100% |

All manner of amazing health "benefits" are attributed to the coconut, but I do not recommend using food as therapy for any purpose. Coconut meat is nearly all fat, the vast majority of which (80%) is saturated. If you eat a healthful low-fat raw vegan diet and live healthfully, you will not need the "benefits" of coconut or any other food.

I suggest eating and drinking fresh coconuts when you visit the tropics, but otherwise reserving them only for an occasional indulgence. Aside from fresh, organic young coconut "jelly" or coconut water, this luscious treat is, unfortunately, not the best choice for your health—or your waistline.

## *Oils Supplant Foods*

Many raw fooders believe that when they eat a large salad, they are consuming a low-fat meal. However, this is true only when the salad includes no oil-based dressing or other high-fat ingredients. Just one liquid ounce (2 tablespoons) of any salad oil transforms an innocent, seemingly healthy salad into a high-fat fiasco. It is no longer diet food, and it is no longer health food.

The simple salad example presented below includes 150 calories from vegetables and vegetable fruits, accompanied by a dressing containing 2 tablespoons of oil. Note that even this small quantity of oil increases the calorie count to nearly 400, and the calories from fat to 64%. In contrast, the same salad with no dressing, or perhaps with a blended fruit dressing, contains just under 10% of calories from fat, which is right on target.

Many raw fooders consume more vegetables *and* more oil in their "typical" salads. In addition, they add nuts, seeds, avocado, olives, and other fatty accompaniments. In this case, both the total calories and the percentage of calories from fat always increase.

| How to Make a High-Fat Green Salad | | | |
|---|---|---|---|
| **Item** | **Cals** | **Fat Cals** | **% Fat** |
| Lettuce: 1 small head (8 oz.) | 35 | 4 | 15% |
| Tomatoes: 3 medium (13 oz.) | 70 | 6 | 9% |
| Cucumber: 1 medium (10.5 oz.) | 45 | 3 | 6% |
| Total calories in vegetables | 150 | 13 | 9% |
| Olive oil: 2 tablespoons | 240 | 240 | 100% |
| Lemon juice: 2 tablespoons | 7 | 0 | 0% |
| Total calories in dressed salad | 397 | 253 | 64% |

Fortunately, there is an easy alternative. We can double the size of our salad and replace the fat with a fruit-based dressing, such as raspberries blended with celery. A fruit-based dressing adds enough calories to the salad to make it a substantial meal, while keeping the total calories from fat right where we want them. This simple dressing adds beautiful color to the salad, and most folks tell me they love it.

| Salad, Take 2: The Low-Fat Alternative | | | |
|---|---|---|---|
| **Item** | **Cals** | **Fat Cals** | **% Fat** |
| Lettuce: 1 large head (16 oz.) | 70 | 8 | 15% |
| Tomatoes: 3 large (19 oz.) | 100 | 9 | 9% |
| Cucumber: 2 medium (21 oz.) | 90 | 5 | 6% |
| Total calories in vegetables | 260 | 22 | 9% |
| Raspberries: 1 pint (11 oz.) | 155 | 14 | 10% |
| Celery: 3 stalks (7 oz.) | 25 | 3 | 10% |
| Total calories in dressed salad | 440 | 39 | 9% |

### *Fatty Fruits—and Lots of Them*

Most fruits have very little fat, usually less than ten percent of total calories. A few "fatty fruits," notably the avocado and the olive, derive about three-quarters of their calories from fat.

Proponents of low-carbohydrate diets and many raw food programs suggest that we eat these high-fat foods in unlimited quantities because they are so low in carbohydrates. We are told that the fats in these fruits have the right S/P ratio and should be considered "good" for us.

However, when we eat a large quantity of fatty fruits, we cannot possibly consume enough carbohydrates. If you like being lulled into lethargy both physically and mentally by your food, then eat fatty fruits in unlimited quantity. If you prefer feeling energized and sharp minded, go for the sweet fruits instead. On days that you choose fatty fruits, be sure that they represent your total fat consumption for the day.

Worthy of special mention because of its increasing popularity in raw food circles is the moderately fatty durian. Running 20 to 30% fat, depending on whose numbers you use, the durian can be a wonderful addition to the 80/10/10 diet on occasion, making a delicious and satisfying meal, all by itself. This large, spiky, exotic pod, whose rich, aromatic fruit is reminiscent of sweet custard, is considered a prime delicacy in Southeast Asia.

Eaten infrequently, durian will create a slight blip on your fat radar screen for a day or two … nothing to be concerned about. As an occasional indulgence, you could do a lot worse.

In higher volume, I would be more concerned with lack of freshness and chemical contamination than I would be with the fat content of this sweet treat. Most durian available in the West is imported frozen from Thailand and therefore cannot be considered fresh food. And sadly, the durian supply is notorious for its heavy treatment with unnecessary agrochemicals.

If you want truly fresh, safe durian, travel to Southern California, Florida, or a tropical location and find a farmer who is willing to share his or her cultivation practices in detail.

**Fatty Fruits at a Glance**

| Item | Cals | Fat Cals | % Fat |
|---|---|---|---|
| Avocado, California (1 large = 8 oz.) | 380 | 290 | 77% |
| Avocado, Florida (1 medium = 11 oz.) | 375 | 265 | 70% |
| Olives, canned (small to x-large, 8 oz.) | 260 | 200 | 78% † |
| Durian (½ to ⅓ of a typical fruit, 8 oz.) | 335 | 100 | 20-30% ‡ |
| Akee (creamy Jamaican fruit, 8 oz.) | 340 | 290 | 84% |

† Olives are inedible off the tree, which should be an indication that they are not human food. Just picked, they contain a bitter-tasting compound called oleuropein. Olives must be cured in oil, water, brine, salt, or lye in order to remove the oleuropein.

‡ The USDA data reflects a 30% fat content for durian. Other sources, including Thailand's Chanthaburi Horticultural Research Center, show durian's fat content to be 20%. In any case, durian is far higher in fat than most sweet fruits, which generally range 2 to 10% fat.

## What Raw Fooders Are Actually Eating

At the 2004 International Festival of Raw and Living Foods in Portland, Oregon, we analyzed a typical day's food intake for a curious young lady from Hawaii who attended one of my lectures. She observed that, living in the tropics, she seemed to eat more fruit (and thus less fat) than other raw fooders she knew. Still, she suspected that she was eating more fat than she realized.

Sure enough, when we ran the numbers, we found that on her average day, she consumed a total of 2,400 calories, 45% from fat. In her "typical" day, she described eating 2 oranges, 6 bananas, 1 papaya, and two salads. The oil, nuts, seeds, and avocado interspersed within these meals caused her fat to total more than four times the maximum 10% target. Here is the breakdown:

**An Actual "Low-Fat" Raw Food Day (45% fat)**

| Item | Cals | Fat Cals | % Fat |
|---|---|---|---|
| **Breakfast** | | | |
| 2 oranges | 126 | 6 | 5% |
| 2 bananas | 200 | 6 | 3% |
| 1 T olive oil | 120 | 120 | 100% |
| 2 oz. walnuts | 371 | 309 | 83% |
| Breakfast total | 817 | 441 | 54% |
| **Lunch** | | | |
| 1 papaya | 119 | 4 | 3% |
| 4 bananas | 420 | 13 | 3% |
| Lunch total | 539 | 16 | 3% |
| **Dinner** | | | |
| 20 oz. lettuce | 96 | 13 | 13% |
| 2 tomatoes | 44 | 4 | 9% |
| 10 oz. avocado | 454 | 344 | 75% |
| ¼ cup sunflower seeds | 205 | 150 | 73% |
| Dinner total | 799 | 502 | 63% |
| Grand total for the day: | 2,155 | 959 | 45% |

## A 75% Fat Salad Is Not Unusual!

Most folks tell me that they eat at least one "healthy" salad every day. They eagerly want to believe that they are really not eating that much fat. A "large" green salad, including a 12-oz. medium-sized head of romaine lettuce, 3 medium tomatoes, and 1 cucumber would contain 169 calories, 17 of which would come from fat (our calculations say that vegetables average about 10% of calories from fat, and this example verifies the assertion).

A dressing that blends three tablespoons of oil (360 calories), ¼ cup of pine nuts (229 calories), and some cilantro, salt, and lemon juice would supply 590 calories—555 of them from fat. Dice in a 6-oz. avocado (284 calories), and the resulting 1,042-calorie meal would provide 194 calories from carbohydrates, 61 from protein, and 791—more than 75%—of its calories from fat! The caloronutrient ratio would be roughly 18/6/76, the exact opposite of what we are looking for. This much fat cannot ever make for a balanced or nutritious meal.

Let's suppose that this 75%-fat salad provided half of your daily calories, the other half coming from two smaller meals plus several snacks. By day's end, even if all your other meals contained zero fat (a theoretical impossibility), you would end up with 38% fat overall. More likely, however, if you are on a raw diet, you will eat a handful of nuts now and then, add a bit of oil to a smoothie or avocado to a raw soup, have a few olives or some durian, or perhaps break open a coconut. All of these foods add substantial fat to your day, and there you have it—60% or even (much) more of your calories coming from fat ... every day.

Even if you eat eight or ten pieces of fruit per day with such a salad, on a 2,000 calorie diet, such a program would probably send your caloronutrient ratio for the day into the range of 50%+ calories from fat.

# Chapter 9
# Stabilizing Body Weight

We have been able to determine our percentage of body fat fairly accurately since that fateful day over 2,000 years ago when Archimedes ran naked through the streets of his hometown yelling "Eureka!" having discovered while bathing a valid method of pyknometry—the science of measuring and comparing the densities or specific gravities of liquids or solids. However, it wasn't until the last few decades that this issue became important to anyone but world-class athletes.

Today, as monitoring our weight has become a national pastime, more and more people are becoming aware of the relationship between body fat and total body weight. Still, the misconceptions and misunderstandings about body composition are widespread.

## What People Don't Know About Body Composition

Undoubtedly, weight control and its implications are issues of huge importance. The side effects of obesity are innumerable, and they spill over into every realm of our private and social lives. As our weight progresses beyond healthy, normal levels, we compromise our mental health, self-image, fitness, personal hygiene, job performance, relationships, and many other things. But what constitutes our body mass, and how does understanding this aid us in achieving our weight goals?

Three elements comprise our total weight: water, lean tissue, and fat. Water makes up as much as 70% of our total mass.[69] Lean tissue includes our bones, muscle, and other nonfatty mass. Fat constitutes the rest of our weight. Lean tissue holds more water and is denser than fat. The high water content of lean tissue easily transmits electrical signals, a fact underlying the most common method of measuring body-fat percentage, the bioimpedance monitor.[70]

***In the last 50 years obesity has gone from relatively unheard of to an epidemic.***

In the not-so-distant past, when virtually everyone carried a relatively low body-fat percentage and harbored little excess water weight, weight alone served as a fairly accurate predictor of a person's shape. Today, as obesity consumes more than half of the population, weight alone is no longer an adequate indicator of what we might look like.

In order to better understand the nuances of body composition and the relationships among water, lean tissue, and fat, we must look deeper into the science of weight loss and weight gain. Consider the following:

### We Can Gain Water Weight While Losing Fat

Loss of fat is typically accompanied by a loss of weight, but not always. It is possible to gain muscle and/or water weight while losing fat. We can very easily gain more in water weight than we lose in fat, yielding a net gain in weight. This is true because water weighs much more than fat, volume for volume, so that a little gain in water weight can equal or exceed the amount lost in conjunction with a considerable amount of body fat.

**A high-fat diet compromises our absorption of nutrients.**

Even if you are steadily losing fat, the simple addition of a little extra salt in the diet can negate any potential weight loss. The great volume of water that the body must take on to dilute the toxins in salt, in any form, results in a net weight gain. (See "Is eating sea salt all right?" on page 260.)

### We Can Also Gain Muscle Weight While Losing Fat

It is possible, but not as common—since muscle growth tends to be fairly slow—to exercise enough so that you gain more weight in muscle than you lose in fat, resulting in an overall weight gain. When all other factors remain equal, however, fat loss does result in weight loss.

### We Can Be "Too Skinny" and Overfat at the Same Time

When thin people have a desire to gain weight, they usually fail to recognize that they need to gain *muscle*, not fat. Almost every client who has ever come to me wanting to curtail their weight loss because they thought that they were getting "too skinny" actually still needed to lose some fat. In more than twenty years of advising people on matters of health, nutrition, and athletic performance, I have known only two individuals who actually wanted *and* needed to gain fat.

What really happens when people begin eating healthfully is that the fat starts falling off and they think they are losing muscle, because they never realized how little muscle they actually carry. People in this situation need to gain muscle while continuing to lose fat. This requires exercise.

One client, a high-end fashion model, came to me saying she would do whatever I suggested in order to extend her youthful beauty, but she could not afford to lose any more weight. She was long and lanky and looked skinny to be sure, but she was undermuscled. When we measured her body fat, she was shocked to discover that it was almost 29%—at least 10% above what I would consider healthy. She did not need to lose weight; she needed to lose fat while gaining muscle. She did just that, and she continued her modeling career for many more years.

### Gorging on Fat Is Not a Strategy for Weight Gain

Many people who eat a lot of fat lose a great deal of weight. How can this be? Consuming a diet that is low in carbohydrates and rich in fat can leave people with a depressed appetite, which leads them to eat fewer calories.[71] Also, although some people can handle dietary fat fairly efficiently (and still consume many calories), most of us do not digest or assimilate it very well. This means that even when we consume the same number of calories in high-fat food as we would on a lower-fat diet, we can experience an effective net reduction in caloric intake. Of course, the heavy fat interferes with nutrient absorption, as well. This is a compound problem, because a high-fat diet is already nutrient poor.

***People in perfect health simply do not drop dead.***

### Overfat People Are Malnourished

We cannot be healthy when we are overfat, since our health cannot be better than its weakest link. To the degree that we are overfat, we are also typically malnourished: the more fat, the more malnourished. The obese person who eats only fruits and vegetables is virtually unheard of; we get fat when we eat foods that are less than optimally nutritious—foods that are nutritionally poor and impair our assimilation of nutrients. Hence, fatness and malnutrition are inseparably linked.

### Overfat People Cannot Be "Perfectly Healthy"

We like to think of ourselves as perfectly healthy, even when we know that we are not. We say things like, "Except for my diabetes, I am perfectly healthy," or "Other than his darned asthma and needing to lose 80 pounds, he is perfectly healthy." We are shocked when someone we deemed perfectly healthy dies suddenly from a heart attack or stroke. But take note: *people in perfect health simply do not drop dead.* While perfect health is our natural state, it occurs only when we take perfect care of ourselves.

## How Much Body Fat Is Healthy?

In order to live healthfully throughout a lifetime, we must learn to maintain both our weight and our body-fat percentage. For men, a healthy body-fat percentage runs in the single digits. For women, the ideal range is about ten points higher. (It is certainly possible for women to drop too low in body fat, despite what the glamour magazines would have us believe. Women can develop infertility, osteoporosis, eating disorders, hormonal imbalances, and other serious conditions when their body fat drops into the single digits.)

Most mainstream guidelines from medical or fitness professionals run significantly higher than my recommendations, as the following table illustrates.[72]

**Body Fat Recommendations for Men and Women**

| Men (Conventional) | Men (Dr. Graham) | Women (Conventional) | Women (Dr. Graham) |
|---|---|---|---|
| Underfat 0–13% | Healthy/ Athletic 3–9% | Underfat 0–24% | Healthy/ Athletic 13–19% |
| Healthy 8–25% | Marginal/ Sedentary 10–14% | Healthy 21–36% | Marginal/ Sedentary 20–24% |
| Overfat 19–30% | Unhealthy 15%+ | Overfat 33–42% | Unhealthy 25% |

This discrepancy results from the fact that I equate health with fitness and athleticism, essentially viewing the two as inseparable. In contrast, government, fitness, and medical "experts" distinguish the athlete from the healthy individual, giving them separate classifications, as if it were possible to be healthy and not athletic. Although we can indeed feel good and live free of symptoms for several years as a sedentary individual, this strategy is sure to fail over time. We should not fool ourselves into believing that anything resembling true health is possible without regular, vigorous exercise.

## Strategies for Increasing Muscle Mass

Increasing muscle mass is one way to decrease overall body fat percentage. As the percentage of lean tissue increases, the percentage of fat tissue automatically decreases. If you are thin but still carry a higher-than-healthful body fat percentage, this is an excellent way to achieve your ideal body composition, because increasing muscle mass has the secondary effect of facilitating fat loss. How does this occur? When we add muscle, we increase our body's caloric requirements. For many of us, there is a time lapse while we become accustomed to eating more food. During this lag time, our bodies commonly utilize stored fats to make up for the deficit in calories, reducing our body-fat percentage.

Unfortunately, muscle mass is easily lost. The phrase "use it or lose it" definitely applies, as muscles must be used on an ongoing basis in order to grow and maintain size. Day to day, muscle loss rarely accounts for even one-hundredth of one percent of our body-weight fluctuations. Muscle loss can account for a fair amount of weight loss, however, if an active person becomes totally sedentary, as in the case of the extended bed rest that is required in instances of extreme sickness or recovery from a debilitating accident. We can measure muscle atrophy within twenty-four hours of the initiation of complete rest. Fortunately, muscles regain their prior size with relative ease when we resume normal activities, even after months of convalescence or weeks of water fasting. Of course, if we are active and then become unexpectedly sedentary and continue eating as much or more than we did before, we will gain fat, as the body stores excess calories as fat, not muscle.

***It is impossible to be truly healthy without being athletic.***

Gaining muscle is the only truly healthful way to gain weight and increase size without running the risk of creating hormonal imbalances that result from harboring excess body fat. The only way to gain muscle weight is by "asking" your body to build through the demands of strength-training activities. Pure strength training is technically defined as "one repetition maximum," or "1RM," meaning you can lift that particular weight a maximum of one time before muscular fatigue results. More often, people train for strength by lifting weights in not more than four sets of one to five repetitions each. Strength training a few times per week is all that is necessary to develop your new, lean body.

## Losing or Gaining Fat ... the Right and Wrong Way

The simplest method of losing fat is to consume fewer total calories each day than the amount you use. Estimating calories consumed versus calories used can provide a very good assessment of your potential overall rate of weight loss. (See Appendix D. "Resources for Diet Analysis" on page 335.) Given that a pound of fat contains 3,500 calories, if you expend 115 calories per day more than you consume, you will fairly reliably lose one pound per month. Such calculations are not necessary on an ongoing basis; typically you only need to figure calories in versus calories out to develop an understanding and a routine. Once you establish healthful daily habits, tracking your diet and exercise will become a thing of the past.

Another way to achieve a net loss of calories for weight reduction is to make a commitment to add regular exercise into your daily routine. You must be patient about it, however, as briskly walking a mile per day only yields on average about a one-pound weight loss over the course of a month. This assumes, of course, that all other factors, including total calorie intake, remain relatively constant during that time.

***Rapid weight changes always represent losses or gains in water weight.***

## *The Truth Behind Detoxification*

The tendency among raw fooders to attribute magical powers, such as "cleansing" properties, to foods is nothing short of misguided. Raw foods do not cleanse; they are simply the foods we are designed for. Consuming them provides the body the necessary energy to relieve itself of toxins that have been held in suspension with water. The body does this through its normal mechanisms—the organs of elimination and detoxification.

Our liver and kidneys are always working to detoxify us. When we consume the standard American diet, these organs work overtime just to keep up, because we are constantly ingesting as many toxins as we eliminate (or more). When we switch to raw food, the liver and kidneys have a chance to catch up. They can finally make progress in detoxifying the body, reducing its toxic load.

One pint of water weighs one pound, so weight loss can be dramatic when we are losing water as a result of reducing the body's toxic load. I have seen people lose twenty-five and even as much as forty pounds in the first week of switching to an all-raw diet. Rarely does more than a pound or so of this weight loss actually represent a loss of fat. As a rule, rapid weight changes always represent water weight losses or gains. Under no circumstances can anybody lose a pound of fat per day, on any diet. Programs that promise we will "lose up to 10 pounds in the first 48 hours" are deceptive. It is possible to lose ten pounds of water in just a few hours, but only an extremely active person could realistically lose much more than a pound of fat per week.

### Sudden Weight Loss in New Raw Fooders

Several notable experiences are quite common when people start eating raw foods, especially when they switch to a diet that is exclusively raw from one that was primarily cooked. The first dramatic change that people frequently notice is a rapid and dramatic loss of weight. This does not always happen, but it happens more often than not. Usually, people perceive this as a good thing, because they have excess weight to lose. After they lose the initial water weight in the first week or two on the raw diet, many people find that they continue to lose weight, though much more slowly. It is likely that this subsequent weight loss represents a loss of fat. Of course, at some point, even these losses must be brought to a stop, or the person will simply fade away.

***No diet exists that results in muscle loss or muscle gain.***

### "I Thought I Had More Muscle!"

Most folks, after a few weeks or months of raw eating, are certain that their diet is causing them to lose muscle. They have never seen themselves so thin. What actually happens during weight loss is that we lose much of the padding (fat) around our muscles and also the fat marbled within our muscles. In addition, on a raw diet, we begin to lose the water that we once retained to dilute toxins. This water also added to the appearance of inflated muscles. Many people mistake this excess fat and water as part of their muscle.

Often, people tell me that in a week or two on a raw diet they lost all their muscle. This is an absolute physiological impossibility. In spite of what we have all heard, no diet of any kind results in (any detectible) muscle loss—or muscle gain, for that matter. If there were a diet that resulted in muscle gain, bodybuilders would be found in the kitchen, instead of the gym. We lose or gain muscle due to variations in our physical fitness programs, not through dietary shifts. In spite of what we have all been told, consuming protein (or any other nutrient) will not assist in the muscle-building process.[73] If you believe such hype, you have been sold a bill of goods.

If they understood body composition, and were honest with themselves, these people would more accurately say, "I thought I had much more muscle than I actually do. Then when I lost the excess water that was inflating my muscles, I was forced to accept the reality that I am not as well muscled as I thought I was."

## Dehydration and Body Weight

Dehydration is considered a contributor to more diseases of lifestyle than any other single factor except fat. When our toxin-to-water ratio is skewed in the direction of toxins, cellular function is compromised. This toxicity affects virtually every function in the body. Correcting dehydration oftentimes remedies weight-loss difficulty, as organ function and energy levels greatly improve.

The dehydration coin has two sides: is it literally a state of "not enough water" or is it a condition of "too much toxin"? The correct answer is, "both." When a man is about to die from dehydration, the toxins within his body have become too concentrated for his body to cope with. The amount of toxins do not increase; they are simply less diluted, and therefore, more concentrated.

Few people would argue that dry-cooked foods (those not steamed or boiled) are low in water. After all, if we put toast through a juicer, no liquid comes out. If we put a pot of water in the oven at 400 degrees for an hour, most if not all of the water evaporates off. The same thing happens to the water in food when it is dry-cooked (and to a lesser extent when wet-cooked). The oven works just like a dehydrator. Most of us just don't realize how critical this issue is for our health.

## Four Ways We Become Dehydrated

Hydration is an important factor in all aspects of our health, and even our weight. When using a bioimpedance scale to measure body fat, we must consider our level of hydration to obtain accurate readings. Both dehydration and water retention skew our readings. Hydration also goes beyond the amount of water we consume, since dehydration occurs for a variety of reasons.

***Humans are not designed to drink water. It's already in our natural foods.***

### *Increased Toxic Load*

The most common way that we become dehydrated is when our toxin intake rises relative to our intake of water. Cooking produces many toxins that cause the body to require additional water. Among the most virulent of these are the acrolein produced by deep frying and the polycyclic aromatic hydrocarbons released during barbecuing and other cooking methods that blacken or char our foods.

Two common products found in most households may in fact, be the most toxic substances popularly consumed. Plain table salt is so toxic that even when extremely diluted, as it is in sea water, it is still deadly. All sailors know that if they drink seawater they will die of dehydration. Salt must be greatly diluted with water before the body can tolerate it. Alcohol, the second deadly household poison, has a similar toxicity. It acts as a diuretic and causes substantial water loss. Few substances dehydrate and impair us as effectively as alcohol.

### Low Water Intake vs. Toxic Load

The second way that we can become dehydrated is when water intake is low relative to toxin intake. If we are to (correctly) assume that the necessary amount of water is in our fresh plant foods before we cook them, we can be certain that an insufficient quantity is left after we cook them.

Cooking removes water from food. This explains why a baked potato weighs so much less than the same potato when it was raw. (Granted, cooking can be utilized as a method of hydrating dry foods, as is the case when we boil rice or lentils, but this is the exception, not the rule.) By driving off water, cooking effectively changes the water-to-toxin ratio in food to favor toxins, while also raising the level of toxins in the food. So cooking food results in a double whammy—not only does it remove water, but a great many toxins are created in the process, increasing our need for water.

*Humans are the causes of their own thirst.*

Unfortunately, it is not part of human nature to drink water; we must learn to do so. Let me explain. In nature, at various times throughout the day, many animals will visit the "water hole" to drink. Some animals, especially the grazers, are notorious for drinking huge quantities of water. The anthropoid apes, however, (biologically, humans are classed as anthropoid apes) are rarely observed to drink water, but they can do so if necessary. Their tongues are not designed to lap water the way carnivores do, so they have to suck water if they must drink. Imagine the position they would have to assume in order to drink: essentially, they would be blinded to enemies as they held down their heads and shoulders while vulnerably exposing their private parts.

Drinking water is simply not necessary for the anthropoids. Except for humans, they do not cause their own thirst. They do not participate in the activities, nor do they eat the foods, that result in thirst. Remember, these animals live in the tropics, often in intense heat, where we would expect that they would need to drink copious quantities of water. It is certain that the anthropoids get plenty of exercise and are quite fit; we have all seen films of them climbing straight up and down trees and vines effortlessly.

In fact, pound for pound, they are about five times stronger than humans. They spend most of their day in the shade. They rest during the midday heat. They eat a low-fat raw diet composed primarily of whole, fresh, ripe, organic, fruits and vegetables. (About 1% of the anthropoid diet is composed of insects, small reptiles, and other flesh foods.)

### Increased Endogenous Toxin Production

The third way we become dehydrated is when our "endogenous" toxin production rises relative to our water intake. Every cell in the body produces toxic waste products as a result of its own metabolism, and many tissues, glands, and organs also produce toxins as a result of their metabolism. These internally produced toxins are referred to as endogenous toxins. (In contrast, toxins that come from outside the body are referred to as exogenous toxins. These are the ones that come from our food, the air, and other aspects of our environment.)

As our levels of physical activity or stress rise, so does the quantity of endogenous toxins we produce, as cellular output increases. This is one of the reasons that we are told to drink water before, during, and after exercise and other physical pursuits—to dilute the toxins we produce.

### High Water Output

When we lose water more rapidly than we replace it, we can also become dehydrated. Altitude, heat, sunshine, wind, humidity, and exercise are among the primary factors that can cause us to lose water. Sometimes, these water losses are not obvious to us. For instance, in conditions of high heat and low humidity, especially if the wind is blowing, our perspiration can evaporate as rapidly as we produce it (compared to conditions of high humidity, where dripping sweat grabs our attention). In low humidity, our skin and clothing remain cool and dry, even though we are perspiring freely.

We can lose far more water than we realize in an airplane, where the air is pressurized to an altitude of 6,000 feet and incredibly dry. Such insidious water loss is sometimes considered more dangerous than the overt sweating incurred with exercise in conditions of high humidity. In both instances, however, we must replace the water that we lose.[74]

***Diagnosable dehydration occurs when we lose just 5% of our weight as water.***

We do not have a high tolerance for variations in our ratio of water to toxins. The average American experiences symptoms of dehydration after losing just 1% of body weight as water (about 2% of normal water volume).[75] For a two-hundred-pound man, that equates to just two pounds, or one quart, of water. Medically diagnosable mild dehydration begins at the level of 5% fluid loss, and 15% is considered severe.[76]

In many major fitness competitions, contestants are weighed periodically throughout the event. Since all rapid weight changes almost exclusively represent water weight, fairly accurate levels of dehydration can be assessed simply through the weighing process. Should an athlete show a 5% loss of weight, he or she is considered to be so dangerously dehydrated as to be removed from the competition. For the one-hundred-pound female triathlete, a five-percent weight loss amounts to only five pounds (equal to five pints, or ten cups) of water.

The medical community tells us that we should drink 8 to 12 eight-ounce glasses of water daily. Although they don't express it as such, this recommendation is necessary to make up for the dehydration caused by the toxins in our foods. Interestingly, the example above shows us that an athlete will be removed from competition for being as dehydrated as the average American! If this degree of dehydration is so hazardous to conditioned athletes (people who spend much of their lives adapting to extremes), imagine how dangerous it is to the less-fit individual.

It makes much more sense to remove the cause of the problem, rather than to continue the cause and introduce a remedy. Drinking huge quantities of water after causing extreme dehydration is not the healthiest option. It does not matter whether the cause is the consumption of cooked, salted, or dehydrated foods or exogenous toxins. Although "the solution to pollution is dilution," it is far better to avoid the pollution in the first place.

People can become dehydrated when making dietary changes if they are not aware that such a problem could arise. Troublingly, some dietary programs include such dehydrating practices as consuming a lot of salt and drinking minimal water. It should be stressed that dehydration is dangerous, and it impairs all other functions in the body. Avoid any dietary regimen that induces a state of dehydration, at all costs.

## Are You Dehydrated?

Approximately 75% of the population is chronically dehydrated and simply doesn't know it, because their symptoms seem normal to them.[77] Having lived with their symptoms for so long, they do not even know what a healthful level of hydration would feel like. When they finally achieve normal, healthy levels of hydration as a result of improvements in lifestyle, people sometimes think there is a problem; they have never before experienced proper hydration.

Although dehydration has many symptoms, one of the most common is fatigue. Of course, many factors can result in fatigue, but if you are fatigued, consider whether dehydration might be the cause. Other clear indicators of dehydration include the following:

- Your urine is deep yellow or dark, rather than almost clear.
- You urinate fewer than six times in twenty-four hours. Eight to twelve times per day is considered a healthy frequency.
- You would describe the volume of urine that you void as "scanty" rather than "satisfactory."

If you are curious about the effects of chronic dehydration, the table below outlines some of the consequences of fluid loss on the body:[78]

**Physiological Effects of Dehydration**

| % Body Weight Lost as Sweat | Effect |
|---|---|
| 2% | Impaired performance |
| 4% | Capacity for muscular work declines |
| 5% | Heat exhaustion |
| 7% | Hallucinations |
| 10% | Circulatory collapse and heat stroke |

# Chapter 10
# Overcoming the Challenges of Going Raw

Only a few people have continually maintained a completely raw diet over a period of years or decades. For many folks, the raw diet is an experiment that fails rapidly. Initial results are deemed positive, when a person has weight to lose, but for those who are already thin, the first response tends to be very negative, due to rapid weight loss and subsequent fatigue. Of course, everyone blames the diet, ignoring how they actually applied it. The old adage "practice makes perfect" rings true, but it should be amended to say, "perfect practice makes perfect," for those who fail early tend to give up rather than persist and pull through.

## Calories Per Bite

A crucial stepping stone for success in a healthy raw diet is understanding the concept of "calories per bite," or caloric density. Raw fruits and vegetables yield far fewer calories per bite than cooked foods or fatty foods, so we must eat more bites in order to consume sufficient calories. Just as a bodybuilder trains to lift more weight or a runner trains to run longer races, in order to succeed on the 80/10/10 diet, we must train our bodies and minds, over time, to eat the kind of volume we would eat in our natural environment.

Every once in a while, we hear an isolated fact about what an animal in the wild eats. The volume is always staggering to our imagination. Animals such as sea otters eat 30% of their weight in food each day.[79] Lions have been known to eat eighty pounds of meat in one meal.[80] I have watched little capuchin monkeys (the type that organ grinders used to train) eat banana after banana after banana. Our perspective of "normal" volume has been skewed by the low-water, low-fiber, high-fat meals we have been eating all our lives.

### *Cooking Reduces Volume*

Due to the reduced water and fiber found in cooked foods, we are accustomed to eating small-volume meals. By eating cooked foods our whole lives, our stomachs never developed their potential elasticity.[81] However, it is not too late. For the new fruit eater, the unnaturally poor flexibility of the stomach muscle causes a feeling of fullness after eating a relatively small volume of fruit and calories. Upon adopting a raw program, many people attempt to solve this problem by adding fat in order to make a meal more sustaining and more calorically dense. They add oil to their fruit smoothies, nuts and seeds to their fruit desserts, and avocados and other fats to their vegetable salads.

To give you a sense of the magnitude of the divergence in calories per bite between cooked and raw foods, let's take an extreme example. A slice of a large pan crust Round Table "Montague's All Meat Marvel" pizza contains 350 calories. At an estimated six bites per slice, that's about 60 calories per bite, the same number of calories as a 12-ounce head of lettuce. If four slices of pizza filled you up, it would take about the same (very small) volume of lettuce to also fill you up, in terms of sheer bulk. But the lettuce wouldn't be satiating, because it would have provided only perhaps one hundredth of the calories. To actually eat the same number of calories from lettuce that you got from eating the four slices of pizza, you would have to eat six heads of lettuce per slice of pizza, or one head of lettuce per bite! When we do the math on this example, we get a staggering result: we would have to eat 24 heads of lettuce to consume the same number of calories in four slices of pizza!

***Water dilutes, but it does not cleanse or detoxify us. The body does all the work.***

## *Dehydrated Foods*

One of the reasons that people like cooked food is that cooking intensifies flavors. Many people new to the raw food diet gravitate toward dehydrated foods, because the dehydrator functions quite similarly to the oven and produces dishes reminiscent of those cooked in an oven. Water deficient, these foods are more condensed calorically, and in terms of flavor, than their raw counterparts.

Dehydrated foods take up less space than the same foods eaten whole. As with cooked foods, their compact size disrupts our natural satiety triggers, which respond (in part) to volume. Dehydrated foods also take longer to digest because of their complexity and dryness. For both of these reasons, we tend to overeat dehydrated or cooked foods before we realize we are full. A similar thing happens with dried fruits, which, in addition to being low in volume, also release their sugars more slowly. These two factors contribute to our tendency to overeat them, a phenomenon not common among people who eat whole, fresh fruit.

We compound these problems when we add the various fats (oils, avocados, nuts, seeds, olives, coconut meat, and the like) used freely among raw foodists to make their dehydrated dishes look and taste similar to their cooked food counterparts. Added to low-calorie vegetable recipes, fat becomes the overwhelming caloronutrient in the entire dish. Many dehydrated raw entrées such as lasagna, pizza, and chili offer 50 to 80% of their calories from fat, sometimes even more.

Dishes of this sort slow digestion, forcing foods to be delayed in the stomach and giving us that "stuffed" feeling we have come to associate with satiation, even though they do not contain the volume that our stomachs are designed to handle. The fact is that most people consume their food in an extremely condensed form—cooked, dehydrated, and fatty—and are eating a far smaller volume of food than is truly healthy. This concentration of our food is part of the reason we tend to overeat in terms of total calories.

***Dehydrated veggies are still "just veggies" and leave us hungry after eating them.***

Contrary to popular mythology, there is no reason to think of dehydrated fruits or vegetables as "super" or "special" in terms of nutrition. Certainly they are not as nutritious as their fresh counterparts, in any quantity. Supplement vendors publish convincing literature to convince you that their green powders or "whole-food-based" supplements supply concentrated nutrition in amounts you could not get from fresh fruits and vegetables. But taking them can serve only to imbalance you, as even in deficiency conditions, we do not need more of any nutrient than we can get in a variety of whole, fresh, ripe, raw plants eaten in sufficient quantity to maintain our body weight.

Of course, low-temperature dehydration causes less nutrient damage than cooking, but dehydrated foods are nutritionally far inferior to fresh food, regardless of processing method. Not only that, but eating them dehydrates *us*, increasing relative bodily toxicity, and requiring yet more water to be consumed to maintain proper hydration. The eight to twelve glasses of water we are told to drink every day are a good indicator of how low in water—or if you prefer, how toxic—our diets really are.

### *More Bites and Raw Success!*

The challenge of eating more bites is often one that people are not prepared for, as evidenced by the considerable weight loss common among new raw fooders. After initial water weight losses, if a person still loses weight regularly, he or she is very likely undereating in terms of total calories. (Digestive, absorptive, or assimilative problems could also contribute to the problem, but these must be considered the exception, not the rule.) While a huge percentage of the Western world's population is suffering from impaired digestion and compromised absorption,[82] these conditions tend to self-correct when the causes (high-fat, cooked, processed, toxic foods unsuited to our physiological design) are eliminated.

Eventually, most people agree that eating more food per day is not a hardship, but one of the many rewards of healthful eating. The 80/10/10 diet is among just a handful of *healthful* plans that allows you to eat as much of the recommended foods as you care for.

### How Do I Eat That Much Fruit?

With 80/10/10 firmly in mind, we return to the question of how to obtain the calories we need, now that high-fat, low-fiber, low-water foods are removed from the diet. To get 80% of your calories from the carbohydrates in fruit, you will have to create some dramatic new eating habits, perhaps more dramatic than any dietary change you have ever made. As you drop the fat from your diet, you must significantly increase your daily fruit consumption, a habit that takes practice to develop. The good news is that your health and your waistline will show you immediate results to let you know you are heading in the desired direction.

One tactic to achieve more bites, and to support our caloric needs, is to start with several fruit meals per day, approximately four. Over time, depending on your exercise program and other healthful habits, you will be able to reduce this number of meals down to three and then possibly even two. Also, make a practice of eating just one or two bites more at each meal than you otherwise would. The elasticity of your stomach will promptly accommodate the extra bites, just as all of your other muscles would elongate if you were to adopt a yoga practice. I must stress: the goal here is not to eat until you hurt but to gently encourage your digestive system to regain its flexibility.

**On average, Americans take only 50 to 100 bites per day.**

You don't have to make this transition all at once, either. If you are not ready to eat just fruit for your breakfast and lunch meals, it is perfectly acceptable to simply begin your meals with fruit. You can eat all the fruit you care for at the start of the meal, and then follow the fruit with other foods. Over time, the amount of fruit you desire at the beginning of the meal will increase. Eventually, you will be able to eat a satiating and calorie-sufficient meal from fruit that will hold you all the way until the next mealtime comes around.

## Satiation—Satisfying Hunger and Appetite

Hunger is a sensation we are all familiar with, but it is often confused with other aspects of eating. The goal of hunger is to satisfy a nutritional requirement for carbohydrates, fats, proteins, vitamins, minerals, enzymes, coenzymes, and all other nutrients. We are driven to eat to fill this need and rewarded by the pleasure of it. Because hunger is the general desire for food, when one is truly hungry, any food will be acceptable.

Appetite, on the other hand, is specific—we desire a specific food or foods. Appetite is also the socially acceptable word for craving, which in turn is the socially acceptable word for addiction. An example of the difference between appetite and hunger goes as follows: When a person says, "I am hungry" and you offer him lettuce, he is likely to say, "I am not hungry for lettuce, but I do have an appetite for chocolate. Do you have any chocolate?" If this person were truly hungry, the lettuce would have been perfectly acceptable. Their wording is accurate: what they really have is appetite… or I might suggest, addiction.

Malnutrition is also a powerful appetite trigger.[83] When we lack essential nutrients, we crave food. Unfortunately, malnourished individuals often eat more of the wrong foods in a vain attempt to control their appetites. For example, obese people, who are always malnourished due to eating unhealthful foods, generally seek to satisfy their cravings with the same foods that caused their malady, and they do this over and over again. The nutritional density of fruit is yet another factor that makes it so satiating and all but impossible to overeat.

Satiation, defined as full satisfaction, is what we truly desire from our food. To fully satisfy yourself at mealtime is a more challenging task than you might think, for there are many aspects to this issue. Are we simply talking nutrition, or do we consider emotional facets as well? Is satiation simply about quantity (bulk), or is quality also a factor?

We know one thing for certain: whether you eat in a restaurant, at a friend's house, or at home, typically a dessert is offered as the last course of any meal. Desserts are known to be satiating; the carbohydrates ensure this effect.[84] We can avoid appetite triggers by choosing the right foods, for the right reasons, for true hunger.

### Can Fats Ever Satisfy?

Fat is a very difficult nutrient to digest. It passes through the stomach and intestinal tract more slowly than other nutrients. Because of this, it is easy to overeat fat, and in the process, stress your digestive capacities beyond their limits. A stuffed feeling results, if you are lucky. The less fortunate end up with digestive ailments of varying severity. Almost every digestive disorder is related to the overconsumption of fat.

#### Emotional Eating

One of the primary ways we handle painful emotions is to literally "eat ourselves numb," with dense, hard-to-digest foods—the so-called "comfort foods." This is effective because of the nature of our nervous systems. Our bodies have a finite amount of nerve energy at any given time. The digestion of food and the conduction of emotions each demand so much energy that they cannot be performed simultaneously.

A classic example to demonstrate this property of our nervous system is a funeral, where some people are grieving so intensely they cannot eat at all, while others cannot stop eating.

As we lighten our diets to vegetarian, vegan and eventually raw, we quite commonly become more aware of our emotional selves. When we commit to eating a raw diet, we gravitate toward fatty foods to provide emotional numbing, as most fresh fruits are not sufficient sedatives to overcome emotional distress. Usually this leads to the consumption of exorbitant amounts of nuts or seeds, which are easy to overeat, because they do not quickly trigger satiation. Digestive distress and undue suffering result from this behavior.

The answer to all this lies not in consuming food at all, but in maintaining emotional poise and developing the ability to fully feel our emotions.

Fats have several factors working against them when it comes to satiety. First, fats pack many calories into tiny packages. Because volume is one of the key factors in experiencing satiation, it is difficult to eat enough volume of a fatty food to feel satiated, without feeling sick first.

Second, the brain monitors blood-sugar levels constantly as a method of determining hunger. As blood-sugar levels rise, hunger decreases. No corollary rapid hunger reaction occurs in the case of blood fat, and even if it did, dietary fat takes a relatively long time to reach the bloodstream, often requiring twelve to twenty-four hours from the time it is eaten. If you eat an entire meal of fatty foods, you still won't be satiated. You will very likely resort to eating a sweet dessert at the end of the meal to finally satisfy your appetite. The idea that eating fat keeps you satiated is simply untrue.

### *Sweet Fruits Win Every Time!*

When we eat sweet fruits, which are rich in simple sugars, the blood-sugar level rises gently, almost immediately, as we discussed in Chapter 2. The sweetness of these highly nutritious foods makes them difficult to overeat. And because of their copious water and fiber content, fruits supply relatively high volume in a low-calorie package, further making it difficult to eat too much of them. We have all been taught that sweets will satiate us, and we have come to rely upon this fact by choosing to eat our sweet desserts at the end of our meals.

*When we eat sweet desserts at the end of our meals, it indicates two things:*

- No matter how much food we ate, it likely did not satisfy our appetite, or else we would not have been tempted by a sweet dessert.
- We ate insufficient simple carbohydrates during the meal, leaving us craving those very carbohydrates at the end of the meal. This is evidence of our natural and substantial need for simple carbohydrates.

Had we eaten sufficiently of fruit at the start of the meal, it is likely that we would not have desired other foods. No other food group matches the ability of fruit to satiate us.

### Monomeals: Eating One Food at a Time

Eating a single-ingredient "monomeal" of fruit is an extremely pleasurable experience quite simply because it is so satiating and yet, so uncomplicated. The minimalism of the meal runs counter to our habitual multiple-food approach, with its accompanying titillation of the tastebuds, thereby allowing us to avoid addiction to stimulation and overeating.

Judging from the way most people eat, I feel safe in saying that addiction stems from variety. Because the mono-fruit meal does not excite the body, and is easily digested, it does not leave us dulled and fatigued after eating, but rather engaged and clear of mind. We are left both perfectly satisfied and mentally poised.

At first attempt, the monomeal may seem "boring," because we are so accustomed to the stimulation of eating multi-ingredient meals. Over time, the simplicity of mono-fruit meals improves digestion and heightens your senses, so that you can pick up the nuances of every bite of raw plant foods. As an added benefit, you will be able to better recognize when you are actually satisfied.

### Am I Supposed to Feel Full?

Given that the key to eating for fullness while simultaneously consuming the right number of calories for our bodies is to eat high-volume, nutrient-rich, simple-carbohydrate foods, then which foods should predominate? The truth is, the human body has only a certain capacity. While it is possible to get adequate nutrition from a variety of different food sources, it is more easily obtained from some foods than from others. For instance, lettuce is highly nutritious in terms of nutrients per calorie, but it would be extremely difficult—essentially impossible due to the finite nature of our digestive capacity—to consume sufficient lettuce to meet our caloric requirements. (At 50 calories for a 10-ounce head, we would have to eat 40 heads a day to consume 2,000 calories).

At the opposite end of the spectrum, it is possible to put the micronutrients required to meet our total daily nutrient requirements into a single small pill. (Of course, our macronutrient needs—water, fiber, carbohydrate, protein, and fat—do not lend themselves to consumption in pill form.) Were you to eat such a pill, however, the lack of volume or bulk would result in a tremendous and unyielding sense of hunger that could only be satisfied by the consumption of more volume.

How do we get volume, nutrients, and simple sugars, all at the same time? We eat sweet fruit. Because of its high water and fiber content, fruit provides more volume with fewer calories than any food category except vegetables. Hence, we can meet our caloric needs without exceeding them, while fulfilling our innate desire to consume foods in large volume. Because of its high volume, low calories, and abundance of nutrients including simple sugars, eating a sweet meal predominated by fruit is bound to be satiating every time.

# Chapter 11
# 80/10/10 in Practice

How does your daily diet differ when you learn to eat the low-fat raw vegan way? On most days, you will eat juicy fruit for breakfast, sweeter fruit for lunch, and all the acid fruit you care for before a vegetable-based dinner. It is really that simple.

Most raw fooders, and anyone else who has been taught to avoid fruit or to eat it in somewhat limited quantities, are initially dumbfounded by this formula. Responses range from "I could never do that" to the full range of nutritional questions that have already been covered in this text.

For people transitioning from a more mainstream diet, the concept of eating fruits and vegetables makes a lot of sense. After all, fruits and vegetables are the true health foods. With the state of human health at its absolute all time lowest, isn't it time that we started eating fruits and vegetables as if our very lives depended upon them?

While people also tend to intuitively sense the wisdom of a low-fat diet, the idea of committing to a completely vegan diet may seem a bit mentally or emotionally challenging at first. But it makes more sense all the time, and the number of vegans is rising every day.

## Slow and Steady

Once people educate themselves about a new positive behavior and become convinced that they desire to incorporate it into their lives, I always encourage them to do so as quickly as possible. Yet, you can be easy on yourself when adopting the 80/10/10 way of life. A gradual transition may be the best that you can hope for if you have amassed a collection of mental, emotional, or habitual blocks that would make a sudden and total switchover difficult.

Direction is more important than speed for most people when it comes to successful transition. Imposing upon yourself the unnecessary pressure to make "all or nothing" changes often leads to frustrating failure. When people stretch themselves too quickly, they often "snap back" into their prior habits.

By decreasing the fat percentage in your diet even one point per week, you can achieve the full benefits of 80/10/10 in less than a year. After that, you have the rest of your life to reap the harvest of health that you have sown. This is not a diet program to be used temporarily, but a healthful eating program for life.

I wrote this book to guide people to a low-fat plant-based *raw foods* diet. No other program exists for this purpose. However, many other low(er)-fat plant-based diet programs exist. Some people choose to transition more gradually by consuming fruit for breakfast and lunch, with a simple low-fat cooked meal plus a raw salad at night. Over a period of months, the salad and other raw dishes nudge out the cooked components, until 100% raw is achieved. If you are interested in such a path, don't feel guilty about it. Give yourself permission to take advantage of the myriad of resources available to support your health in the most appropriate way for you right now.

For some folks, there is a greater sense of urgency than for others, as health issues can impose themselves powerfully. If that is the case, feel free to transition your diet as rapidly as you can. There is no danger in converting to 80/10/10 immediately. One 89-year-old man I worked with went from standard eating to 80/10/10 overnight, and never looked back.

You do not have to think of yourself as becoming a vegetarian, vegan, or raw fooder to be an 80/10/10 fan. Just keep decreasing the fat and increasing the amount of fruits and vegetables you add into your already-existing program.

### Actual Stories of Transition to 80/10/10

The following are actual posts (slightly edited for space) from my VegSource discussion board.

**From:** turtle (dialup-4.243.137.125.dial1.sanfrancisco1.level3.net)

**Subject:** transition from high fat raw to low fat raw

**Date:** December 17, 2004 at 8:40 am PST

I have been doing the high fat … nuts, seeds, and oils raw food way of eating and would like to transition over to the low-fat fruit-based 811. Is there a good way to transition? I would like to hear people's experiences with this … so if any of you have any suggestions, I am all ears!

I know that I am eating way too many nuts and seeds and that this has not supported my well being. I have found it difficult to let go of the nuts and seeds on an every meal basis. Thanks for your help.

ഗ ഗ ഗ

**From:** Janie (66.180.141.217)

**Subject:** Re: transition from high fat raw to low fat raw

**Date:** December 17, 2004 at 7:39 pm PST

Since it seems that you have already been attempting to go cold turkey and it hasn't been working out, it seems that transitioning may be the way for you. I did a low-fat transition myself at first by keeping my overt fats to 10% of my calories or less, which translated to about 20% or less of the amount of calories I was eating at the time. Later I brought it down to 10% or less overall.

The way I would approach transitioning from where you are to a lower fat way would be to try to do two adjustments:

- I would try to eat more caloric-dense fruits
- I would also try to move my nuts or seeds eating to my evening meal only

Then after that, I would work on decreasing the fat from the nuts and seeds overall so that I approach 10% or less, more and more often, until I'm doing it all the time (on average).

I would approach it as a transition, and be easy on yourself psychologically with your slip-ups (if you have them) by just letting them go and realizing that you have another opportunity to get going again towards your goals coming up as early as your next meal choice. You may find as I did with going 100% raw again, that the transition period ends up being shorter than you thought it would be. ;-)

Aloha!

ꟹ ꟹ ꟹ

**From:** Jaime (ip68-4-209-131.oc.oc.cox.net)

**Subject:** Re: transition from high fat raw to low fat raw

**Date:** December 17, 2004 at 12:20 pm PST

I found that my ideal was to go cold turkey, but I ended up transitioning, as 811 involves more than just diet, in my opinion.

My transition began months before, if not years. I read the posts of others on this board, took note of how my body reacted to particular foods, noted what worked and what didn't, and then practiced what worked more and more. I cut out supplements, gourmet raw food and dehydrated food, frozen food, spices and salt, onions and garlic, raw dairy, and juice (even raw juice).

I used to think raw juice wasn't so bad, then I'd have it and would feel so imbalanced I'd eat some raw vegan sushi or raw cheese, then I'd be off 811 completely. I'd say I played this back-and-forth game for a year or more. I would think 811 doesn't work, but really I was not doing it completely. So I decided to incorporate everything I knew that worked.

For me what works is: getting loads of sleep (up to 12 hours a night) as this helps with 811 immensely, exercising before eating (I used to exercise after), eating one or two meals per day, waiting until 11 a.m. or noon to eat, having only one type of fruit per meal, and following that with one type of green such as celery or lettuce, no raw juice, raw vegan food only, no dates or bananas unless they are ripe and fresh picked, and eating whole foods.

I did not add all of these things at once. It took me about a month to add them and I still consider myself in transition. So I guess what I am saying is 811 is more than just percentages and involves whole foods, rest, exercise, fresh air, sunlight, etc. Once I set my intention for how I was going to follow 811 it took time to actually put it into practice. Also, I am constantly learning what is useful and what is not and make adjustments accordingly. So I think this whole thing is a process, and intentions of "cold turkey" do not manifest, at least not for me.

∽ ∽ ∽

**From:** Dr. Doug Graham (http://forum.foodnsport.com)
**Subject:** Another way
**Date:** December 17, 2004 at 1:17 pm PST

*(Author's note: I posted this message to offer another perspective to Jaime's message above, which emphasizes giving up certain foods. Approaching* 80/10/10 *with a focus toward the foods and other practices to add into your life, rather than those to eliminate, can make all the difference in your success with—and enjoyment of—the* 80/10/10 *plan.)*

I recommend that the transition from standard American raw to 811 be done as follows:

- Increase the percentage of whole, fresh, ripe, raw, organic plants in your diet, at each meal.
- Increase the percentage of fruit in your diet, at the beginning of each meal.
- Increase the total carbs in your diet, at each meal.

- Increase the quantity of fresh whole ripe raw organic greens in your diet until you reach close to 3% of total daily calories or slightly more.
- Increase the amount of sleep you get until you can honestly say that you are getting "enough" each night.
- Increase the amount of physical activity you perform until it accounts for a minimum of 2/5 (40%) of your total calories used.

Hope this helps,
Dr. D.

## The Formula

So, what are we talking about in terms of foods? 80/10/10 works out easily and naturally if your calories break down approximately as follows:

- 90 to 97% from sweet and nonsweet fruits.
- 2 to 6% from tender, leafy greens and celery.
- 0 to 8% from everything else (other vegetables like cabbage and broccoli, plus fatty fruits, nuts, and seeds).

You can generally accomplish this with two or three large fruit meals during the day, plus a large salad in the evening. Fruit predominates heavily, yet you consume as many greens as you like.

### Average Caloronutrient Ratios by Food Category

Here is a rough estimate of the average caloronutrient ratio for various whole raw food categories, expressed in terms of percentage of calories from carbohydrates, protein, and fat (C/P/F):

- Fruits average 90/5/5
- Vegetables average 70/20/10
- Nuts average 10/10/80
- Seeds average 18/12/70
- Avocados average 20/5/75

## How Much Overt Fat?

When contemplating reducing your fat consumption to 10% or less of total calories consumed, you must remember that somewhere around 5% of your calories will likely come from fat even if you eat only fruits and vegetables. Thus, as a rule of thumb, you should plan on having about 5% of your calories in the form of nuts, seeds, avocados, nut butters, and the like. On a 2,000-calorie diet, you should be shooting for overt fat consumption in the neighborhood of 100 calories (5% of 2,000 = 100).

What does this mean in terms of food? It means that in a single day, an average person endeavoring to follow the 80/10/10 plan would consume in the neighborhood of:

- 1/3 of a medium-sized avocado (6-ounces edible portion), or
- 0.6 ounces of almonds (about 15 nuts), or
- 20 medium olives, or
- less than 1 tablespoon of oil.

There is another option, however. You could choose to eat no overt fats at all for a day or two, or longer, relying exclusively upon eating a sufficient quantity of fruits and vegetables to meet your calorie need. By doing so, you will have effectively "saved up" for a day when you could eat a moderate quantity of fatty food without feeling guilt or that you had gone off of the program. If you average your caloronutrient intake for the week you should still be able to achieve 80/10/10 in this fashion.

Of course, if you really overdo it on fatty foods, you will notice it right away and likely again the next morning. The tiredness, foul mouth, slowed digestion and elimination, and other sensations are too pronounced to ignore. They are great motivating factors to bring you right back to the joys of the straight and narrow 80/10/10.

## How Many Calories?

In the beginning, most people do not eat enough raw foods to obtain their necessary daily calories, because they are used to eating concentrated cooked foods. As I described in Chapter 10, you will have to eat a much larger volume of whole fresh fruits and vegetables to obtain the same number of calories that you would from cooked meats and starches, because raw fruits and vegetables are not as calorically dense. They contain a large amount of water and fiber—essential nutrients to be sure, but these two items add a great deal of volume to our food.

Another obstacle most people must overcome in order to succeed with the 80/10/10 raw diet, is the fear of consuming fruit for the major portion of their calories. In general, fruits are considerably higher in calories than vegetables and leafy greens. So it makes sense that most of the raw food diet be made up of fruit, complemented by large salads to provide essential minerals such as sodium, potassium, calcium, and magnesium.

Determining caloric needs is not an exact science. There is room for a fair amount of flexibility, especially on a day-to-day basis. Averaged over a year's time, we will likely find that people who maintain their weight consume a predictable range of calories based upon their size, muscularity, and activity level.

### *10 Times Body Weight = BMR*

Below I offer two guidelines for estimating the number of calories you should consider eating each day. Both of them begin by multiplying your body weight (or your ideal/desired body weight) by 10. This provides a very rough estimate of your resting basal metabolic rate (BMR)—the number of calories required to operate your brain, organs, and all essential functions.

For example, if you weigh 150 pounds, you can estimate that you need somewhere around 1,500 calories per day, plus or minus about 10%, just to maintain your basic metabolism at rest. Then, depending on your activity level, I offer the following calculations.

### *Calorie Guidelines for Healthy (Athletic) People*

My optimal calorie-consumption guideline is likely to be different than the advice you may find elsewhere, and somewhat higher than the American average. This is because I base my recommendation upon a healthful (high) level of physical activity—the level that humans would have to maintain in order to obtain sufficient food in a more natural setting.

Nature intended humans to have to cover large expanses of ground on foot, to climb trees, and even to swim when necessary in order to obtain food and warmth. The resulting fitness level would be considerably higher than that of the average American, as would the average calorie output. As more food would be consumed, so would a greater number of nutrients be available. Good nutrition literally hinges upon us being fit enough to be healthy.

With the above in mind, I suggest that a healthy athletic person should utilize at least as many calories in physical endeavors as they use for their resting BMR. (Resting BMR is equivalent to 10 times your ideal body weight). This means, for instance, that a 150-pound man who uses 1,500 calories as his baseline should also use at least another 1,500 calories in his activities for the day, on average, for a total of 3,000 calories.

Using the 80/10/10 diet, nutritional intake would be vastly better than the American average for all nutrients. Fitness levels would need to be increased, of course, in order to achieve that level of activity, but this can be done gradually.

### Calorie Guidelines for Less-Active People

To be abundantly clear, I would like to reiterate: Good nutrition literally hinges upon us being fit enough to be healthy. By this I mean to say that even the most "perfect" diet will never result in true health unless it is accompanied by high-level fitness and all of the other essential elements of healthful living (see sidebar entitled "Fundamental Elements of Health" on page 11). I cannot recommend highly enough that you exert at least as much attention and effort into upleveling your level of fitness as you do into learning about and achieving optimal nutrition.

That said, if you are a less-active person wending your way toward fitness and health, here are some guidelines for caloric intake.

If your work and the rest of your day is relatively sedentary, add another 200 calories to the BMR estimate described above. Then add calories for exercise, perhaps 300–600 calories per session. It could be more or less, depending upon the frequency, intensity, and duration of your fitness sessions. If you also have a physically demanding job, you might require another 800 to 1,600 additional calories or more.

Thus, a sedentary woman who weighs 130 pounds must eat about 1,300 calories simply to maintain her body weight. Let us suppose that she needs another 260 calories (an additional 20%) per day to meet her physical needs such as puttering around the house, going up stairs, or to the mailbox, etc. This hypothetical woman would need to eat food that supplied about 1,560 calories per day.

A large man of 280 pounds, who is fit and not fat, who participates in sports and works in construction, would require roughly 2,800 calories for basal metabolism. Add to that the 1,500 calories he expends at work each day and the 2,000 he needs for his daily sports training. This active man needs to eat sufficient food to supply him with approximately 6,250 calories per day. He has to consume four times as many calories as the sedentary woman in our first example.

### Calorie Comparison: 8 Ounces of Selected Foods

This chart demonstrates the tremendous range of caloric density among high-water versus high-fat whole foods in the 80/10/10 program. In each case, the food item weighs eight ounces. *(Note that you would have to eat 42 servings of 8 ounces of lettuce, or 21 large heads, to get the same number of calories as one 8-ounce portion of macadamia nuts!)*

| | |
|---|---|
| **Lettuce** | 39 calories (1 small head romaine) |
| **Cucumber** | 27 calories (½ medium) |
| **Tomato** | 41 calories (2 medium) |
| **Peach** | 89 calories (2 medium) |
| **Apple** | 109 calories (2 small) |
| **Mango** | 147 calories (1 medium) |
| **Banana** | 202 calories (2 medium) |
| **Avocado** | 362 calories (1 large) |
| **Cashews** | 1,254 calories (1.7 cups) |
| **Sunflower seeds** | 1,293 calories (1.5+ cups) |
| **Almonds** | 1,318 calories (1.7 cups or 200 nuts) |
| **Walnuts** | 1,483 calories (2+ cups, or 57 nuts) |
| **Macadamias** | 1,628 calories (1.8 cups, or 88 nuts) |

## How Much to Eat

To give you an example of the volume of fruits and vegetables required, let's say you need about 2,000 calories per day. A medium-sized banana has 105 calories; a large honeydew melon has 461 calories; a medium peach has 39 calories; and a large simple salad may have 175 calories (a large 20-oz. head of lettuce runs about 96 calories, and a pound of nonsweet fruits has about 75 calories).

To consume 2,000 calories from raw foods, you would need to eat something like a large honeydew melon for breakfast (461 calories), a 12-banana smoothie for lunch (1,260 calories), 4 peaches before dinner (153), and a large salad for dinner (175). This would provide 2,026 calories, with a 90/6/4 caloronutrient ratio (90% carbohydrates, 6% protein, and 4% fat). If you didn't have any physical activity that day, you might eliminate two bananas and one of the peaches.

If it was a physical day, you could add half of a 6-oz. California avocado to the salad. It would provide about 145 more calories, 111 of which would be from fat. The caloronutrient ratio for the day would then be 86/6/9. Adding a whole avocado would take the fat percentage for the day up to 13% … not a big deal, but it would be better to add a few pieces of fruit to meet the extra caloric requirements of your exercise routine.

### The Diet for a Lifetime

Just like the rings on a tree, life is about growth, which often requires change. The 80/10/10 diet may seem like a huge shift in your lifestyle in the beginning, but as the rewards for taking care of your body unfold, you will come to see that the benefits of living this way far outweigh the cost. Developing 80/10/10 as a lifestyle will enhance every moment of your life to come. I applaud you for taking the first step to the new you.

# Appendix A
# Sample Menu Plans

This appendix contains four seasonal sample menus for the 80/10/10 lifestyle, broken into one-week sections (seven days of meals for summer, autumn, winter, and spring). Each two-page spread includes a day's worth of recipes on the left-hand side and a corresponding caloronutrient analysis chart on the right.

Each day's menu plan includes a breakfast, lunch, and three-course dinner, hand-selected for seasonal freshness and designed to total approximately 2,000 calories. You can easily increase or decrease the quantity of any ingredient, to adjust the recipes in the direction of your desired caloric intake.

The smoothies, fruit salads, soups, dressings, vegetable salads, and slaws in this section demonstrate the abundance of whole fruit and vegetable meals available on the 80/10/10 plan. This guide emphasizes fruits in season, when they are freshest and least expensive. The 80/10/10 motto is, "simplicity at mealtime, variety throughout the year." As you become accustomed to this lifestyle, you will discover the joy of eating seasonally and anticipating the taste sensations each new bounty of fruits brings. Feel free to experiment! Use this guide as an inspirational tool to help you discover your own favorite combinations.

Some recipes contain additional information, indicated by a dagger symbol (†), to help answer your questions and smooth your transition to this way of eating. These include helpful tidbits about fruit varieties and their availability, ideas for recipe variations, and tips on buying, preparing, and eating the foods.

Don't worry about your caloronutrient ratio at each meal, or even each day. The 80/10/10 guideline (at least 80% of calories from carbohydrates and at most 10% fat and protein) is intended as an average—something to strive for over time. Thus, as you page through the menu plan, you will see higher-fat days and lower-fat days ... but by the end of the week, the numbers all come out to 80/10/10, more or less.

The best way to really understand the caloronutrient ratio and get a true sense of the level of fat in your own diet, is to weigh your food and enter numbers in an online diet-analysis program for about a week. We used Nutridiary.com as a basis for creating this recipe guide.

Note that no two fruits are nutritionally identical. Each crop of produce (sometimes even each piece) differs in caloronutrient ratio from the next, depending on such factors as ripeness, soil quality, shipping environment, and time since harvest.

In addition, any attempt to standardize measures like "one apple" or "one head of lettuce" (although we do so in the upcoming ingredient conversion charts) is subjective at best, given the regional variability of produce. Thus, the only way to accurately compare food quantities is to list ingredients by weight, rather than by the piece. All weights refer to edible portions only, so be sure to remove peels, stems, cores, seeds, and pits before you weigh your food.

Remember that each individual's digestive capacity is different, as is their level of exercise. Both of these factors affect our ability to absorb nutrients efficiently. As you mature in this lifestyle, your natural digestive "fire" will increase.

For these reasons and others, the numbers in these charts are rough approximations at best. Use them to steer your diet in a low-fat direction, but track your numbers in the aggregate, and don't get too hung up on the details.

## Seasonal Availability of Produce

The following table offers an overview of domestic availability for common fruits and vegetable fruits. It is a broad, general list, showing the greatest number of months these foods are commonly obtainable at market nationwide, regardless of variety or where they are grown.

For example, the papaya, shown to be available all year, includes several varieties, from Florida, California, Hawaii, Mexico, and Central America—each of which produces papayas at different times. Modern distribution and storage technologies allow us access to many of these foods throughout the year (sometimes at great cost to our pocketbooks, our health, and our natural resources).

During the *pre* and *post* seasons, you may be able to find these foods domestically grown, but they tend to come at a higher price and reduced quality. To achieve maximum freshness, I strongly encourage you to choose locally grown, organic produce in season whenever possible.

| Food | Peak Season | Pre/Post Season |
|---|---|---|
| **Sweet Fruits** | | |
| **Apples** | September-October | August/November |
| **Apricots** | July | June/August |
| **Avocado** | May-November | April/December |
| **Banana** | January-December | N/A |
| **Blackberry** | July-August | May-June/September |
| **Blueberry** | July-August | June/September |
| **Cherries** | June | May/July |
| **Dates** | September-October | August/November |
| **Figs** | July-September | June/October |
| **Grapes** | July-September | June/October |
| **Kiwi** | December-February | November/March |
| **Mango** | May-August | April/September |
| **Melon** | June-August | May/September |
| **Nectarines** | June-September | July/August |
| **Oranges** | December-April | November/May |
| **Papayas** | January-December | N/A |
| **Peaches** | July-September | June/October |
| **Pears** | August-September | July/October |
| **Persimmons** | October-November | September/December |
| **Pineapples** | June-August | May/September |
| **Plums** | August-September | July/October |
| **Pomegranates** | October-November | September/December |
| **Raspberries** | July-August | June/September |
| **Strawberries** | April-May/October | March/June & September/November |
| **Tangerines** | November-March | October/April |
| **Vegetable Fruits** | | |
| **Cucumbers** | July-August | June/September |
| **Bell Peppers** | September-October | August/November |
| **Tomatoes** | July-October | June/November |
| **Yellow Squash** | July-August | June/September |
| **Zucchini** | July-August | June/September |

## If You Don't Own a Scale...

We have listed the ingredients in the menu plan in terms of ounces and pounds, in order to provide an accurate caloronutrient breakdown. If you do not have a scale at home, the charts below can help you measure out the quantities called for. Eventually you will become proficient in estimating weights and average caloric content of various foods, a skill that will pay dividends in saved kitchen time.

| Portion Equivalents: Sweet Fruits (1 lb.) | |
|---|---|
| Apples | 4 cups sliced, 3.5 medium |
| Apricots | 2.75 cups sliced, 13 medium |
| Bananas | 3 cups sliced, 4 medium |
| Blackberries | 3 cups |
| Blueberries | 3 cups |
| Cantaloupe Melon | 2.75 cups cubed |
| Casaba Melon | 2.5 cups cubed |
| Cherries, sweet | 4 cups with pits, 64 medium |
| Dates | 12.5 cups pitted, 19 medjool, 56 deglet |
| Figs | 9 medium |
| Grapefruits | 2 cups sectioned, 2 medium |
| Grapes | 3 cups |
| Honeydew | 2.75 cups diced |
| Kiwis | 2.5 cups, 6 medium |
| Mangos | 2.75 cups sliced, 2 medium |
| Nectarines | 2 cups sliced, 3 medium |
| Oranges | 2.5 cups sectioned, 3.5 medium |
| Papayas | 3 cups cubed, 1.5 medium |
| Peaches | 2.7 cups sliced, 4.5 medium |
| Pears | 2.75 cups sliced, 2.5 medium |
| Persimmons | 2.75 medium |
| Pineapples | 3 cups, 1 medium |
| Plums | 2.75 cups sliced, 7 medium |
| Raisins | 3 cups |
| Raspberries | 3.5 cups |
| Strawberries | 2.5 cups sliced, 38 medium |

| Tangerines | 2 cups sections, 2 medium |
|---|---|
| Watermelon | 3.75 cups, 1/4 of a large melon> |
| **Portion Equivalents: Vegetables (1 lb.)** | |
| Bell peppers | 3 cups chopped, 4 medium |
| Broccoli | 5 cups chopped, 0.75 bunch |
| Butter leaf lettuce | 2.75 cups chopped |
| Cabbage | 5 cups chopped, 0.5 medium head |
| Cauliflower | 4.5 cups chopped, 1 head |
| Celery | 4.5 cups chopped, 11 medium stalks |
| Cucumbers, peeled | 3 cups sliced, 2.5 medium |
| Green/Red leaf lettuce | 12.5 cups shredded, 1 large head |
| Romaine lettuce | 9.5 cups shredded, 1 large head |
| Spinach | 15 cups, 1 bunch |
| Tomatoes | 2.5 cups chopped, 3.5 medium |
| Tomatoes, cherry | 3 cups |
| **Portion Equivalents: Overt Fats (specified below)** | |
| Avocado (6–7 ounces) | 1 medium |
| Almonds (1oz.) | 23 kernels |
| Hemp seeds (1oz.) | 4 tablespoons |
| Macadamia nuts (1 oz.) | 10–12 kernels |
| Pecans (1 oz.) | 20 halves |
| Pine Nuts (1 oz) | 140 nuts |
| Pistachios (1 oz.) | 49 kernels |
| Sesame seeds (1 oz.) | 3.5 tablespoons |
| Sunflower seeds (1 oz.) | 5 tablespoons |
| Tahini (1 oz.) | 2 tablespoons |
| Walnuts (1 oz.) | 14 halve |

## Summer Menu Plan: Day One

### *Breakfast:* Watermelon

4 lbs. watermelon

***Directions:*** *Slice melon in half and sit outside and bask in summer's glory while you spoon this delightful fruit!*

### *Lunch:* Peachy Keen

1 lb. bananas, 1 lb. peaches

***Directions:*** *Blend with 16 oz. water. Adjust water for desired consistency.*

### *Dinner:*

### *Course One:* Mango Lime Delight!

1 lb. mangos, Juice of ½ a lime

***Directions:*** *Peel and slice mangos into a bowl. Drizzle with lime juice.*

† 300 varieties of mangos are cultivated and studied in Florida alone. The U.S. market sees roughly six varieties widely distributed: Haden, Tommy Atkins, kent, keitt, ataulfo (also called honey, champagne, Manila, Asian, or yellow), and Haitian mangos.

### *Course Two:* Sweet Tomatoes

8 oz. mango, 8 oz. heirloom tomatoes

***Directions:*** *Blend ¾ of the mango with ¾ of the tomato. Cut the remaining mango and tomato into small chunks, toss in and stir.*

### *Course Three:* Mango Red-Pepper Salad

1 lb. romaine lettuce, 8 oz. each: cucumbers, mangos, and red peppers, 4 oz. tomatoes

***Directions:*** *Chop the lettuce into a large bowl. Peel the cucumber if you prefer. Thinly slice the cucumber and slice tomato into wedges; toss with salad greens. Peel and pit the mango, core the pepper, and blend together as a dressing.*

| Summer Menu Plan: Day One | | | |
|---|---|---|---|
| **Watermelon** | **Carb** | **Protein** | **Fat** |
| Grams | 137 | 11 | 3 |
| Calories | 483 | 39 | 22 |
| % total calories | 89 | 7 | 4 |
| **Total calories for this course** | **544** | | |
| **Peachy Keen** | **Carb** | **Protein** | **Fat** |
| Grams | 147 | 9 | 3 |
| Calories | 527 | 33 | 21 |
| % total calories | 90 | 6 | 4 |
| **Total calories for this course** | **581** | | |
| **Mango Lime Delight** | **Carb** | **Protein** | **Fat** |
| Grams | 79 | 2 | 1 |
| Calories | 283 | 9 | 10 |
| % total calories | 94 | 3 | 3 |
| **Total calories for this course** | **302** | | |
| **Sweet Tomatoes** | **Carb** | **Protein** | **Fat** |
| Grams | 49 | 3 | 1 |
| Calories | 173 | 11 | 11 |
| % total calories | 88 | 6 | 6 |
| **Total calories for this course** | **195** | | |
| **Mango Red Pepper Salad** | **Carb** | **Protein** | **Fat** |
| Grams | 77 | 11 | 3 |
| Calories | 269 | 39 | 27 |
| % total calories | 80 | 12 | 8 |
| **Total calories for this course** | **335** | | |
| **Daily Totals** | **Carb** | **Protein** | **Fat** |
| Grams | 489 | 36 | 11 |
| Calories | 89 | 7 | 5 |
| **Caloronutrient ratio for the day** | **89** | **7** | **5** |
| **Total calories for today** | **1957** | | |

## Summer Menu Plan: Day Two

### *Breakfast:* Watermelon

4 lbs. watermelon

***Directions:*** *The other half of the large watermelon awaits you! Spoon the fruit into a blender for a refreshing morning drink! Seeds can be avoided, as they will sink to the bottom of the glass.*

### *Lunch:* Just Bananas!

2 lbs. bananas

***Directions:*** *Blend into a smoothie with 16 oz. water, or enjoy them as they are.*

† If you have a hard time eating very many bananas, it is likely they are not at peak ripeness. The common variety of banana, the cavendish, is ripe when it is generously speckled with brown spots and smells sweet. Prior to this state, they contain more starch and are harder to digest. Proper fruit ripeness is essential to adequate nutrition and assimilation.

### *Dinner*

### *Course One:* Summer Berry Salad

4 oz. blueberries, 4 oz. raspberries, 8 oz. peaches

***Directions:*** *Mix in a bowl and enjoy!*

### *Course Two:* Peach Heirloom Tomato Soup

8 oz. peaches, 8 oz. heirloom tomatoes

***Directions:*** *Blend ¾ of the peaches with ¾ of the tomato. Thinly slice the remaining ingredients and stir them into the soup for added texture.*

### *Course Three:* Blackberry Sesame Salad

1 lb. lettuce, 4 oz. tomatoes, 8 oz. blackberries, 2 tbsp. raw, mechanically hulled tahini.

***Directions:*** *Finely chop the lettuce into a large bowl. Slice the tomato into wedges and toss with lettuce. Dress with a blend of blackberries and tahini.*

| Summer Menu Plan: Day Two | | | |
|---|---|---|---|
| **Watermelon** | **Carb** | **Protein** | **Fat** |
| Grams | 137 | 11 | 3 |
| Calories | 483 | 39 | 22 |
| % total calories | 89 | 7 | 4 |
| **Total calories for this course** | | **544** | |
| **Just Bananas!** | **Carb** | **Protein** | **Fat** |
| Grams | 207 | 10 | 3 |
| Calories | 747 | 36 | 24 |
| % total calories | 93 | 4 | 3 |
| **Total calories for this course** | | **807** | |
| **Summer Berry Salad** | **Carb** | **Protein** | **Fat** |
| Grams | 52 | 4 | 2 |
| Calories | 184 | 15 | 13 |
| % total calories | 87 | 7 | 6 |
| **Total calories for this course** | | **212** | |
| Peach Heirloom Tomato Soup | Carb | Protein | Fat |
| Grams | 32 | 4 | 1 |
| Calories | 112 | 14 | 10 |
| % total calories | 83 | 10 | 7 |
| **Total calories for this course** | | **136** | |
| Blackberry Sesame Salad | Carb | Protein | Fat |
| Grams | 48 | 15 | 19 |
| Calories | 171 | 53 | 149 |
| % total calories | 46 | 14 | 40 |
| **Total calories for this course** | | **373** | |
| Daily Totals | Carb | Protein | Fat |
| Grams | 476 | 44 | 28 |
| Calories | 1697 | 157 | 218 |
| **Caloronutrient ratio for the day** | **82** | **8** | **11** |
| **Total calories for today** | | **2072** | |

## Summer Menu Plan: Day Three

### *Breakfast:* Honeydew Melon

3 lbs. honeydew melon

### *Lunch:* Figgy Delicious

1 lb. figs, 1 lb. bananas

***Directions:*** *Blend with 16 oz. water, or to desired consistency.*

### *Dinner*

### *Course One:* Mango and Raspberry

8 oz. mango, 8 oz. raspberries

***Directions:*** *Slice or cube the mango into a bowl and sprinkle with raspberries.*

### *Course Two:* Delightfully Cool Cukes

8 oz. mango, 8 oz. cucumbers

***Directions:*** *Thinly slice ¼ of the cucumber. Blend the rest with the mango, and mix in sliced cucumber. Enjoy!*

### *Course Three:* Raspberry Salad

1 lb. green-leaf lettuce, 8 oz. cucumber, 8 oz. mango, 8 oz. raspberries

***Directions:*** *Chop the lettuce into a bowl. Peel and slice the cucumber, and mix with salad. Peel and pit the mango, then blend with raspberries to dress the salad.*

† Another way to serve this is to slice the mango over the top and drop whole raspberries over the salad.

| Summer Menu Plan: Day Three | | | |
|---|---|---|---|
| **Honeydew Melon** | **Carb** | **Protein** | **Fat** |
| Grams | 124 | 7 | 2 |
| Calories | 447 | 27 | 16 |
| % total calories | 91 | 6 | 3 |
| **Total calories for this course** | | **490** | |
| **Figgy Delicious** | **Carb** | **Protein** | **Fat** |
| Grams | 191 | 8 | 3 |
| Calories | 686 | 30 | 23 |
| % total calories | 93 | 4 | 3 |
| **Total calories for this course** | | **739** | |
| **Mango and Raspberry** | **Carb** | **Protein** | **Fat** |
| Grams | 66 | 4 | 2 |
| Calories | 234 | 14 | 17 |
| % total calories | 89 | 5 | 6 |
| **Total calories for this course** | | **265** | |
| **Delightfully Cool Cukes** | **Carb** | **Protein** | **Fat** |
| Grams | 43 | 2 | 1 |
| Calories | 158 | 9 | 8 |
| % total calories | 90 | 5 | 5 |
| **Total calories for this course** | | **175** | |
| **Raspberry Salad** | **Carb** | **Protein** | **Fat** |
| Grams | 83 | 11 | 3 |
| Calories | 296 | 40 | 25 |
| % total calories | 82 | 11 | 7 |
| **Total calories for this course** | | **361** | |
| **Daily Totals** | **Carb** | **Protein** | **Fat** |
| Grams | 507 | 32 | 4 |
| Calories | 1821 | 120 | 89 |
| **Caloronutrient ratio for the day** | **90** | **6** | **4** |
| **Total calories for today** | | **2030** | |

## Summer Menu Plan: Day Four

### *Breakfast* : Cherries

2 lbs. sweet cherries

### *Lunch:* Sweet Peach Salad

1 lb. bananas, 1 lb. peaches, 8 oz. blueberries

***Directions:*** *Slice the bananas and peaches into a bowl. Sprinkle the blueberries on top. Enjoy!*

### *Dinner*

### *Course One:* Apricot Blueberry Salad

1 lb. apricots, 8 oz. blueberries

***Directions:*** *Cut the apricots into large chunks and place them in a bowl. Blend the blueberries into a sauce and pour over the apricots.*

### *Course Two:* Mango Fennel Soup

1 lb. mangos, 1 large sprig of fennel

***Directions:*** *Blend 3/4 of the mangos and the bottom 3/4 of the fennel sprig. Pour into a bowl. Cut the remaining mango into small chunks and mix into the soup. Garnish with the top of the fennel sprig. Delicious!*

### *Course Three:* Apricot Celery Salad

1 lb. butter lettuce, 4 oz. tomato, 4 oz. celery, 1 lb. apricots

***Directions:*** *Chop the lettuce into a bowl. Slice tomato and mix with the lettuce. Blend apricots with celery and pour over the salad.*

| Summer Menu Plan: Day Four | | | |
|---|---|---|---|
| **Cherries** | **Carb** | **Protein** | **Fat** |
| Grams | 145 | 10 | 2 |
| Calories | 522 | 35 | 15 |
| % total calories | 91 | 6 | 3 |
| **Total calories for this course** | **572** | | |
| **Sweet Peach Salad** | **Carb** | **Protein** | **Fat** |
| Grams | 180 | 11 | 3 |
| Calories | 644 | 39 | 27 |
| % total calories | 91 | 5 | 4 |
| **Total calories for this course** | **710** | | |
| **Apricot Blueberry Salad** | **Carb** | **Protein** | **Fat** |
| Grams | 83 | 8 | 3 |
| Calories | 298 | 29 | 20 |
| % total calories | 86 | 8 | 6 |
| **Total calories for this course** | **347** | | |
| **Mango Fennel Soup** | **Carb** | **Protein** | **Fat** |
| Grams | 77 | 2 | 1 |
| Calories | 277 | 8 | 10 |
| % total calories | 94 | 3 | 3 |
| **Total calories for this course** | **295** | | |
| **Apricot Celery** | **Carb** | **Protein** | **Fat** |
| Grams | 69 | 14 | 3 |
| Calories | 241 | 49 | 26 |
| % total calories | 76 | 16 | 8 |
| **Total calories for this course** | **316** | | |
| **Daily Totals** | **Carb** | **Protein** | **Fat** |
| Grams | 554 | 45 | 12 |
| Calories | 1982 | 160 | 98 |
| **Caloronutrient ratio for the day** | **89** | **7** | **4** |
| **Total calories for today** | **2240** | | |

## Summer Menu Plan: Day Five

### *Breakfast :* Cantaloupe

3 lbs. cantaloupe

### *Lunch:* Mango and Banana

1 lb. bananas, 1 lb. mangos

***Directions:*** *Slice, mix into a bowl, and devour!*

### *Dinner*

### *Course One:* Apricots

1 lb. apricots

### *Course Two:* Orange Pepper Tomato Soup

8 oz. romaine lettuce, 8 oz. tomatoes, 8 oz. yellow or orange bell pepper, parsley sprig

***Directions:*** *Blend lettuce, ¾ of the tomatoes, and 3/4 of the bell pepper. Slice one tomato, and stir into the soup. Garnish with the remaining bell pepper sliced into rings, and the chopped parsley.*

### *Course Three:* Heirloom Avocado Salad

8 oz. romaine lettuce, 8 oz. cucumber, 12 oz. tomatoes, 6 oz. California avocado, ¼ cup cilantro

***Directions:*** *Peel and slice the cucumber into a bowl with the lettuce, chopped. Separately, chop the tomato and avocado into chunks and stir together with finely chopped cilantro until well blended, and then pour over salad.*

| Summer Menu Plan: Day Five | | | |
|---|---|---|---|
| **Cantaloupe** | **Carb** | **Protein** | **Fat** |
| Grams | 111 | 11 | 3 |
| Calories | 401 | 41 | 21 |
| % total calories | 86 | 9 | 5 |
| **Total calories for this course** | | **463** | |
| **Mango and Banana** | **Carb** | **Protein** | **Fat** |
| Grams | 181 | 7 | 3 |
| Calories | 651 | 26 | 21 |
| % total calories | 93 | 4 | 3 |
| **Total calories for this course** | | **698** | |
| **Apricots** | **Carb** | **Protein** | **Fat** |
| Grams | 50 | 6 | 2 |
| Calories | 181 | 23 | 14 |
| % total calories | 83 | 11 | 6 |
| **Total calories for this course** | | **218** | |
| **Orange Pepper Tomato Soup** | **Carb** | **Protein** | **Fat** |
| Grams | 32 | 7 | 2 |
| Calories | 109 | 24 | 14 |
| % total calories | 74 | 16 | 10 |
| **Total calories for this course** | | **147** | |
| **Heirloom Avocado Salad** | **Carb** | **Protein** | **Fat** |
| Grams | 43 | 10 | 28 |
| Calories | 155 | 38 | 229 |
| % total calories | 37 | 9 | 54 |
| **Total calories for this course** | | **422** | |
| **Daily Totals** | **Carb** | **Protein** | **Fat** |
| Grams | 417 | 41 | 38 |
| Calories | 1497 | 152 | 299 |
| **Caloronutrient ratio for the day** | **77** | **8** | **15** |
| **Total calories for today** | | **1948** | |

## Summer Menu Plan: Day Six

### *Breakfast:* Apricots

2 lbs. apricots

### *Lunch:* Banana Romaine Smoothie

2 lbs. bananas
8 oz. romaine lettuce

**Directions:** *This equates to approximately 8 medium-sized bananas, weighed without the peel. Blend and serve. It is surprisingly delicious!*

### *Dinner:*

### *Course One:* Blackberry-Smothered Peaches

8 oz. peaches, 8 oz. blackberries

**Directions:** *Slice peaches into a bowl. Blend blackberries into a sauce and pour onto the slices.*

### *Course Two:* Berry Green Soup

8 oz. blueberries, 8 oz. blackberries, 8 oz. raspberries, 8 oz. romaine lettuce

**Directions:** *Blend all ingredients. Pour into a serving bowl.*

† For added texture leave some of the berries whole.

### *Course Three:* Crushed Berry Salad

8 oz. baby spinach, 4 oz. tomato, 4 oz. cucumber, 4 oz. blackberries, 4 oz. raspberries, 4 oz. peaches

**Directions:** *Place the spinach into a bowl. Peel the cucumber and slice, along with the tomato, and mix with the spinach. Pour berries into a separate bowl. and mash with a fork. Cut the peach into small pieces and mix with the berries. Pour over the salad.*

| Summer Menu Plan: Day Five | | | |
|---|---|---|---|
| **Apricots** | **Carb** | **Protein** | **Fat** |
| Grams | 101 | 13 | 4 |
| Calories | 360 | 46 | 29 |
| % total calories | 82 | 11 | 7 |
| **Total calories for this course** | | **435** | |
| **Banana Romaine Smoothie** | **Carb** | **Protein** | **Fat** |
| Grams | 215 | 13 | 4 |
| Calories | 770 | 46 | 30 |
| % total calories | 91 | 5 | 4 |
| **Total calories for this course** | | **846** | |
| **Blackberry Smothered Peaches** | **Carb** | **Protein** | **Fat** |
| Grams | 43 | 5 | 2 |
| Calories | 154 | 19 | 13 |
| % total calories | 83 | 10 | 7 |
| **Total calories for this course** | | **186** | |
| **Berry Green Soup** | **Carb** | **Protein** | **Fat** |
| Grams | 89 | 10 | 4 |
| Calories | 314 | 37 | 32 |
| % total calories | 82 | 10 | 8 |
| **Total calories for this course** | | **383** | |
| **Crushed Berry Salad** | **Carb** | **Protein** | **Fat** |
| Grams | 51 | 12 | 3 |
| Calories | 177 | 42 | 23 |
| % total calories | 73 | 17 | 10 |
| **Total calories for this course** | | **242** | |
| **Daily Totals** | **Carb** | **Protein** | **Fat** |
| Grams | 499 | 53 | 17 |
| Calories | 1775 | 190 | 127 |
| **Caloronutrient ratio for the day** | **85** | **9** | **6** |
| **Total calories for today** | | **2092** | |

## Summer Menu Plan: Day Seven

### *Breakfast:* Casaba Melon

4 lbs. casaba melon

### *Lunch:* Mango Salad

2 lbs. mango, 8 oz. butter lettuce

***Directions:*** *Chop the lettuce into a bowl. Dice mango into cubes and arrange over the lettuce and serve.*

† Add a squeeze of lime for a little variation and tang.

### *Dinner*

### *Course One:* Tropical Peach Smoothie

12 oz. mangos, 12 oz. peaches

***Directions:*** *Blend with 8 oz. water.*

† The mango is sometimes called a tropical peach, or the peach called a temperate mango. Both fruits are at their peak in the summer months and are favorites in their respective regions. Enjoy this blend of tropical and temperate fruit. Feel free to eat as a fruit salad, if you prefer.

### *Course Two:* Tomato Basil Soup

1 lb. tomatoes, 5 sun-dried tomato halves, fresh basil to taste

***Directions:*** *Soak sun-dried tomatoes for 10 minutes. Blend ¾ of the tomatoes, basil and sun-dried tomatoes. Pour into a bowl. Chop the remaining tomato into chunks, and place in the center of the soup. Garnish with one fresh basil leaf.*

### *Course Three:* Heirloom Tomato Heaven!

1 lb. heirloom tomatoes, 9 oz. baby mixed greens, 2 tbsp. hemp seeds

***Directions:*** *Place the mixed greens into a bowl. Cut the tomatoes into wedges. Mix the tomatoes and hemp seeds and use to top the salad.*

| Summer Menu Plan: Day Seven | | | |
|---|---|---|---|
| **Casaba Melon** | **Carb** | **Protein** | **Fat** |
| Grams | 119 | 20 | 2 |
| Calories | 423 | 71 | 14 |
| % total calories | 83 | 14 | 3 |
| **Total calories for this course** | | **508** | |
| **Mango Salad** | **Carb** | **Protein** | **Fat** |
| Grams | 159 | 8 | 3 |
| Calories | 568 | 27 | 24 |
| % total calories | 92 | 4 | 4 |
| **Total calories for this course** | | **619** | |
| **Tropical Peach Smoothie** | **Carb** | **Protein** | **Fat** |
| Grams | 90 | 5 | 2 |
| Calories | 323 | 17 | 14 |
| % total calories | 91 | 5 | 4 |
| **Total calories for this course** | | **354** | |
| **Tomato Basil Soup** | **Carb** | **Protein** | **Fat** |
| Grams | 29 | 6 | 2 |
| Calories | 97 | 20 | 15 |
| % total calories | 74 | 15 | 11 |
| **Total calories for this course** | | **132** | |
| **Heirloom Tomato Heaven!** | **Carb** | **Protein** | **Fat** |
| Grams | 36 | 18 | 12 |
| Calories | 127 | 67 | 107 |
| % total calories | 42 | 22 | 36 |
| **Total calories for this course** | | **301** | |
| **Daily Totals** | **Carb** | **Protein** | **Fat** |
| Grams | 433 | 52 | 21 |
| Calories | 1538 | 202 | 174 |
| **Caloronutrient ratio for the day** | **80** | **11** | **9** |
| **Total calories for today** | | **1914** | |
| **Weekly totals** | **Carb** | **Protein** | **Fat** |
| **Caloronutrient ratio for the week** | **84** | **8** | **8** |

## Autumn Menu Plan: Day One

### *Breakfast:* Grapes

1.5 lbs. black grapes

### *Lunch:* Banana with Fig Sauce

1 lb. bananas, 1 lb. figs

***Directions:*** *Blend figs with enough water to make a thick sauce. Slice the bananas, and pour fig sauce over the slices.*

### *Dinner*

### *Course One:* Pomegranate Orange Juice

2 cups orange juice, 1 cup fresh pomegranate juice

***Directions:*** *Use a citrus press or electric citrus reamer to juice the oranges and the pomegranate. Cut the pomegranate in half, and juice it like an orange. Mix and devour!*

### *Course Two:* Tomato Cucumber Soup

8 oz. tomatoes, 8 oz. cucumbers, 8 oz. yellow bell peppers

***Directions:*** *Peel the cucumber. Blend ¾ of the tomato, all of the cucumber, and ¾ of the pepper. Dice remaining tomato and pepper to use as a garnish.*

### *Course Three:* Pistachio Cucumber Salad

1 lb. red-leaf lettuce, 8 oz. tomatoes, 8 oz. cucumbers, 1 oz. pistachios

***Directions:*** *Chop lettuce into a bowl. Peel and slice ½ of the cucumber. Dice the tomato. Blend the other half with pistachios and cucumber for the dressing.*

| Autumn Menu Plan: Day One | | | |
|---|---|---|---|
| **Black Grapes** | **Carb** | **Protein** | **Fat** |
| Grams | 123 | 5 | 1 |
| Calories | 442 | 18 | 9 |
| % total calories | 94 | 4 | 2 |
| **Total calories for this course** | | **469** | |
| **Banana with Fig Sauce** | **Carb** | **Protein** | **Fat** |
| Grams | 191 | 8 | 3 |
| Calories | 686 | 30 | 23 |
| % total calories | 93 | 4 | 3 |
| **Total calories for this course** | | **739** | |
| **Pomegranate Orange Juice** | **Carb** | **Protein** | **Fat** |
| Grams | 91 | 6 | 2 |
| Calories | 342 | 21 | 14 |
| % total calories | 90 | 6 | 4 |
| **Total calories for this course** | | **377** | |
| **Tomato Cucumber Soup** | **Carb** | **Protein** | **Fat** |
| Grams | 30 | 6 | 2 |
| Calories | 104 | 19 | 13 |
| % total calories | 76 | 14 | 10 |
| **Total calories for this course** | | **136** | |
| **Pistachio Cucumber Salad** | **Carb** | **Protein** | **Fat** |
| Grams | 34 | 15 | 15 |
| Calories | 126 | 56 | 123 |
| % total calories | 42 | 18 | 40 |
| **Total calories for this course** | | **305** | |
| **Daily Totals** | **Carb** | **Protein** | **Fat** |
| Grams | 469 | 40 | 23 |
| Calories | 1700 | 144 | 182 |
| **Caloronutrient ratio for the day** | **84** | **7** | **9** |
| **Total calories for today** | | **2026** | |

## Autumn Menu Plan: Day Two

### *Breakfast:* Plums

2 lbs. plums

### *Lunch:* Fuyu Persimmon

2 lbs. fuyu persimmon

***Directions:*** *For those who may not be familiar with the persimmon, the fuyu is a nonastringent variety that can be eaten relatively hard or soft, depending on your preference. The peel is edible, though some people prefer to eat the fruit without it.*

† Fuyus are ready to eat when the four-leaf-clover-shaped top pulls off readily without excessive breakage to the leaves. The fuyu is smaller in size than its relative the hachiya, so it takes more of them to equate to the same calories.

### *Dinner*

### *Course One:* Blended Grapes

1 lb. red seedless grapes

***Directions:*** *Pull grapes off the stem and blend them into a grape drink.*

† Blend in a stalk or two of celery for a salty twist, but make sure you blend the celery first and then add the grapes. Doing this ensures that the fibers of the celery get broken up well. If you'd like to make it even smoother, then chop the celery into small pieces before you blend it.

### *Course Two:* Kiwi Cucumber Soup

1 lb. kiwis, 8 oz. cucumbers, 2 oz. pomegranate seeds

***Directions:*** *Peel the kiwi and the cucumber. Blend 10 oz. kiwi and all the cucumber to form the soup base. Slice the remaining kiwi, and stir it into the soup or arrange on top for garnish. Sprinkle pomegranate seeds on top for a splash of flavor, texture, and color.*

### *Course Three:* Kiwi Strawberry Salad

1 lb. red-leaf lettuce, 8 oz. cucumbers, 8 oz. strawberries, 8 oz. kiwi

***Directions:*** *Prep the lettuce and slice cucumber into a bowl. Peel the kiwi. Remove the strawberry tops ( if desired, or blend them in as well). Blend the kiwi and strawberry, and dress your salad.*

| Autumn Menu Plan: Day Two | | | |
|---|---|---|---|
| **Plums** | **Carb** | **Protein** | **Fat** |
| Grams | 104 | 6 | 3 |
| Calories | 373 | 23 | 21 |
| % total calories | 89 | 6 | 5 |
| **Total calories for this course** | | **417** | |
| **Fuyu Persimmon** | **Carb** | **Protein** | **Fat** |
| Grams | 169 | 5 | 2 |
| Calories | 602 | 19 | 14 |
| % total calories | 95 | 3 | 2 |
| **Total calories for this course** | | **635** | |
| **Blended Grapes** | **Carb** | **Protein** | **Fat** |
| Grams | 82 | 3 | 1 |
| Calories | 295 | 12 | 6 |
| % total calories | 94 | 4 | 2 |
| **Total calories for this course** | | **313** | |
| **Kiwi Cucumber Soup** | **Carb** | **Protein** | **Fat** |
| Grams | 81 | 7 | 3 |
| Calories | 293 | 25 | 24 |
| % total calories | 86 | 7 | 7 |
| **Total calories for this course** | | **342** | |
| **Kiwi Strawberry Salad** | **Carb** | **Protein** | **Fat** |
| Grams | 66 | 11 | 3 |
| Calories | 242 | 42 | 27 |
| % total calories | 77 | 14 | 9 |
| **Total calories for this course** | | **311** | |
| **Daily Totals** | **Carb** | **Protein** | **Fat** |
| Grams | 502 | 32 | 12 |
| Calories | 1805 | 121 | 92 |
| **Caloronutrient ratio for the day** | **89** | **6** | **5** |
| **Total calories for today** | | **2018** | |

## Autumn Menu Plan: Day Three

### ***Breakfast:*** **Papaya**

2 lbs. red papaya

### ***Lunch :*** **Banana Romaine Smoothie**

2 lbs. bananas, 8 oz. romaine lettuce

***Directions:*** *Blend bananas and romaine with as much water as desired for preferred consistency.*

### *Dinner*

### *Course One: Strawberries*

2 lbs. strawberries

***Directions:*** *Eat fresh or blend into a refreshingly tart drink.*

### *Course Two: Celery Red Pepper Soup*

8 oz. celery, 8 oz. red bell peppers, 8 oz. tomatoes

***Directions:*** *Blend the celery and red pepper to make the soup base. Dice the tomatoes and add to the top.*

### *Course Three: Strawberry Fennel Salad*

8 oz. romaine lettuce, 8 oz. fennel bulb, 2 lbs. strawberries

***Directions:*** *Chop the lettuce into a bowl. Thinly slice the fennel bulb, and strawberries, and mix them with the salad greens.*

| Autumn Menu Plan: Day Three | | | |
|---|---|---|---|
| **Papaya** | **Carb** | **Protein** | **Fat** |
| Grams | 89 | 6 | 1 |
| Calories | 324 | 20 | 10 |
| % total calories | 91 | 6 | 3 |
| **Total calories for this course** | | **354** | |
| **Banana Romaine Smoothie** | **Carb** | **Protein** | **Fat** |
| Grams | 215 | 13 | 4 |
| Calories | 770 | 46 | 30 |
| % total calories | 91 | 5 | 4 |
| **Total calories for this course** | | **846** | |
| **Strawberries** | Carb | Protein | Fat |
| Grams | 70 | 6 | 3 |
| Calories | 246 | 22 | 22 |
| % total calories | 84 | 8 | 8 |
| **Total calories for this course** | | **290** | |
| **Celery Red Pepper Soup** | **Carb** | **Protein** | **Fat** |
| Grams | 31 | 6 | 2 |
| Calories | 105 | 19 | 14 |
| % total calories | 76 | 14 | 10 |
| **Total calories for this course** | | **138** | |
| **Strawberry Fennel Salad** | **Carb** | **Protein** | **Fat** |
| Grams | 94 | 12 | 4 |
| Calories | 328 | 41 | 30 |
| % total calories | 82 | 10 | 8 |
| **Total calories for this course** | | **399** | |
| **Daily Totals** | **Carb** | **Protein** | **Fat** |
| Grams | 499 | 43 | 14 |
| Calories | 1773 | 148 | 1066 |
| **Caloronutrient ratio for the day** | **87** | **7** | **5** |
| **Total calories for today** | | **2027** | |

## Autumn Menu Plan: Day Four

### *Breakfast:* Banana Milk

1 ¼ lb. bananas

***Directions:*** *Blend bananas with enough water to make a "milky" consistency.*

† Add a tablespoon of raw carob powder to the mix for a carob milk treat!

### *Lunch* : Hachiya Persimmon

2 lbs. hachiya persimmons

***Directions:*** *The hachiya is best eaten by pulling the top clover leaf off and sucking the insides out. The skin of this fruit is edible and thinner than the fuyu. No peeling is necessary or even possible with the hachiya persimmon.*

† Unlike the fuyu, the hachiya is an astringent variety of persimmon. When unripe, the tannins of this fruit will leave you with a chalky feeling in your mouth. You know this fruit is ripe when it feels so soft it that is seems it should fall apart in your hands. However, it can take anywhere from a couple of weeks to a couple of months for this fruit to reach its peak. I like to say, "buy them at Thanksgiving and eat them at Christmas." You may find that some have black spots on the outside. This is the result of external sun damage, but it does not affect the fruit's quality.

### *Dinner*

### *Course One: Plums*

1.5 lbs. plums

### *Course Two: Cabbage Red Pepper Soup*

8 oz. red cabbage, 8 oz. red peppers, 8 oz. cucumbers

***Directions:*** *Peel the cucumber. Blend everything, and enjoy!*

### *Course Three: Tomato Fennel Slaw*

8 oz. red cabbage, 1 lb. tomatoes, 1 frond of fennel for garnish and flavor

***Directions:*** *Chop all ingredients and stir together in a bowl.*

† If the flavor of fennel is not palatable to you, substitute any mild herb you enjoy, such as basil or cilantro.

| Autumn Menu Plan: Day Four | | | |
|---|---|---|---|
| **Banana Milk** | **Carb** | **Protein** | **Fat** |
| Grams | 207 | 10 | 3 |
| Calories | 747 | 36 | 24 |
| % total calories | 93 | 4 | 3 |
| **Total calories for this course** | | **807** | |
| **Hachiya Persimmon** | **Carb** | **Protein** | **Fat** |
| Grams | 169 | 5 | 2 |
| Calories | 602 | 19 | 14 |
| % total calories | 95 | 3 | 2 |
| **Total calories for this course** | | **635** | |
| **Plums** | **Carb** | **Protein** | **Fat** |
| Grams | 78 | 5 | 2 |
| Calories | 281 | 17 | 15 |
| % total calories | 90 | 5 | 5 |
| **Total calories for this course** | | **313** | |
| **Cabbage Red Pepper Soup** | **Carb** | **Protein** | **Fat** |
| Grams | 35 | 7 | 1 |
| Calories | 121 | 24 | 11 |
| % total calories | 78 | 15 | 7 |
| **Total calories for this course** | | **156** | |
| **Tomato Fennel Slaw** | **Carb** | **Protein** | **Fat** |
| Grams | 38 | 7 | 2 |
| Calories | 128 | 24 | 14 |
| % total calories | 78 | 14 | 8 |
| **Total calories for this course** | **166** | | |
| **Daily Totals** | **Carb** | **Protein** | **Fat** |
| Grams | 527 | 34 | 10 |
| Calories | 1879 | 34 | 10 |
| **Caloronutrient ratio for the day** | **90** | **6** | **4** |
| **Total calories for today** | | **2077** | |

## Autumn Menu Plan: Day Five

### *Breakfast:* Grapes

2 lbs. green grapes

### *Lunch: Sweet Bananas!*

1 lb. bananas, 4 oz. dates

**Directions:** *Pit the dates and place in a blender. Pour just enough water to allow the dates to blend into a paste. Peel the bananas and blend them in with the date purée, using as much water to reach your desired consistency.*

### *Dinner*

### *Course One: Fresh-Squeezed Orange Juice*

16 oz. fresh-squeezed orange juice

### *Course Two: Orange Pepper Cucumber Soup*

8 oz. orange bell peppers, 8 oz. cucumbers, 4 oz. strawberries

**Directions:** *Blend the peppers and cucumbers. Garnish with sliced strawberries for color and texture.*

### *Course Three: Orange Pecan Salad*

1 lb. baby spinach, 4 oz. broccoli florets, 4 oz. fresh-squeezed orange juice, 1 oz. pecans

**Directions:** *Tear the spinach into a bowl. Chop the broccoli and mix with greens. Blend the orange juice with the pecans for the dressing. Enjoy!*

| Autumn Menu Plan: Day Five | | | |
|---|---|---|---|
| **Green Grapes** | **Carb** | **Protein** | **Fat** |
| Grams | 164 | 7 | 1 |
| Calories | 591 | 23 | 12 |
| % total calories | 94 | 4 | 2 |
| **Total calories for this course** | | **626** | |
| **Sweet Bananas!** | **Carb** | **Protein** | **Fat** |
| Grams | 189 | 7 | 2 |
| Calories | 679 | 25 | 14 |
| % total calories | 95 | 3 | 2 |
| **Total calories for this course** | | **718** | |
| **Fresh-Squeezed Orange Juice** | **Carb** | **Protein** | **Fat** |
| Grams | 47 | 3 | 1 |
| Calories | 184 | 12 | 8 |
| % total calories | 90 | 6 | 4 |
| **Total calories for this course** | | **204** | |
| **Orange Pepper Cucumber Soup** | **Carb** | **Protein** | **Fat** |
| Grams | 28 | 4 | 1 |
| Calories | 100 | 16 | 9 |
| % total calories | 80 | 13 | 7 |
| **Total calories for this course** | | **125** | |
| **Orange Pecan Salad** | **Carb** | **Protein** | **Fat** |
| Grams | 40 | 20 | 23 |
| Calories | 138 | 70 | 177 |
| % total calories | 36 | 18 | 46 |
| **Total calories for this course** | | **385** | |
| **Daily Totals** | **Carb** | **Protein** | **Fat** |
| Grams | 468 | 41 | 28 |
| Calories | 1692 | 146 | 220 |
| **Caloronutrient ratio for the day** | **82** | **7** | **11** |
| **Total calories for today** | | **2058** | |

## Autumn Menu Plan: Day Six

### *Breakfast :* Grapes

2 lbs. red grapes

### *Lunch:* Figs

2 lbs. figs

### *Dinner*

### *Course One: Pineapple Strawberry Drink*

1 lb. pineapple, 1 lb. strawberries

***Directions:*** *Peel and core the pineapple. De-stem the strawberries. Blend pineapple and strawberries until they make a smoothie.*

### *Course Two: Pineapple Red Pepper Soup*

1.5 lbs. pineapple, 8 oz. red bell peppers, 8 oz. tomatoes

***Directions:*** *Peel and core the pineapple, core the pepper and blend. Dice the tomato and stir into the soup, or sprinkle on top as garnish.*

### *Course Three: Strawberry Parsley Salad*

1 lb. red-leaf lettuce, 8 oz. cherry tomatoes, 8 oz. strawberries, 1 oz. parsley

***Directions:*** *Chop the lettuce into a bowl. Blend the strawberries and parsley as the dressing.*

| Autumn Menu Plan: Day Six | | | |
|---|---|---|---|
| **Red Grapes** | **Carb** | **Protein** | **Fat** |
| Grams | 164 | 7 | 1 |
| Calories | 591 | 23 | 12 |
| % total calories | 94 | 4 | 2 |
| **Total calories for this course** | | **626** | |
| **Figs** | **Carb** | **Protein** | **Fat** |
| Grams | 174 | 7 | 3 |
| Calories | 625 | 24 | 22 |
| % total calories | 93 | 4 | 3 |
| **Total calories for this course** | | **671** | |
| **Pineapple Strawberry Drink** | **Carb** | **Protein** | **Fat** |
| Grams | 88 | 6 | 2 |
| Calories | 313 | 20 | 16 |
| % total calories | 89 | 6 | 5 |
| **Total calories for this course** | | **349** | |
| **Pineapple Red Pepper Soup** | **Carb** | **Protein** | **Fat** |
| Grams | 105 | 8 | 2 |
| Calories | 367 | 28 | 18 |
| % total calories | 89 | 7 | 4 |
| **Total calories for this course** | | **413** | |
| **Strawberry Parsley Salad** | **Carb** | **Protein** | **Fat** |
| Grams | 40 | 10 | 3 |
| Calories | 144 | 37 | 22 |
| % total calories | 71 | 18 | 11 |
| **Total calories for this course** | | **203** | |
| **Daily Totals** | **Carb** | **Protein** | **Fat** |
| Grams | 571 | 38 | 11 |
| Calories | 2040 | 132 | 90 |
| **Caloronutrient ratio for the day** | **90** | **6** | **4** |
| **Total calories for today** | | **2259** | |

## Autumn Menu Plan: Day Seven

### *Breakfast:* Concord Grapes

2 lbs. concord grapes

### *Lunch :* Figgy Bliss

1 lb. bananas, 1 lb. figs, 16 oz. young coconut water

***Directions:*** *Blend and savor.*

### *Dinner*

### *Course One:* Papaya

1 lb. papaya

### *Course Two:* Grapefruit Tomato Soup

8 oz. grapefruit, 8 oz. tomatoes, 8 oz. cucumbers

***Directions:*** *Blend the grapefruit, cucumber, and ½ of the tomatoes for the soup base. Chop, slice, or dice the remaining tomato for color and texture.*

### *Course Three:* Orange Avocado Slaw

8 oz. celery, 8 oz. cabbage, 4 oz. California avocado, 8 oz. fresh-squeezed orange juice

***Directions:*** *Grate the cabbage and celery with a food processor, or cut very fine. Place into a bowl. Dice the avocado into a separate bowl, stir in the orange juice, and mix with a fork until it becomes a chunky sauce. Stir into the cabbage mixture until evenly coated.*

| Autumn Menu Plan: Day Seven | | | |
|---|---|---|---|
| **Concord Grapes** | **Carb** | **Protein** | **Fat** |
| Grams | 117 | 4 | 2 |
| Calories | 422 | 15 | 19 |
| % total calories | 93 | 3 | 4 |
| **Total calories for this course** | **456** | | |
| **Figgy Bliss** | **Carb** | **Protein** | **Fat** |
| Grams | 207 | 12 | 4 |
| Calories | 753 | 42 | 31 |
| % total calories | 91 | 5 | 4 |
| **Total calories for this course** | **826** | | |
| **Papaya** | **Carb** | **Protein** | **Fat** |
| Grams | 44 | 3 | 1 |
| Calories | 162 | 10 | 5 |
| % total calories | 91 | 6 | 3 |
| **Total calories for this course** | **177** | | |
| **Grapefruit Tomato Soup** | **Carb** | **Protein** | **Fat** |
| Grams | 40 | 5 | 1 |
| Calories | 141 | 18 | 11 |
| % total calories | 83 | 11 | 6 |
| **Total calories for this course** | **170** | | |
| **Orange Avocado Slaw** | **Carb** | **Protein** | **Fat** |
| Grams | 55 | 9 | 19 |
| Calories | 201 | 32 | 154 |
| % total calories | 52 | 8 | 40 |
| **Total calories for this course** | **387** | | |
| **Daily Totals** | **Carb** | **Protein** | **Fat** |
| Grams | 463 | 33 | 27 |
| Calories | 1679 | 117 | 220 |
| **Caloronutrient ratio for the day** | **83** | **6** | **11** |
| **Total calories for today** | **2016** | | |
| **Weekly totals** | **Carb** | **Protein** | **Fat** |
| **Caloronutrient ratio for the week** | **87** | **6** | **7** |

## Winter Menu Plan: Day One

### *Breakfast*

### *Banana Milk*

2 lb. bananas

***Directions:*** *Blend bananas with enough water to make a "milky" consistency.*

### *Lunch*

### *Hachiya Persimmon*

2 lbs. hachiya persimmons

### *Dinner*

### *Course One: Orange Papaya Smoothie*

8 oz. papaya, 8 oz. fresh-squeezed orange juice

***Directions:*** *De-seed the papaya and then peel or simply scoop out the flesh with a spoon. Blend with the orange juice.*

### *Course Two: Orange Verde Soup*

8 oz. romaine lettuce, 8 oz. Valencia oranges

***Directions:*** *Blend lettuce and ¾ of the oranges together. Break apart the remaining orange into segments for garnish.*

### *Course Three: Orange-Walnut Salad*

8 oz. romaine lettuce, 4 oz. oranges, 1 oz. walnuts

***Directions:*** *Chop the lettuce into a bowl. Peel the oranges, cut them into small pieces, and place in a separate bowl along with chopped walnuts. Stir and pour over lettuce. Simply delicious*

| Winter Menu Plan: Day One | | | |
|---|---|---|---|
| **Banana Milk** | **Carb** | **Protein** | **Fat** |
| Grams | 207 | 10 | 3 |
| Calories | 747 | 36 | 24 |
| % total calories | 93 | 4 | 3 |
| **Total calories for this course** | **807** | | |
| **Hachiya Persimmon** | **Carb** | **Protein** | **Fat** |
| Grams | 169 | 5 | 2 |
| Calories | 602 | 19 | 14 |
| % total calories | 95 | 3 | 2 |
| **Total calories for this course** | **635** | | |
| **Orange Papaya Smoothie** | **Carb** | **Protein** | **Fat** |
| Grams | 48 | 3 | 1 |
| Calories | 181 | 12 | 7 |
| % total calories | 90 | 6 | 4 |
| **Total calories for this course** | **200** | | |
| **Orange Verde Soup** | **Carb** | **Protein** | **Fat** |
| Grams | 34 | 5 | 1 |
| Calories | 121 | 18 | 11 |
| % total calories | 81 | 12 | 7 |
| **Total calories for this course** | **150** | | |
| **Walnut Orange Salad** | **Carb** | **Protein** | **Fat** |
| Grams | 25 | 8 | 20 |
| Calories | 90 | 30 | 160 |
| % total calories | 32 | 11 | 57 |
| **Total calories for this course** | **280** | | |
| **Daily Totals** | **Carb** | **Protein** | **Fat** |
| Grams | 483 | 31 | 27 |
| Calories | 1741 | 115 | 216 |
| **Caloronutrient ratio for the day** | **84** | **6** | **10** |
| **Total calories for today** | **2072** | | |

## Winter Menu Plan: Day Two

### *Breakfast:* Citrus Salad

8 oz. grapefruit, 1 lb. Valencia oranges, 1 lb. sweet tangerines

***Directions:*** *Peel the fruits and cut them into a bowl. Enjoy the contrasting flavors.*

† Experiment with all the different varieties of oranges and tangerines. Blood oranges make an excellent addition or substitution to this "salad."

### *Lunch:* Banana Celery Smoothie

2 lbs. bananas, 4 oz. celery

***Directions:*** *Cut the celery into small pieces to sever the fibers, making them easier to blend. Blend banana and celery with as much water as needed for desired consistency.*

### *Dinner*

### *Course One:* Fresh-Squeezed Orange Juice

16 oz. fresh-squeezed orange juice

### *Course Two:* Cabbage Tomato Soup

8 oz. fresh-squeezed orange juice, 8 oz. cabbage, 4 oz. romaine lettuce, 4 oz. tomatoes

***Directions:*** *Blend orange juice, cabbage, and lettuce. Pour purée into a large serving bowl, and sprinkle with diced tomato. Voilà!*

### *Course Three:* Orange Fennel Slaw

8 oz. cabbage, 1 lb. oranges, 1 shoot of fennel top

***Directions:*** *Finely chop the cabbage and fennel into a bowl. Chop the oranges into small pieces, and stir into the cabbage-fennel mix.*

| Winter Menu Plan: Day Two | | | |
|---|---|---|---|
| **Citrus Salad** | **Carb** | **Protein** | **Fat** |
| Grams | 138 | 10 | 2 |
| Calories | 496 | 35 | 18 |
| % total calories | 91 | 6 | 3 |
| **Total calories for this course** | **549** | | |
| **Banana Celery Smoothie** | **Carb** | **Protein** | **Fat** |
| Grams | 211 | 11 | 3 |
| Calories | 759 | 38 | 26 |
| % total calories | 92 | 5 | 3 |
| **Total calories for this course** | **823** | | |
| **Fresh-Squeezed Orange Juice** | **Carb** | **Protein** | **Fat** |
| Grams | 47 | 3 | 1 |
| Calories | 184 | 12 | 8 |
| % total calories | 90 | 6 | 4 |
| **Total calories for this course** | **204** | | |
| **Cabbage Tomato Soup** | **Carb** | **Protein** | **Fat** |
| Grams | 47 | 7 | 1 |
| Calories | 171 | 26 | 12 |
| % total calories | 82 | 12 | 6 |
| **Total calories for this course** | **209** | | |
| **Orange Fennel Slaw** | **Carb** | **Protein** | **Fat** |
| Grams | 70 | 8 | 1 |
| Calories | 250 | 27 | 7 |
| % total calories | 88 | 10 | 2 |
| **Total calories for this course** | **284** | | |
| **Daily Totals** | **Carb** | **Protein** | **Fat** |
| Grams | 513 | 39 | 8 |
| Calories | 1860 | 138 | 71 |
| **Caloronutrient ratio for the day** | **90** | **7** | **3** |
| **Total calories for today** | **2069** | | |

## Winter Menu Plan: Day Three

### *Breakfast:* Papaya

2 ½ lbs. red papaya

### *Lunch:* Bananas with Date Sauce

1 lb. bananas
4 oz. dates

***Directions:*** *Slice the bananas into a bowl. Pit the dates and blend them with just enough water to make a thick sauce. Pour over the bananas and devour!*

### *Dinner*

### *Course One:* Pineapple Orange Drink

12 oz. pineapple, 16 oz. fresh-squeezed orange juice

***Directions:*** *Peel and core the pineapple. Blend. Cheers!*

### *Course Two:* P.L.T. Soup

12 oz. pineapple, 8 oz. romaine lettuce, 4 oz. tomatoes

***Directions:*** *Peel and core the pineapple. Blend with the lettuce, then pour into a bowl. Dice the tomato and pour over the soup.*

### *Course Three:* Pineapple Tahini Salad

8 oz. romaine lettuce, 8 oz. cucumbers, 4 oz. pineapple, 1 oz. raw, mechanically hulled tahini

***Directions:*** *Chop the lettuce into a bowl. Peel and slice the cucumber, and mix with the lettuce. Peel and core the pineapple. Blend with the tahini and dress the salad.*

| Winter Menu Plan: Day Three | | | |
|---|---|---|---|
| **Papaya** | **Carb** | **Protein** | **Fat** |
| Grams | 111 | 7 | 2 |
| Calories | 404 | 25 | 13 |
| % total calories | 91 | 6 | 3 |
| **Total calories for this course** | **442** | | |
| **Bananas with Date Sauce** | **Carb** | **Protein** | **Fat** |
| Grams | 189 | 7 | 2 |
| Calories | 679 | 25 | 14 |
| % total calories | 95 | 3 | 2 |
| **Total calories for this course** | **718** | | |
| **Pineapple Orange Drink** | **Carb** | **Protein** | **Fat** |
| Grams | 92 | 5 | 1 |
| Calories | 344 | 20 | 12 |
| % total calories | 92 | 5 | 3 |
| **Total calories for this course** | **376** | | |
| **P.L.T. Soup** | **Carb** | **Protein** | **Fat** |
| Grams | 56 | 6 | 1 |
| Calories | 194 | 20 | 12 |
| % total calories | 86 | 9 | 5 |
| **Total calories for this course** | **226** | | |
| **Pineapple Tahini Salad** | **Carb** | **Protein** | **Fat** |
| Grams | 34 | 10 | 15 |
| Calories | 125 | 36 | 121 |
| % total calories | 44 | 13 | 43 |
| **Total calories for this course** | **282** | | |
| **Daily Totals** | **Carb** | **Protein** | **Fat** |
| Grams | 482 | 35 | 21 |
| Calories | 1746 | 126 | 172 |
| **Caloronutrient ratio for the day** | **85** | **6** | **8** |
| **Total calories for today** | **2044** | | |

## Winter Menu Plan: Day Four

### *Breakfast:* Pineapple Kiwi Smoothie

1 lb. pineapple, 1 lb. kiwi

***Directions:*** *Blend and enjoy. Add water for a thinner consistency if desired.*

### *Lunch :* Dates and Cucumber

10 oz. medjool dates, 1 lb. cucumbers

***Directions:*** *Peeled cucumber works best for this recipe. Pit the dates and thickly slice the cucumber. Place one date on each cucumber slice and devour. It's sweet, juicy, and crunchy!*

† Nutritional information is only available for the two major varieties of dates, medjool and deglet noor. Countless other varieties exist that you may prefer. Several mail-order providers from Southern California specialize in rare and exotic varieties and will ship them to just about anywhere in the U.S. Enjoy dates when they are the freshest in late fall and early winter.

### *Dinner*

### *Course One:* Satsuma Tangerines

1 lb. tangerines

### *Course Two:* Grapefruit Cucumber Soup

8 oz. cucumbers, 8 oz. grapefruit, 8 oz. tomatoes

***Directions:*** *Blend and enjoy.*

### *Course Three:* Satsuma Cucumber

1 lb. baby spinach, 8 oz. satsuma tangerines, 8 oz. cucumbers, ½ oz. pine nuts

***Directions:*** *Tear the spinach into a bowl. Blend the tangerines and cucumber into a dressing. Sprinkle with pine nuts.*

| Winter Menu Plan: Day Four | | | |
|---|---|---|---|
| **Pineapple Kiwi Smoothie** | **Carb** | **Protein** | **Fat** |
| Grams | 124 | 8 | 3 |
| Calories | 444 | 27 | 23 |
| % total calories | 90 | 5 | 5 |
| **Total calories for this course** | **494** | | |
| **Dates and Cucumber** | **Carb** | **Protein** | **Fat** |
| Grams | 226 | 8 | 1 |
| Calories | 809 | 30 | 10 |
| % total calories | 95 | 4 | 1 |
| **Total calories for this course** | **849** | | |
| **Satsuma Tangerines** | **Carb** | **Protein** | **Fat** |
| Grams | 61 | 4 | 1 |
| Calories | 216 | 13 | 11 |
| % total calories | 90 | 5 | 5 |
| **Total calories for this course** | **240** | | |
| **Grapefruit Cucumber Soup** | **Carb** | **Protein** | **Fat** |
| Grams | 40 | 5 | 1 |
| Calories | 141 | 18 | 11 |
| % total calories | 83 | 11 | 6 |
| **Total calories for this course** | **170** | | |
| **Satsuma Cucumber** | **Carb** | **Protein** | **Fat** |
| Grams | 38 | 17 | 12 |
| Calories | 133 | 59 | 95 |
| % total calories | 46 | 21 | 33 |
| **Total calories for this course** | **287** | | |
| **Daily Totals** | **Carb** | **Protein** | **Fat** |
| Grams | 489 | 42 | 18 |
| Calories | 85 | 7 | 7 |
| **Caloronutrient ratio for the day** | **85** | **7** | **7** |
| **Total calories for today** | **2040** | | |

## Winter Menu Plan: Day Five

### *Breakfast:* Satsuma Tangerines

2 lbs. Satsuma tangerines

### *Lunch:* Just Bananas!

2 lbs. bananas

***Directions:*** *Blend the bananas into a smoothie or eat them straight. The choice is all yours!*

### *Dinner:*

### *Course One:* Papaya Pineapple Drink

1 lb. papaya, 8 oz. pineapple

***Directions:*** *Blend and serve. For a thinner drink add as much water as you desire.*

### *Course Two:* Papaya Lime Soup

1 lb. papaya, 8 oz. romaine lettuce, 1 oz. lime juice

***Directions:*** *Blend all ingredients and pour into a bowl. Splendid!*

### *Course Three:* Orange Hemp Seed Salad

1 lb. red-leaf lettuce, 8 oz. Valencia oranges, 2 tbsp. hemp seeds

***Directions:*** *Chop the lettuce into a bowl. Peel the oranges and place them in a separate bowl. Stir in the hemp seeds, and pour the mixture over the lettuce.*

## Winter Menu Plan: Day Five

| Satsuma Tangerines | Carb | Protein | Fat |
|---|---|---|---|
| Grams | 121 | 7 | 3 |
| Calories | 432 | 26 | 23 |
| % total calories | 90 | 5 | 5 |
| **Total calories for this course** | | **481** | |
| **Just Bananas!** | **Carb** | **Protein** | **Fat** |
| Grams | 207 | 10 | 3 |
| Calories | 747 | 36 | 24 |
| % total calories | 93 | 4 | 3 |
| **Total calories for this course** | | **807** | |
| **Papaya Pineapple Drink** | **Carb** | **Protein** | **Fat** |
| Grams | 73 | 4 | 1 |
| Calories | 265 | 14 | 7 |
| % total calories | 93 | 5 | 2 |
| **Total calories for this course** | | **286** | |
| **Papaya Lime Soup** | **Carb** | **Protein** | **Fat** |
| Grams | 30 | 4 | 1 |
| Calories | 104 | 15 | 8 |
| % total calories | 82 | 12 | 6 |
| **Total calories for this course** | | **127** | |
| **Orange Hemp Seed Salad** | **Carb** | **Protein** | **Fat** |
| Grams | 44 | 19 | 11 |
| Calories | 165 | 75 | 90 |
| % total calories | 50 | 23 | 27 |
| **Total calories for this course** | | **259** | |
| **Daily Totals** | **Carb** | **Protein** | **Fat** |
| Grams | 475 | 44 | 19 |
| Calories | 1713 | 166 | 152 |
| **Caloronutrient ratio for the day** | **84** | **8** | **7** |
| **Total calories for today** | | **2031** | |

## Winter Menu Plan: Day Six

### *Breakfast:* Kiwi Orange Drink

1 lb. kiwi, 16 oz. fresh-squeezed orange juice

***Directions:*** *Peel the kiwi and blend with the orange juice.*

### *Lunch:* Banana Wraps

1 ¾ lbs. bananas, 8 oz. romaine lettuce

***Directions:*** *Peel the bananas and wrap in whole lettuce leaves.*

### *Dinner*

### *Course One:* Tangerine Pineapple Blend

8 oz. tangerines, 12 oz. pineapple

***Directions:*** *Peel and core the pineapple. Blend with the tangerines for a thick smoothie.*

### *Course Two:* Tangerine Celery Soup

8 oz. tangerines, 4 oz. celery, 4 oz. red bell peppers

*Directions: Blend and pour into a bowl.*

† It helps to use a sweet and seedless variety of tangerine for this recipe. Oranges can also substitute well for the tangerines.

### *Course Three:* Pineapple Red Pepper Salad

1 lb. butter lettuce, 4 oz. pineapple, 4 oz. red bell peppers, 1 oz. sliced almonds

***Directions:*** *Prep the lettuce into a bowl. Blend the pineapple and red pepper to dress your salad. Garnish with almonds.*

| Winter Menu Plan: Day Six | | | |
|---|---|---|---|
| **Kiwi Orange Drink** | **Carb** | **Protein** | **Fat** |
| Grams | 118 | 9 | 3 |
| Calories | 440 | 32 | 28 |
| % total calories | 88 | 6 | 6 |
| **Total calories for this course** | | **500** | |
| **Banana Wraps** | **Carb** | **Protein** | **Fat** |
| Grams | 189 | 11 | 3 |
| Calories | 677 | 41 | 27 |
| % total calories | 90 | 6 | 4 |
| **Total calories for this course** | | **745** | |
| **Tangerine Pineapple Blend** | **Carb** | **Protein** | **Fat** |
| Grams | 73 | 4 | 1 |
| Calories | 262 | 13 | 9 |
| % total calories | 92 | 5 | 3 |
| **Total calories for this course** | | **284** | |
| **Tangerine Celery Soup** | **Carb** | **Protein** | **Fat** |
| Grams | 40 | 4 | 1 |
| Calories | 143 | 13 | 10 |
| % total calories | 86 | 8 | 6 |
| **Total calories for this course** | | **166** | |
| **Pineapple Red Pepper Salad** | **Carb** | **Protein** | **Fat** |
| Grams | 37 | 14 | 16 |
| Calories | 132 | 49 | 126 |
| % total calories | 43 | 16 | 41 |
| **Total calories for this course** | | **307** | |
| **Daily Totals** | **Carb** | **Protein** | **Fat** |
| Grams | 457 | 42 | 24 |
| Calories | 1654 | 148 | 200 |
| **Caloronutrient ratio for the day** | **8** | **7** | **10** |
| **Total calories for today** | | **2002** | |

## Winter Menu Plan: Day Seven

### *Breakfast:* Papaya Banana Salad

8 oz. papaya, 1 lb. banana

***Directions:*** *Cut fruits into a bowl and mix.*

### *Lunch:* Dates and Celery

10 oz. dates, 16 oz. celery

***Directions:*** *Eat them together, or one at a time.*

### *Dinner*

#### *Course One: Fresh Squeezed Orange Juice*

16 oz. fresh-squeezed orange juice

#### *Course Two: Orange Broccoli Soup*

8 oz. broccoli, 8 oz. oranges

***Directions:*** *Blend both ingredients into a delicious soup.*

#### *Course Three: Grapefruit Tahini Salad*

1 lb. romaine lettuce, 4 oz. broccoli, 4 oz. grapefruit, 1 oz. raw mechanically hulled tahini

***Directions:*** *Finely chop the lettuce and broccoli into a bowl. Blend the grapefruit and the tahini to dress the salad.*

| Winter Menu Plan: Day Seven | | | |
|---|---|---|---|
| **Papaya Banana Salad** | **Carb** | **Protein** | **Fat** |
| Grams | 126 | 6 | 2 |
| Calories | 454 | 23 | 15 |
| % total calories | 92 | 5 | 3 |
| **Total calories for this course** | | **492** | |
| **Dates and Celery** | **Carb** | **Protein** | **Fat** |
| Grams | 226 | 8 | 1 |
| Calories | 809 | 30 | 10 |
| % total calories | 95 | 4 | 1 |
| **Total calories for this course** | | **849** | |
| **Fresh-Squeezed Orange Juice** | **Carb** | **Protein** | **Fat** |
| Grams | 47 | 3 | 1 |
| Calories | 184 | 12 | 8 |
| % total calories | 90 | 6 | 4 |
| **Total calories for this course** | | **204** | |
| **Orange Broccoli Soup** | **Carb** | **Protein** | **Fat** |
| Grams | 42 | 9 | 2 |
| Calories | 146 | 30 | 12 |
| % total calories | 78 | 16 | 6 |
| **Total calories for this course** | | **188** | |
| **Grapefruit Tahini Salad** | **Carb** | **Protein** | **Fat** |
| Grams | 42 | 15 | 16 |
| Calories | 149 | 52 | 124 |
| % total calories | 46 | 16 | 38 |
| **Total calories for this course** | | **325** | |
| **Daily Totals** | **Carb** | **Protein** | **Fat** |
| Grams | 483 | 41 | 22 |
| Calories | 1742 | 174 | 169 |
| **Caloronutrient ratio for the day** | **85** | **7** | **8** |
| **Total calories for today** | | **2058** | |
| **Weekly totals** | **Carb** | **Protein** | **Fat** |
| **Caloronutrient ratio for the week** | **85** | **7** | **8** |

# Spring Menu Plan: Day One

## *Breakfast:* Papaya with Kiwi Sauce

2.5 lbs. papaya, 8 oz. kiwi

***Directions:*** *De-seed and peel the papaya. Cut into a bowl. Blend the kiwi and pour over the papaya.*

## *Lunch:* Banana Celery Smoothie

1 ¾ lbs. bananas
4 oz. celery

***Directions:*** *Cut the celery into small pieces to sever the fibers, making them easier to blend. Blend banana and celery with as much water as needed for desired consistency.*

## *Dinner*

### *Course One:* Pineapple Kiwi Drink

8 oz. pineapple
8 oz. kiwi

***Directions:*** *Peel and core the pineapple. Peel the kiwi, and then blend the two ingredients.*

### *Course Two:* Pineapple Fennel Soup

8 oz. pineapple, 4 oz. celery, 4 oz. cucumber, 1 oz. fennel fronds

***Directions:*** *Blend the pineapple, celery, and fennel, and pour into a bowl. Cut the cucumber into small chunks and use to garnish the top of the soup.*

### *Course Three:* Pineapple Macadamia Salad

1 lb. green-leaf lettuce, 4 oz. tomatoes, 4 oz. pineapple, 1 oz. macadamia nuts

***Directions:*** *Chop the lettuce into a bowl. Slice the tomato and toss with the greens. Blend the pineapple and macadamia nuts for a scrumptious dressing!*

| Spring Menu Plan: Day One | | | |
|---|---|---|---|
| **Papaya with Kiwi Sauce** | **Carb** | **Protein** | **Fat** |
| Grams | 144 | 10 | 3 |
| Calories | 524 | 34 | 23 |
| % total calories | 90 | 6 | 4 |
| **Total calories for this course** | **581** | | |
| **Banana Celery Smoothie** | **Carb** | **Protein** | **Fat** |
| Grams | 185 | 9 | 3 |
| Calories | 665 | 34 | 23 |
| % total calories | 92 | 5 | 3 |
| **Total calories for this course** | **722** | | |
| **Pineapple Kiwi Drink** | **Carb** | **Protein** | **Fat** |
| Grams | 62 | 4 | 1 |
| Calories | 221 | 14 | 12 |
| % total calories | 89 | 6 | 5 |
| **Total calories for this course** | **247** | | |
| **Pineapple Fennel Soup** | **Carb** | **Protein** | **Fat** |
| Grams | 37 | 3 | 1 |
| Calories | 130 | 11 | 6 |
| % total calories | 88 | 7 | 4 |
| **Total calories for this course** | **147** | | |
| **Pineapple Macadamia Salad** | **Carb** | **Protein** | **Fat** |
| Grams | 36 | 10 | 23 |
| Calories | 130 | 36 | 184 |
| % total calories | 37 | 10 | 53 |
| **Total calories for this course** | **350** | | |
| **Daily Totals** | **Carb** | **Protein** | **Fat** |
| Grams | 464 | 36 | 31 |
| Calories | 1670 | 129 | 248 |
| **Caloronutrient ratio for the day** | **8** | **6** | **12** |
| **Total calories for today** | **2047** | | |

## Spring Menu Plan: Day Two

### *Breakfast:* Bananas with Carob Sauce

1 lb. bananas, 1 oz. medjool dates, 1 oz. raw carob powder

***Directions:*** *Slice most of the bananas into a bowl, reserving ½ of one banana for the sauce. Blend the dates, ½ banana, and carob with just enough water to make a sauce. Pour over the sliced banana.*

### *Lunch:* Banana Milk

2 lbs. bananas

***Directions:*** *Blend bananas with enough water to make a "milky" consistency.*

### *Dinner*

### *Course One:* Strawberry Pineapple Drink

8 oz. strawberries, 8 oz. pineapple

***Directions:*** *Prep both ingredients and blend.*

### *Course Two:* Strawberry Yellow Pepper Soup

1 lb. strawberries, 8 oz. yellow bell peppers, 8 oz. romaine lettuce

***Directions:*** *Chop all ingredients into a blender, except for 1 strawberry, and blend. Pour into a bowl and garnish with the reserved strawberry, thinly sliced.*

### *Course Three:* Strawberry Red Pepper Salad

1 lb. romaine lettuce, 4 oz. red bell peppers, 8 oz. strawberries

***Directions:*** *Finely chop the lettuce into a bowl. Blend the red peppers and strawberries into a dressing. Pour over the salad.*

| Spring Menu Plan: Day Two | | | |
|---|---|---|---|
| **Bananas with Carob Sauce** | **Carb** | **Protein** | **Fat** |
| Grams | 150 | 7 | 2 |
| Calories | 509 | 23 | 13 |
| % total calories | 93 | 4 | 3 |
| **Total calories for this course** | | **545** | |
| **Banana Milk** | **Carb** | **Protein** | **Fat** |
| Grams | 207 | 10 | 3 |
| Calories | 747 | 36 | 24 |
| % total calories | 93 | 4 | 3 |
| **Total calories for this course** | | **807** | |
| **Pineapple Strawberry Drink** | **Carb** | **Protein** | **Fat** |
| Grams | 44 | 3 | 1 |
| Calories | 157 | 10 | 8 |
| % total calories | 89 | 6 | 5 |
| **Total calories for this course** | | **175** | |
| **Strawberry Yellow Pepper Soup** | **Carb** | **Protein** | **Fat** |
| Grams | 57 | 8 | 3 |
| Calories | 197 | 28 | 20 |
| % total calories | 81 | 11 | 8 |
| **Total calories for this course** | | **245** | |
| **Strawberry Red Pepper Salad** | **Carb** | **Protein** | **Fat** |
| Grams | 39 | 8 | 2 |
| Calories | 133 | 28 | 18 |
| % total calories | 74 | 16 | 10 |
| **Total calories for this course** | | **179** | |
| **Daily Totals** | **Carb** | **Protein** | **Fat** |
| Grams | 497 | 36 | 11 |
| Calories | 1743 | 125 | 83 |
| **Caloronutrient ratio for the day** | **89** | **6** | **4** |
| **Total calories for today** | | **1951** | |

## Spring Menu Plan: Day Three

### *Breakfast:* Citrus Celebration!

8 oz. pineapple, 8 oz. kiwi, 8 oz. strawberries, 8 oz. red grapefruit, 8 oz. oranges

***Directions:*** *Prep all ingredients, chop, and mix together into a bowl.*

### *Lunch:* Ataulfo Mangos

2 lbs. ataulfo mangos

† This Mexican variety of mango begins its season in late April. Also known as honey, champagne, Manila, Asian, or yellow mango, it is a smaller-than-average mango, with a pale yellow color and a virtually fiberless flesh and sweet flavor, which makes it a leader of the imported varieties. While imported mangos are subject to hot-water treatment (unless you live in areas where they are grown locally, such as South Florida and Southern California), they are sometimes the only varieties available. It is always a good idea to visit areas where tropical fruits are grown.

### *Dinner*

### *Course One:* Kiwi Strawberry

1 lb. kiwi, 1 lb. strawberries

***Directions:*** *Slice, dice, and enjoy.*

### *Course Two:* Strawberry Cucumber Soup

1 lb. strawberries, 8 oz. cucumbers

***Directions:*** *Peel and slice the cucumber and blend the strawberries, leaving a little of each for garnish. Blend, pour into a bowl, and decorate.*

### *Course Three:* Strawberry Almond Salad

1 lb. red-leaf lettuce, 4 oz. cucumbers, 4 oz. strawberries, 1 oz. almonds

***Directions:*** *Chop the lettuce into a large bowl. Peel and slice the cucumber and mix with the lettuce. Blend the strawberries and almonds for a dressing.*

| Spring Menu Plan: Day Three | | | |
|---|---|---|---|
| **Citrus Celebration** | **Carb** | **Protein** | **Fat** |
| Grams | 130 | 9 | 3 |
| Calories | 467 | 33 | 22 |
| % total calories | 90 | 6 | 4 |
| **Total calories for this course** | | **522** | |
| **Ataulfo Mangos** | **Carb** | **Protein** | **Fat** |
| Grams | 154 | 5 | 2 |
| Calories | 553 | 17 | 20 |
| % total calories | 94 | 3 | 3 |
| **Total calories for this course** | | **590** | |
| **Kiwi Strawberry** | **Carb** | **Protein** | **Fat** |
| Grams | 101 | 8 | 4 |
| Calories | 363 | 29 | 30 |
| % total calories | 86 | 7 | 7 |
| **Total calories for this course** | | **422** | |
| **Strawberry Cucumber Soup** | **Carb** | **Protein** | **Fat** |
| Grams | 40 | 4 | 2 |
| Calories | 142 | 16 | 14 |
| % total calories | 83 | 9 | 8 |
| **Total calories for this course** | | **172** | |
| **Strawberry Almond Salad** | **Carb** | **Protein** | **Fat** |
| Grams | 27 | 13 | 16 |
| Calories | 101 | 51 | 134 |
| % total calories | 35 | 18 | 47 |
| **Total calories for this course** | | **286** | |
| **Daily Totals** | **Carb** | **Protein** | **Fat** |
| Grams | 452 | 39 | 27 |
| Calories | 1626 | 146 | 220 |
| **Caloronutrient ratio for the day** | **8** | **7** | **11** |
| **Total calories for today** | | **1992** | |

## Spring Menu Plan: Day Four

### *Breakfast :* Orange Juice

4 cups fresh-squeezed orange juice

### *Lunch :* Banana and Ataulfo Smoothie

1 lb. bananas, 1 lb. ataulfo mangos

**Directions:** *Blend and devour!*

### *Dinner:*

### *Course One:* Papaya Strawberry Boats

1 lb. papaya, 1 lb. strawberries

**Directions:** *Deseed the papaya, and fill with sliced strawberries. Arm yourself with a spoon and enjoy!*

### *Course Two: Celery Orange Soup*

8 oz. celery, 8 oz. red bell peppers, 8 oz. Valencia oranges

**Directions:** *Blend the celery, orange, and ¾ of the red pepper. Pour into a bowl and decorate with the remaining red pepper, finely chopped.*

### *Course Three: Orange Red Pepper Salad*

1 lb. red-leaf lettuce, 4 oz. oranges, 2 oz. red bell peppers, 1 oz. Brazil nuts

**Directions:** *Tear the lettuce into a bowl. Use the pulse setting on your blender to turn the oranges, bell pepper, and Brazil nuts into a chunky dressing.*

| Spring Menu Plan: Day Four | | | |
|---|---|---|---|
| **Orange Juice** | **Carb** | **Protein** | **Fat** |
| Grams | 94 | 6 | 2 |
| Calories | 367 | 25 | 16 |
| % total calories | 90 | 6 | 4 |
| **Total calories for this course** | | **408** | |
| **Banana and Ataulfo Smoothies** | **Carb** | **Protein** | **Fat** |
| Grams | 181 | 7 | 3 |
| Calories | 651 | 26 | 22 |
| % total calories | 93 | 4 | 3 |
| **Total calories for this course** | | **699** | |
| **Papaya Strawberry Boats** | **Carb** | **Protein** | **Fat** |
| Grams | 79 | 6 | 2 |
| Calories | 285 | 21 | 16 |
| % total calories | 88 | 7 | 5 |
| **Total calories for this course** | | **322** | |
| **Celery Orange Soup** | **Carb** | **Protein** | **Fat** |
| Grams | 47 | 6 | 2 |
| Calories | 166 | 22 | 14 |
| % total calories | 82 | 11 | 7 |
| **Total calories for this course** | | **202** | |
| **Orange Red Pepper Salad** | **Carb** | **Protein** | **Fat** |
| Grams | 31 | 12 | 20 |
| Calories | 114 | 44 | 171 |
| % total calories | 35 | 13 | 52 |
| **Total calories for this course** | | **329** | |
| **Daily Totals** | **Carb** | **Protein** | **Fat** |
| Grams | 432 | 37 | 29 |
| Calories | 1538 | 138 | 239 |
| **Caloronutrient ratio for the day** | **81** | **7** | **12** |
| **Total calories for today** | | **1961** | |

## Spring Menu Plan: Day Five

### *Breakfast:* Sweet-Tart Delight

16 oz. fresh-squeezed orange juice, 8 oz. ataulfo mangos, 8 oz. strawberries

***Directions:*** *Blend everything and try not to drink it too fast... it's that good!*

### *Lunch:* Just Bananas!

2 lbs. bananas

### *Dinner*

### *Course One:* Fresh-Squeezed Orange Juice

16 oz. fresh-squeezed orange juice

### *Course Two:* Spinach Red Pepper Soup

8 oz. spinach, 8 oz. red bell peppers, 8 oz. oranges

***Directions:*** *Blend all of the ingredients and pour into a bowl.*

### *Course Three:* Orange Pistachio Salad

8 oz. baby spinach, 8 oz. red-leaf lettuce, 4 oz. oranges, 1 oz. pistachios

***Directions:*** *Chop the spinach and lettuce into a bowl. Blend the oranges and pistachio, and dress your salad!*

| Spring Menu Plan: Day Five | | | |
|---|---|---|---|
| **Sweet-Tart Delight** | **Carb** | **Protein** | **Fat** |
| Grams | 124 | 5 | 2 |
| Calories | 461 | 20 | 18 |
| % total calories | 92 | 4 | 4 |
| **Total calories for this course** | | **499** | |
| **Just Bananas!** | **Carb** | **Protein** | **Fat** |
| Grams | 207 | 10 | 3 |
| Calories | 747 | 36 | 24 |
| % total calories | 93 | 4 | 3 |
| **Total calories for this course** | | **807** | |
| **Fresh-Squeezed Orange Juice** | **Carb** | **Protein** | **Fat** |
| Grams | 47 | 3 | 1 |
| Calories | 184 | 12 | 8 |
| % total calories | 90 | 6 | 4 |
| **Total calories for this course** | | **204** | |
| **Spinach Red Pepper Soup** | **Carb** | **Protein** | **Fat** |
| Grams | 49 | 11 | 2 |
| Calories | 167 | 37 | 14 |
| % total calories | 77 | 17 | 6 |
| **Total calories for this course** | | **218** | |
| **Orange Pistachio Salad** | **Carb** | **Protein** | **Fat** |
| Grams | 35 | 16 | 14 |
| Calories | 126 | 59 | 115 |
| % total calories | 42 | 20 | 38 |
| **Total calories for this course** | | **300** | |
| **Daily Totals** | **Carb** | **Protein** | **Fat** |
| Grams | 462 | 45 | 22 |
| Calories | 1685 | 164 | 179 |
| **Caloronutrient ratio for the day** | **83** | **8** | **9** |
| **Total calories for today** | | **2028** | |

## Spring Menu Plan: Day Six

### *Breakfast:* Spring Fruit Salad

1 lb. sweet oranges, 1 lb. strawberries, 8 oz. kiwi

***Directions:*** *Cut all the fruits into chunky bite-size pieces, toss, and savor the flavor!*

### *Lunch:* : Ataulfo Strawberry Salad

2 lbs. ataulfo mangos, 1 lb. strawberries

***Directions:*** *Dice the mangos and slice the strawberries into a bowl.*

### *Dinner:*

### *Course One:* Papaya

1.5 lbs. papaya

### *Course Two: Papaya Gazpacho*

1 lb. papaya, 8 oz. tomatoes, 2 oz. fresh basil

***Directions:*** *Deseed the papaya, peel, and cut it into small chunks, or blend it, if you prefer. Dice the tomato and finely chop the basil. Add them both to the papaya mixture. Enjoy!*

### *Course Three: Papaya Salad Wraps*

1 lb. butter lettuce, 1 lb. papaya, juice of 1 lime

***Directions:*** *In a bowl, cut the papaya into small chunks. Mix it with the lime juice until it all melds together. Use the lettuce leaves as wrappers, and use your papaya-lime blend as a filling.*

| Spring Menu Plan: Day Six | | | |
|---|---|---|---|
| **Spring Fruit Salad** | **Carb** | **Protein** | **Fat** |
| Grams | 121 | 10 | 3 |
| Calories | 436 | 36 | 25 |
| % total calories | 88 | 7 | 5 |
| **Total calories for this course** | | **497** | |
| **Ataulfo Strawberry Salad** | **Carb** | **Protein** | **Fat** |
| Grams | 189 | 8 | 4 |
| Calories | 677 | 27 | 31 |
| % total calories | 92 | 4 | 4 |
| **Total calories for this course** | | **735** | |
| **Papaya** | **Carb** | **Protein** | **Fat** |
| Grams | 67 | 4 | 1 |
| Calories | 242 | 15 | 8 |
| % total calories | 91 | 6 | 3 |
| **Total calories for this course** | | **265** | |
| **Papaya Gazpacho** | **Carb** | **Protein** | **Fat** |
| Grams | 57 | 6 | 2 |
| Calories | 204 | 22 | 14 |
| % total calories | 85 | 9 | 6 |
| **Total calories for this course** | | **240** | |
| **Papaya Salad Wraps** | **Carb** | **Protein** | **Fat** |
| Grams | 57 | 9 | 2 |
| Calories | 199 | 31 | 13 |
| % total calories | 82 | 13 | 5 |
| **Total calories for this course** | | **243** | |
| **Daily Totals** | **Carb** | **Protein** | **Fat** |
| Grams | 491 | 37 | 12 |
| Calories | 1758 | 131 | 91 |
| **Caloronutrient ratio for the day** | **89** | **7** | **5** |
| **Total calories for today** | | **1980** | |

## Spring Menu Plan: Day Seven

### *Breakfast:* Strawberries

3 lbs. strawberries

† If you are looking to get a little extra greens, or to save time, you can eat the tops to the strawberries. They do change the texture a bit, but they also add a little green flavor. If you enjoy eating greens with your fruit, then this is a complete package.

### *Lunch:* Banana Romaine Smoothie

2 lbs. bananas, 8 oz. romaine lettuce

***Directions:*** *Blend into a smoothie.*

### *Dinner:*

### *Course One:* Orange Kiwi

1 lb. oranges
8 oz. kiwi

***Directions:*** *Peel the oranges, then cut them into chunks and place in a bowl. Peel the kiwi and cut into slices. Stir into the oranges.*

### *Course Two:* Cauliflower Tomato Soup

8 oz. cauliflower florets, 1 lb. tomatoes

***Directions:*** *Blend cauliflower with ¾ of the tomatoes. Dice the remaining tomato and stir it into the soup or place on top for garnish.*

### *Course Three:* Orange Tahini Salad

8 oz. romaine lettuce, 8 oz. baby spinach, 4 oz. oranges, 1 tbsp. raw mechanically hulled tahini

***Directions:*** *Tear greens into a bowl. Blend orange segments with tahini, and dress.*

| Spring Menu Plan: Day Seven | | | |
|---|---|---|---|
| **Strawberries** | **Carb** | **Protein** | **Fat** |
| Grams | 105 | 9 | 4 |
| Calories | 370 | 32 | 33 |
| % total calories | 85 | 7 | 8 |
| **Total calories for this course** | **435** | | |
| **Banana Romaine Smoothie** | **Carb** | **Protein** | **Fat** |
| Grams | 215 | 13 | 4 |
| Calories | 770 | 46 | 30 |
| % total calories | 91 | 5 | 4 |
| **Total calories for this course** | **846** | | |
| **Orange Kiwi** | Carb | Protein | Fat |
| Grams | 60 | 5 | 1 |
| Calories | 216 | 17 | 12 |
| % total calories | 88 | 7 | 5 |
| **Total calories for this course** | **245** | | |
| **Cauliflower Tomato Soup** | **Carb** | **Protein** | **Fat** |
| Grams | 33 | 8 | 2 |
| Calories | 111 | 28 | 13 |
| % total calories | 73 | 18 | 9 |
| **Total calories for this course** | **152** | | |
| **Orange Tahini Salad** | **Carb** | **Protein** | **Fat** |
| Grams | 36 | 15 | 15 |
| Calories | 129 | 55 | 122 |
| % total calories | 42 | 18 | 40 |
| **Total calories for this course** | **306** | | |
| **Daily Totals** | **Carb** | **Protein** | **Fat** |
| Grams | 449 | 50 | 26 |
| Calories | 1596 | 178 | 210 |
| **Calonutrient ratio for the day** | **80** | **9** | **11** |
| **Total calories for today** | **1984** | | |
| **Weekly totals** | **Carb** | **Protein** | **Fat** |
| **Calonutrient ratio for the week** | **84** | **7** | **9** |

# Appendix B. Frequently Asked Questions

## *Table of Contents*

## What are raw foods?

There are different definitions of raw foods, depending upon whom you ask. For our purposes, we will define raw foods as those foods that are whole and fresh and have not been subjected to cooking of any type. Raw foods are Nature's finished products; they are ready to be consumed, as is. Like the raw materials that construction workers use to build a house, raw foods become the building materials that our bodies use to maintain and reconstruct themselves.

"Raw" is a relative term. Some people would argue that dehydrated or powdered foods are still raw, even though they are not whole. (Water is a profoundly important essential nutrient; once water has been removed from a food, it should no longer be considered "whole.")

There is no need to argue, and there is room for the occasional exception. What you do most of the time will have a big impact in your life. What you do rarely should be considered exceptions. The impact of exceptions does not accrue like the impact of that which you do with regularity. Nonetheless, whole, fresh, raw plant foods with all of their original components intact, including water and fiber, are by far the most healthful.

## What is a raw food diet?

A raw food diet is one that is predominated by foods that have not been cooked. People who adopt this diet are often referred to as "raw fooders" or "raw foodists." Those who eat only raw plants are called "raw food vegans" or "raw vegans."

The healthy raw food diet that I recommend in this book is made up of whole, fresh, ripe, raw, organic plant foods. It is predominated by fruits and allows for all the greens that you care to eat, plus small quantities of nuts, seeds, and fatty fruits.

## What about an all-fruit diet?

I do not recommend an all-fruit diet. In my experience, we must eat vegetables, especially dark leafy greens, in order to experience optimum nutrition and ideal health. I recommend that 2 to 6% of our total calories consumed, on average, come from greens. In terms of volume, this would mean somewhere between 1 and 4 heads of lettuce, or ¼ to 1 pound of kale, or ½ to 2 pounds of spinach, per day (depending on how many calories you normally consume).

## Are all raw food diets the same?

No, there are many approaches to eating a raw diet. Although for some it includes raw meat and other animal products, I do not recommend the consumption of animal-derived foods of any kind (including honey and milk), for reasons of health, ecology, and compassion.

Most raw food diets obtain a high percentage of daily calories from fats, by including oils and significant amounts of avocado, nuts and seeds, and sometimes coconut meat and olives. These diets tend to be unsustainable, since too much fat, even raw fat, causes health problems and results in the underconsumption of carbohydrates. In a vain effort to compensate for the nutritional insufficiencies of these diets, people often resort to the use of supplements and stimulants.

We cannot succeed eating primarily vegetables (even when we include substantial quantities of green drinks), because even impossibly huge amounts do not contain nearly enough calories to fuel us. A sustainable raw food diet, therefore, draws the great bulk of its daily calories from fruits, which are relatively high in calories, along with liberal amounts of vegetables for their high mineral content, plus a (very) small amount of nuts and seeds.

## What about individual differences?

A huge amount of misinformation is being taught in holistic health circles about metabolic typing. "Experts" tell us that people are born as either "fast" or "slow" metabolizers (sometimes called "fast or slow oxidizers"), and that the rate of your metabolism determines the foods that are best suited for you to eat.

Fast metabolizers, so they say, burn through fuel more rapidly than slow metabolizers, making them relatively more efficient at digesting their food.

Actually, the opposite is true. Using an automobile analogy, it's easy to understand that the car that gets more miles to the gallon is more efficient than the car that gets fewer miles to the gallon. Similarly, the person who uses the least fuel to accomplish any particular task, i.e., the slow metabolizer, is the most efficient.

As the "wisdom" of this line of thinking goes, if you are a fast-metabolizing raw fooders, you must consume an exceptionally high percentage of your total calories (60–80%) as fat in the form of nuts, seeds, oils, avocados, olives, and the like. Fruits, it is said, are insufficient for fast metabolizers in terms of fuel density, leaving them constantly hungry, causing them to fall off the raw "wagon," and to suffer from the maladies (mistakenly) associated with the overconsumption of fruit sugars. By eating more fat, it is implied that nutrition will be enhanced.

Only the very slowest metabolizers, they teach, could even hope to have a chance of health when utilizing fruit for fuel. Even so, slow metabolizers are advised to keep fruit to a minimum because it is too high in high-glycemic simple carbohydrates. A few pieces of fruit per week at the very most, are recommended for slow metabolizers. Perhaps, they say, serious athletes who also happen to be very slow metabolizers can eat a bit more fruit. But in general, they argue that fruit consumption should simply be avoided. They claim that it is too easy (and too dangerous) to overeat fruit.

Apparently, according to many teachers, it is a rare individual indeed, who is a slow metabolizer.

### Metabolism

One reason that this theory fails is that many of those who teach it do not know the definition of the word "metabolism." Here are some terms that should be useful in this discussion.

**Fasting BMR:** The "fasting" basal metabolic rate is a measure of the amount of fuel a person utilizes, per unit of time, when awake and totally at rest. It does not include such functions as physical activity, daily household chores, or even digestion. This means no food has been consumed for at least 72 hours and the body requires no digestive energy. Fasting BMR accounts for the use of around 1,000 calories per day for most people, though this number does tend to be slightly affected by body size.

**BMR:** The basal metabolic rate number you are more likely to encounter estimates the calories consumed for people who are awake and resting, but not fasting or abstaining from consuming food. Most people can roughly estimate this number by multiplying their body weight by ten.

**Metabolism:** We use the word "metabolism" to mean BMR plus all the activities of the day. Metabolism is not, in and of itself, a single function, but rather the sum of all of the catabolic and anabolic processes that go on within your body. Anabolic processes are the building activities, those that combine simpler structures to form more complex ones. They include growth, repair, and all of the recombinant chemistry that goes on at the cellular and visceral level. Catabolic processes are those that break complex structures down into simpler ones. Digestion, osteoclastic activity (cells that break down bones), the conversion of glycogen to glucose, and aging are examples of catabolism in action.

When we refer to someone as having a "fast metabolism," we mean that they require more fuel to perform the same number of anabolic and catabolic processes as a person with a slow metabolism. This means that the fast metabolizers are less efficient in their use of fuel.

Either way, however, according to most sports physiology texts, the difference between fast and slow metabolic rates is very small indeed. Most texts agree that the BMR rarely varies much more than about plus or minus 5% from person to person of similar body size and design. Body surface area, scientists have proven, is the biggest factor affecting BMR.[85]

### Activity—not metabolism—governs fuel usage

What truly does affect fuel use is the amount of physical exertion one performs. A sedentary person may use only 200 calories per day in performing their daily functions, whereas someone going for a vigorous four-hour hike could use 2,000 calories. Professional athletes often use 4,000 calories solely for their daily training, and Tour de France riders are known to use 10,000 to 14,000 calories, or more, on the most intense days of this grueling competition. Hence it is easy to see that the differences in BMR, or metabolism, as it is commonly but mistakenly referred to, play an exceptionally small role in total calorie usage.

At most, BMR variations represent less than 100 calories out of the 2,000 to 4,000 that most people eat per day. Textbooks suggest that BMR differences typically account for only one to two per cent of total calories consumed. This is approximately the caloric equivalent of one bite of an apple. This certainly is not enough to make a noticeable difference in fuel consumption or preferred fuel sources between even the fastest and the slowest of metabolizers.

The truly fast metabolizer uses more calories per hour throughout the day, than the average person does. The more calories one utilizes in the course of a day, the faster that person's total metabolism would be.

## An Example

For example, we can reasonably estimate that a moderately active, 110-pound, 5'4" woman might eat about 2,000 calories per day and a lightly active man who is 5'10" tall and 150 pounds uses about 2,400 calories. In this example, the man uses an average of 100 calories per hour.

For the sake of simplicity, we shall call 100 calories per hour (plus or minus 10%) the midrange of metabolic rate. We could therefore assert that a person who uses, on average, more than 110 calories per hour would be termed a fast metabolizer and a person who uses less than 90 calories per hour would be a slow metabolizer. We could assign people progressively faster and slower metabolic designations the more their calorie usage differed from the midrange.

At this point we have come to an unbridgeable contradiction. We are told that fast metabolizers—those people who utilize the most fuel per hour, are supposedly the very people who will thrive on the highest fat levels in their diet. Meanwhile, we are also being told that only slow-metabolizing athletes should attempt to utilize a diet higher in carbohydrates from fruit. Yet we know that athletes are the very people who have the fastest metabolisms, despite any variations in their BMR.

To make matters more confusing, scientific research consistently proves that the more fat you consume, the more your health will suffer. Somewhere, someone must be wrong in these assertions. It is not possible to straddle both sides of this fence. Either a fat-based diet is most healthful or a fruit-based diet is, but it cannot be both; and it cannot be one for some people and the other for other people.

Small cows eat small amounts of food relative to large cows. Active cows eat more food than their sedentary counterparts, yet all cows eat essentially the same food. Fruits and vegetables have been touted as the ultimate health foods for humans for over a century, and they have been the primary food of humankind throughout our existence, up until the recent past.

Whether you are small or large, active or sedentary, fruits and vegetables remain the optimum foods of choice for fulfilling all human nutritional needs. If one person needs to consume a greater number of calories than another person, it simply means that they must eat a greater quantity of food, not completely different foods.

In case the above is not enough of a contradiction to try to puzzle out, work on this one: It has been repeatedly asserted that most people would experience the greatest levels of health using a diet that is composed primarily of fats. This assertion is based on the assumption that most people are fast metabolizers, a premise that cannot be true. Whenever we work with large numbers, the law of averages comes into play. Using the law of averages, a "normal" or "bell" curve is always formed. In the bell curve, only about 5 to 10% of the people would truly be classed as fast metabolizers, 5 to 10% would be slow metabolizers, and the rest, roughly 80%, would fall somewhere in the middle. These would be average metabolizers, not slow and not fast.

Do not be misled by metabolism (or oxidation) mumbo jumbo. Track your fat intake on any given day and see for yourself just exactly what percentage of your calories it comprises. Once you do, you will understand why so many raw fooders are having problems. High fat is also the reason that most scientific studies of raw fooders draw negative conclusions. Is it any wonder that people have trouble staying healthy on their high-fat raw regimens, or that they find cooked carbohydrates so alluring?

Those who convince unsuspecting new raw fooders to steer clear of fruit and gorge on fat do succeed in accomplishing one goal; the creation of nutritional inadequacies. This opens the door for selling us nutritional supplements in a vain attempt to compensate for the very deficiencies that result from consuming a high-fat raw diet. Of course, most newcomers want to learn and are prone to following the advice they are given.

## Can I thrive on only raw foods?

No essential nutrient exists in meat, grains, legumes, or dairy that is not also available in fruits, vegetables, nuts and seeds—and in a form that is easier to digest. Indeed, many vital nutrients, such as soluble fibers and the thousands of phytonutrients, can only be garnered from plants. Fruits, vegetables, and leafy greens not only contain sustainable amounts of carbohydrates, protein, and fat, they also contain them in the percentages, ratios, and forms that are optimum for human health.

People thrive on the raw diet, often telling others how it has improved their health and their lives. When people integrate a proper raw diet with other healthful living practices, they rarely, if ever, develop weight-control problems or chronic (or even short-term) illnesses. Health becomes a fact of life.

For millions of years, most humans, and their ancestors, lived a gatherer lifestyle in a tropical environment where large amounts of easy-to-pick fruit were readily available to meet their nutritional needs. The human diet was likely entirely plant based and eaten without the application of fire or heat.

Accordingly, the human digestive and eliminative tracts developed to process raw fruits and vegetables for fuel and growth. We are biologically designed to obtain our nutrition from uncooked fruits and vegetables.

Only within the last 10,000 years has cereal agriculture allowed humans to trade their frugivorous diets for cooked grain-based fare.[86] People's bodies remained the same, but the food they chose to eat began to vary for the worse. The human body has not had sufficient time, evolutionarily speaking, to alter its digestive system to meet this fundamental dietary change. The likelihood of doing so is slim at best, as heated foods are of lower nutritional quality, and cooking introduces toxic elements. Hence, the adaptation would be a downward one, and would be technically considered a devolution.

## Will eating raw make me healthy?

A proper raw diet will result in improved health, but I must emphasize that the body, not food, creates health. Food does not build; the body builds. Food does not cleanse; the body cleanses. Good health, after all, is the result of a healthy lifestyle.

The raw diet is but one component of healthful living. Adequate rest and sleep, regular, vigorous physical activity, plenty of fresh air, sunlight, a positive outlook on life, and many other factors are also essential to creating good health.

## Why didn't the 80/10/10 diet work for me?

People come to me at times having tried this method of eating unsuccessfully. Upon examination, I have found almost invariably that they were not actually doing what I recommend. As I truly desire to see people succeed, I want to mention here several key factors that people often overlook when adopting the 80/10/10 lifestyle.

*You are not following 80/10/10 if:*

- Less than 2% of your total calories come from vegetables and leafy greens. For true health, I recommend consuming 2 to 6% of calories from leafy greens. For 4% of your calories to come from vegetables on a 2000-calorie diet, you would have to eat roughly a pound of greens per day.
- Your caloric intake is insufficient to maintain your desired body weight.
- You burn less than 40% of your total calories through physical activity (at least 800 calories per day if you average 2,000 calories).

- Your habitual sleep pattern doesn't meet your body's needs.
- You eat all day long rather than one to four meals a day.
- You lack emotional poise (your lifestyle is sufficiently stressful to cause your system ongoing adrenal exertion).
- You expose your fully (or substantially) unclothed skin to moderate sunlight less than 30 minutes per day. (Our bodies require approximately 15 minutes of sunlight exposure per day to produce sufficient vitamin D. I would consider 30 minutes a day a healthful minimum… remember, our species wasn't designed to live indoors.)

## Why do people "fail" on the raw diet?

The most common reason for lack of success with the raw diet is the overall poor health of the new raw fooders who unknowingly obtains most of his or her daily calories from raw fat sources. This occurs even as they eat what they consider a tremendous amount of vegetables, because vegetables contain so few calories.

The components of fatty foods are not a match for human nutritional needs. Eating a high-fat diet paves the way to a wide variety of health issues that have their basis in nutritional insufficiency.

Eating sweet-fruit carbohydrates in insufficient volume to produce a feeling of satiation results predictably in carbohydrate cravings and disordered eating behaviors. Almost every raw fooders who goes back to eating cooked foods find himself eating cooked carbohydrates—bread, rice, pasta, potatoes, corn, lentils, and beans—time and again, until they figure out that they simply are not eating anywhere near enough fruit. If they don't go back to cooked starches (and the fats that make them taste good), they are generally driven to eating concentrated and refined carbohydrates such as candy, chocolate, alcohol, pastries, cookies, or dried fruits. This same scenario—caused by underconsuming the whole-food simple sugars in fruit—is equally true for people on the cooked standard American diet who find themselves suffering from cravings and disordered eating.

The other significant reason that people fail on the raw diet is emotional. Here, I discuss two common variants on the "emotional eating" theme. The first involves using food to suppress our ability to feel. The second involves using food to evoke certain feelings.

Let's take the "numbing out" scenario first. Cooked food does not really comfort us, as we are led to believe, but it certainly does numb us from feeling. Rather than making us feel good, it inhibits our ability to fully feel anything at all.

Unconsciously, we have learned to push down our emotions with heavy foods that require too much nerve energy to allow for both digestion and intense emoting to occur simultaneously. We are not just imagining things: this process of "numbing out" is very real, in a physiological sense. With the exception of strenuous physical activity, the two most energy-expensive tasks our bodies commonly undertake are breaking down foods in combinations that have a high digestive demand and processing intense emotions. In general, we must do one or the other.

We have all had the experience of completely losing our appetite because of an intense emotional upset. This occurs when the emotional component edges out the digestive task. Conversely, when digestion takes priority (which occurs almost every time we eat heavily), we experience an emotional numbing, a lack of feeling. In a world full of emotional pain and physical discomfort, numbness can easily be misinterpreted as comfort.

This might occur when a person gets into an argument and then drowns himself in a pint of ice cream because he is so filled with anger and frustration. A raw fooders in the same scenario may turn instead to nuts and dried fruits, but in both cases what really needs to happen is to bring out and accept these emotions.

As one lightens the digestive load by switching to raw foods, the body suddenly has more nerve energy to conduct emotions, and emotions suppressed over the years begin to emerge. This unexpected challenge proves overwhelming for many people. Until people learn to properly deal with their emotional baggage, it is likely that eating raw foods will allow uncomfortable emotions to surface. They will find themselves going back to eating cooked foods for the emotional "comfort" that they bring.

Emotional acceptance means that without distraction from television, books, friends, music, food, etc. we sit quietly and actually feel the emotion with full intensity where it lies within our body. When instead we try to hide or distract ourselves from painful thoughts and feelings, we only suppress them more deeply, to be felt (generally with greater intensity) at a later date. It is important to realize that without the "negative" emotions, we could experience no "positive" emotions, as they are two sides of the same coin.

They are a part of us like all other parts, and by rejecting them we only turn away from an aspect of ourselves that is demanding our undivided attention.

The second type of emotional eating involves felt attachments to specific cooked foods. Such attachments often originate from an attempt to recreate a past event or moment in our lives that we remember as positive and yearn to experience again. People often find these emotions very difficult to overcome.

In the same way that drug addicts never successfully duplicate the unique "high" of their first drug experience, no matter how many times they try, eating cooked food never quite generates that specific emotional experience we are looking for. Instead, we get disappointed, and then we eat more cooked food to numb our awareness of the disappointment.

It takes a lot of insight to understand that although those emotions are important and the experiences were valuable, eating cooked food will not bring them back. We must let them go and generate new positive experiences in the present moment.

People who are emotionally attached to cooked foods aren't actually addicted to them, since it is physiologically impossible to be addicted to something that is harmful to us. The body simply is not put together that way. It is designed to thrive and cannot become addicted to a harmful substance. The human psyche, however, can become very much addicted to the shift in perception that occurs after we ingest certain substances. A yearning for that shift in perception is the ever-present illusion that lures us to eat cooked foods.

If you eat cooked foods, you stand the risk of becoming an emotional vegetable—someone who becomes evermore dependent upon their cooked food "fix."

### Another One Bites the Dust ...

*The following is an excerpt (slightly edited for space) from an actual post to my online discussion group on VegSource.com. It exemplifies the stories I hear every time I meet someone who tries try to go raw without eating fruit.*

*Predictably, such people experience constant hunger, disordered eating, digestive problems from overeating nuts, intense sweet cravings, a sense of needing to "fill the void" with poorly combined dehydrated sweets, massive overdosing on fats, guilt, low energy, and general dissatisfaction with food—and often bingeing and purging, as well.*

*See if you recognize yourself or someone you know as you read this candid account of a high-fat raw fooders who is desperate to find a program that works. Especially take note of the second paragraph, where the author describes her conception of "a healthy, simple way of eating." The diet she outlines probably totals about 1,600 calories, and a minimum of 40% fat … and her program devolves from there.*

There is much I love about being raw. It makes a lot of sense to me and for the most part I feel much better than I ever did eating cooked foods. What I do not love about the raw food lifestyle is the effect nuts and dehydrated foods have on my system. It is very hard for me to find the right balance. When I do feel like I have found "the right way to eat" for me, an old inner demon creeps in and pushes me off my center, which throws me into a tailspin.

When I began this second stint with 100% raw, it was very easy for me to go back to a healthy, simple way of eating. My diet consisted of apple lemon ginger juice in the morning with powdered green formula, [with four large apples this might be 450 calories—DG] lunch was usually a green salad with avocado and some kind of cultured vegetables, and dinner was some version of the same or maybe a prepared raw meal from the market. [Two large salads combined would likely contain not more than 1,000 calories: 600 from two avocados and up to 400 from vegetables—DG]

I experimented with flaxseed and other dehydrated crackers to find they congested me (I would eat too many and get bloated and constipated.) I started running more in April, and for a while I seemed to find my groove with the food and exercise. I noticed that I started to crave sweets, so I started adding more fruit to my diet like oranges and nectarines. But I am afraid the sugar in the fruit had a negative affect on my body because now I can't get off of the raw sweet snacks. If I have a bag of dates I can easily go through a pound of them, so I stay clear of those as best I can.

I also have a hard time controlling the quantity of nuts I consume. I tried my darnedest to not buy raw dehydrated nuts, nut treats, and raw desserts. But the problem is that now that I allowed myself the sweet fruits and raw desserts I tend to want more. I feel a bit ashamed to admit this, but I pretty much finished off an entire jar of cashew nut butter in one sitting. My willpower feels so small right now. It is amazing how different my personality and attitude can be. It feels like old cooked food demons are creeping in. There is no way for me to keep fun foods in my home for fear that I will consume them all. I know the simpler the diet the better, but often the will is weak and my body suffers.

About a month ago, my attitude went from enthusiastic and cheery to irritable. I felt very fatigued and hot tempered, and my diet started going from clean to not so clean. My running decreased and wasn't as consistent as it had been, and my sleeping habits started getting bad; I can't wake up early anymore. My attitude has not been very positive, and I feel depressed most of the time.

Concerned, I have started adding B12 supplements and hemp seed oil. I can't seem to get back to a clean way of eating. I almost feel like I need to get some sort of blood test to see if I am deficient in any areas or to measure my level of candida. I do not want food to be the deciding factor for how I feel. I really want food to be unimportant. I want to remain raw ... but eating to live, not living to eat. I know that raw can work for me as long as I am able to either stay away from those foods that are difficult to digest or simply consume them in smaller quantities.

## Isn't it hard to go raw?

Learning how to eat a raw food diet properly takes time, patience, and yes, effort. Although I provide a blueprint for doing it healthfully, most people find it challenging to adopt the raw diet 100% the first time out, unless they get professional guidance. It seldom occurs overnight, and in fact, can take years to accomplish.

Because our taste buds have been exposed to, and our brains have experienced the excitement of salt, sugar, and spices, we may miss those tastes initially when they are no longer part of the daily diet. However, most people find that the tradeoff for good health and longevity is more than worth living without a few of the harshest flavoring agents.

Once the taste buds are no longer exposed each day to these stimulants and excitotoxins, they once again develop an appreciation for the taste of fresh fruits and vegetables. You can become an extremely discerning person, with taste buds that can easily recognize the differences among various qualities of fruit.

Of course, it is far more pleasant to be healthy than it is to be sick, and far less expensive, too. Weighing all factors with a longer-term perspective, I would say it is easier to eat raw than eat cooked.

## What advice do you have for new raw fooders?

Those new to the raw food diet often fall victim to their own innocence, coupled with their inquisitive nature. Most people, when trying a new diet, want to find out as much about it as possible, and often as quickly as possible. The raw food diet, which is so radically different from the others, often leaves people bewildered about "what to do." Nutritional and other health concerns can overwhelm them, especially when social pressures about their diet from peers, family, and friends beset them.

Fortunately, there is a huge amount of information available about raw foods on websites, in books, and from counselors. But beware: most of the "leaders" who offer this information have little education, experience, or professional training in nutrition or health creation.

Newcomers do not have enough perspective to be able to discern the valid information from the dangerous or the sound science from the well-marketed infomercial. We can quickly end up with a situation where the blind are being led by the semi-sighted.

My advice is to be certain that you seek guidance from someone who has reached stability in his or her own food program. I recommend increasing the consumption of whole fruits and vegetables and minimizing any use of supplements, super foods, or condiments of all types. Eat simply at each meal, reducing the total number of ingredients while obtaining variety in your diet throughout the seasons.

## Do fruits and vegetables have enough nutrients?

The very best quality water, vitamins, minerals, antioxidants, phytonutrients, enzymes, coenzymes, fiber, protein, carbohydrates, and fats all come from organically grown fruits and vegetables grown in highly composted, living soils. They are complete nutritional packages and provide all the nutrients we need, in the proportions and ratios our bodies require for proper functioning. No man-made vitamin tablet or other supplement can compare with Nature's handiwork.

Of all foods, fruits are richest in vitamins and water, and second richest in minerals and fiber, while vegetables and leafy greens are richest in minerals and fiber, and second richest in vitamins and water. Vegetables supply minerals and fiber so far in excess of our needs that the quantity supplied in fruit actually comes closer to meeting our needs. (As I have stated elsewhere, consuming more than we need of any nutrient is not better, and in fact creates nutritional imbalances, despite marketing hype to the contrary).

Fruits, being far higher in calories than vegetables and thus capable of fueling us adequately, should comprise the majority of our diets. Some fruits, however, do actually fall short in terms of minerals, so it is important to include some vegetables in our diet to make up for the eventual lack that could develop on a fruit-only diet. Nonetheless, in every category, the nutrient content of fruit comes closer to matching human nutritional needs than that of any other food group.

We need small quantities of both proteins and fats. So, although fruits and vegetables are not high in protein and fat content, they still remain their ideal source.

## What about vitamin $B_{12}$?

Almost every health and nutrition professional in the world holds the notion that people must at least supplement their diets with a $B_{12}$ source if they don't eat meat. But the truth is, vitamin $B_{12}$ deficiency is not limited to vegetarians and vegans; it is common among meat eaters as well—not because they don't eat enough $B_{12}$, but because they don't properly produce and absorb it. Let me explain just a bit about how this all works.

As I see it, two primary vegan sources of natural vitamin $B_{12}$ exist for humans, either of which, under ideal conditions, should be sufficient to provide the $B_{12}$ to meet our needs:

- First, vitamin $B_{12}$ is a waste product of a bacteria that can be found in and on the foods we eat (of both animal and plant origin).
- Second, $B_{12}$ is also produced in the intestine and the mucosa of healthy humans.

An alleged but very unlikely third source of $B_{12}$ may be unheated algae, spirulina, chlorella, and other creatures (which are not plants, by the way, and thus not to be considered vegan), and also raw seaweeds like nori, wakame, dulse, kombu, etc. Although these substances apparently do contain some human-active $B_{12}$, they also contain significant amounts of noncobalamin analogs of $B_{12}$, which actually interfere with the absorption of true $B_{12}$. The analog form of $B_{12}$ registers on test results, masquerading as the human nutrient, but the body cannot use it. To compound the problem, analog $B_{12}$ also occupies the body's $B_{12}$ uptake sites or "receptors," thus lowering our ability to utilize true $B_{12}$.

From a health and biological-design perspective, the question of whether the $B_{12}$ in these foods is the kind we need or an analog (or some of both) becomes irrelevant. Regardless of the answer, I do not recommend the consumption of sea life under any circumstances. Humans are terrestrial creatures and as such our digestive capacities and nutritional requirements are adapted to the consumption of plants from the land. Aquatic plants and animals are not our natural foods, nor does their nutritional makeup match our needs.

If you disagree, take yourself to the oceanside one day and collect some of your own fresh algae or seaweed. I think you will find these "foods," as they appear unprocessed in nature, to be abhorrent in taste. Compare this reaction to the sensory thrill that you experience when you see, smell, and taste a perfectly ripe piece of fruit picked fresh from the tree. Your visceral response to these two scenarios should tell you unequivocally which of these items is food for humans.

That said, I return to the first two $B_{12}$ sources mentioned above. If it is true that plant and animal foods can contain $B_{12}$, and that we make it within our bodies as well, then how is it that we find vitamin $B_{12}$ deficiency in humans? This is an extremely complex matter, but I will discuss four reasons for this phenomenon in a very simplified manner.

### *1) Our produce no longer contains vitamin $B_{12}$.*

Since the beginning of time, humans have acquired some of their vitamin $B_{12}$ directly from fruits and vegetables … but they did not know they were doing so. You see, scientists did not discover vitamin $B_{12}$ until the 1950s, and by then our commercially produced plant foods had spent about a decade devoid of vitamin $B_{12}$, a nutrient that had existed plentifully in plant foods since time immemorial.

How did this come about? Well, plants do not make a lot of vitamins. Rather, they soak them up from the soil through their roots. Most of our vitamins are made by bacteria in the soil. Since the advent of modern agriculture in 1942, when Bayer and other chemical manufacturers began diverting leftover chemical weapons from World War II into use as pesticides and fertilizers,[87] farmers have inadvertently sterilized the bacteria out of our soils. The resulting loss of plant-derived dietary vitamin $B_{12}$ is just one of the unintended consequences of "better living through chemistry," an initiative that continues to devastate the balance of nature in ways we are only beginning to comprehend.

Given this historical perspective, it is easy to understand why nutritional researchers generally encounter no vitamin $B_{12}$ in plant foods since they take their samples from among produce grown in dead soils. However, organically grown plants specifically cultivated in highly composted soils rich with organic matter can contain plenty of $B_{12}$ and a host of other nutrients not found (or found in short supply) in industrially grown produce.

Organic matter, defined as anything that rots, is the root of organic farming and the engine that runs the entire web of life on Earth. Fungi and bacteria eat the organic matter, and then they "poop" … in the process contributing complex substances to the soil, including vitamin $B_{12}$ and other nutrients, in profusion. Plants grown in such soils take up these nutrients through their roots.

When we add chemicals to the soil, we destroy not only "pests" and the bacteria that produce vitamin $B_{12}$, but also the entire pyramid of soil life (which begins with organic material, then fungi and bacteria but also includes mites, then predatory mites, springtails, and worms). Most agricultural soil in the United States contains only 1 to 2% organic matter, a level that qualifies it as biologically dead. The practice of farming with chemicals and not returning any organic matter to the soil is now more than sixty years old. The far-reaching devastating side effects of this practice on all forms of life on Earth—and their delicately balanced ecosystems—are too numerous to adequately describe in anything less than a separate book.

Therefore, I recommend getting to know the organic farmers at your local farmer's markets and making sure that they use compost. (I prefer vegan fertilizers and compost that don't contain animal products or manure.) People find this difficult to hear, but I also believe that if you live where farmer's markets and organically grown tropical fruits are not available, you would do well to consider relocating. Of course, growing your own food would be best of all, and I highly recommend doing so, whenever possible.

### *2) We wash our produce.*

A hundred years ago, people tended to bathe once a week or less, on average, and they did not concern themselves with fastidiously washing the surfaces of their fruits and vegetables as they do these days. In part, this is another result of agrochemical food production, as people have been misled to believe that pesticide residues can be adequately washed off by rinsing or scrubbing the outsides of their produce.

In the past, when people ate lettuce, celery, carrots, and other vegetables fresh from the ground, the soil left clinging to the vegetables often contained vitamin $B_{12}$. They also obtained the nutrient from the bacteria-laden dirt that accumulates near the stems of apples, peaches, pears, and other core and stone fruits. But between the chemicals we apply to the soils and our obsessive fear of germs and bacteria, we effectively eliminate this source of the nutrient, as well.

### *3) We cannot absorb the $B_{12}$ we eat.*

Meat eaters easily consume enough $B_{12}$ because the bacteria that make it, live in the digestive tracts of livestock, and it is distributed in the muscle meats of the animals they eat. As described earlier, vegans who eat organically grown plants from richly composted soils, and who don't compulsively wash their produce, should also get plenty of the nutrient.

In both of these cases, vitamin $B_{12}$ deficiency is usually only a problem if you lack a chemical called the "intrinsic factor," which causes people to be unable to absorb $B_{12}$. How does this occur? It seems that intrinsic factor production is reduced as dietary fat increases. This is by far the most common cause of $B_{12}$ deficiency. Doctors can easily test whether a person has a normal ability to absorb $B_{12}$. For those who do not, no amount of the vitamin in the diet will help. Thus, all of us, vegetarians and meat eaters alike, are at risk of $B_{12}$ deficiency.

A high-fat diet increases this risk substantially, for two reasons. First, the colonies of $B_{12}$-producing bacteria in our intestines utilize carbohydrates for fuel. As the amount of fat in our diets goes up, the amount of carbohydrate goes down, thus reducing the quantity of fuel available to the microbe. Less fuel results in a smaller colony and an overall decrease in $B_{12}$ production. Second, the $B_{12}$ uptake sites in our intestines become clogged when there is excess fat in the diet, further reducing $B_{12}$ absorption. When reduced $B_{12}$ production is coupled with impaired absorption, the likelihood of $B_{12}$ deficiency becomes predictable.

### *4) Medical $B_{12}$ standards are artificially high.*

The situation is further complicated by the fact that many refined starchy foods are "enriched" with a synthetic form of vitamin $B_{12}$. When doctors test for "normal" $B_{12}$ levels, their results are skewed towards the high end by the fact that most people eat these foods (mostly grain products—cereals, breads, pasta, cookies, cakes, etc.) on a daily basis. People who eat a grain-free diet not supplemented by this poor imitation of the natural nutrient often test "low" for $B_{12}$ even if their levels are healthy and they are totally asymptomatic. This is because their $B_{12}$ levels are being compared to those of people who are consuming a $B_{12}$ supplement in their food at almost every meal.

## How important is it to eat organically grown food?

Organic produce is always to be preferred, but life is full of compromises and choices. It may be better to eat commercially grown raw vegetables than to eat cooked or steamed organic vegetables, but it is a difficult choice.

Organically grown produce generally contains more vitamins and minerals than conventional produce (see the FAQ "What about vitamin B12?" on page 253), and the fresher it is the better. Organic produce generally contains little or no pesticide residue in comparison with conventional produce; nevertheless, the amounts involved are not usually critical to health, and it is far more important to avoid the pathogenic effects from cooked food.

To concern yourself with pesticide residues while eating cooked food is a proverbial fire and frying pan situation. Neither is good for us. The best solution is to consume only organic raw plants. Otherwise, the decision is much like choosing whether to shoot oneself in the foot or shoot oneself in the hand.

In the case of cooked complex carbohydrates (grains, potatoes, corn, legumes), however, eating them both raw and free of synthetic chemicals has recently become a matter of grave concern. Commercial agroscientists are scrambling to counteract the seriously negative press being caused by a recently discovered DNA-damaging carcinogen and neurotoxin called acrylamide. This potent chemical killer was found in high concentrations in the food supply in 2002 by a Swedish researcher.

Scientists at the World Health Organization and elsewhere originally attributed shockingly high levels of acrylamide (found most prominently in bread, chips, crackers, french fries, and other dry-cooked carbohydrates) to the cooking process itself, because they found none to be present in raw foods. But we have since learned that acrylamide is a building block for polyacrylamide, a surfactant added to enhance the effectiveness of Monsanto's Roundup and other herbicide products used ubiquitously in industrial farming.

Further research is in order to determine whether bread, pastries, and crispy snacks made from organically grown plants contain this lethal chemical, but in any case the presence of acrylamide in these foods presents one more nail in the coffin of the standard American diet. If you still eat these foods, I urge you to do at least some reading about this profoundly toxic chemical. You can begin with the two articles referenced in the endnotes of this book.[88]

## Do I have to do calculations every day?

No. You don't have to calculate percentages every day to make sure you're eating properly. By eating primarily fruit, vegetables, and leafy greens, your diet is automatically close to the ideal of 80/10/10. However, you may want to use a calculator to determine whether you are getting enough calories for the day to meet your basic metabolic and exercise needs.

The tools in Appendix D. Resources for Diet AnalysisAppendix D. Resources for Diet Analysis are especially helpful to the newcomer, because it is common to undereat fruit and overeat fatty foods when beginning the raw vegan diet. I recommend that you input your food information into CRON-O-Meter or on Nutridiary.com, FitDay.com, or another similar website for at least a week, to make sure you have the relevant information about your calories and caloronutrient ratio.

Very often, people simply do not eat enough because their stomachs are used to accepting a certain volume of food each day, and raw foods are not as calorie dense as cooked foods. Therefore, to consume enough calories, you need to train your stomach to accept more food, especially fruits.

## How do I eat so much fruit at once?

It takes some practice to develop the ability to consume what, from the raw perspective, should be thought of as "normal" amounts of food for a human. Somewhere in between "all you care for" and "all you can" there is a happy medium that will enable you to increase the amount you consume without overeating. The stomach is very accommodating in this regard and will stretch quickly to allow you to consume normal/healthy quantities of fruit.

At the same time, your image of what is a healthy amount, and your mindset about quantities of fruit will grow to match your ability to eat it. The more you practice eating meals of just fruit, only fruit, and nothing but fruit, the easier and easier it will become to consume appropriate volumes.

If your fruit meal does not "hold" you until the next meal time, at least three to five hours later, then you did not eat a sufficient quantity of food. With practice, it will get easier. Until then, feel free to add an extra fruit meal between breakfast and lunch, and again between lunch and dinner.

## What does "mono eating" mean?

Mono eating is the practice of eating one particular food for an entire meal, in sufficient quantity to produce satiation until the next meal. This is the way that every nonhuman creature on Earth generally eats. I recommend eating monomeals for optimal digestion, absorption, and assimilation.

A monomeal might consist of four or five bananas for a sedentary beginner or twelve to eighteen bananas for a seasoned raw athlete. Another monomeal might be two or three mangos for the beginner, and four or more for the athlete.

It is important to remember when reading about food volumes that a small inactive woman may only eat a quarter of what an active male could eat. Do not be intimidated when you hear a low-fat raw vegan athlete tell you that he ate a dozen or more bananas for lunch. Four or five may be sufficient to meet your needs if you are a smaller, less active individual.

Variety is obtained over time, throughout the seasons, not at every meal. In nature, if sufficient food is available, animals tend to eat one food at a time until they are full.

## What's wrong with avocados, nuts, and seeds?

Avocados, nuts, and seeds are extremely high in fat content, especially nuts and seeds:

- Avocado (77% fat): 4 ounces (about ½) = 200 calories; 165 fat.
- Almonds (73% fat): 4 ounces (½ cup⁺) = 650 calories; 480 fat.
- Flaxseeds (58% fat): 4 ounces (¾ cup) = 560 calories; 325 fat.

When it comes to fat, the source doesn't matter so much; fat is fat. Fat travels from the lymph system directly into the blood. Too much fat will thicken the blood, causing the red blood cells to clump together so they cannot deliver oxygen to the cells. Excess fat also blocks the action of insulin in bringing sugars to the cells, which leads to diabetes and other blood-sugar problems. (Chapter 2 discusses this in detail.)

It is best to eat only small amounts of avocados, nuts, and seeds (not more than half of an avocado in a day or one ounce of nuts for a sedentary person; twice that for an athlete), and not to eat them daily. Fruits, vegetables, and leafy greens contain adequate high-quality fatty acids (assuming we're getting enough calories) to meet all of our needs.

Eventually, it is best to free yourself from the desire to experience a heavy feeling after a meal, as this is an indicator that the digestive system is being overworked. In order to feel satisfied, it is best to eat large amounts of sweet fruit, which may pass through your stomach quickly, but will satisfy true hunger for hours.

## What do you mean by "true hunger"?

True hunger is a sensation that occurs primarily deep in the low part of the throat, much like the feeling of thirst, but a bit lower, about where the concave "notch" appears between the collar bones, at the bottom of the neck. The sensation might be described as resembling a dull ache.

The stomach sensation we commonly associate with hunger is often the result of its muscular walls shrinking after completing the digestive task of the last meal. If a perceived feeling of hunger is accompanied by feelings of faintness, stomach pangs, headaches, or other discomforts, it is actually a sign of withdrawal from harmful substances.

A healthy person can skip a meal or two with no feelings of weakness or distress. When one is healthy, true hunger signifies no urgency for food, since the body knows it has reserves for its use in time of need. You should be at all times comfortable in your body.

## Is eating sea salt all right?

Extracted sodium chloride, in any form is an irritant and is toxic to the body. It deadens the taste buds' ability to sense sweet, sour, or bitter (which is why salt users often say that food has no taste without salt), retards digestion and excretion, and upsets our critical natural water balance.

We must take care to distinguish here between extracted sodium chloride "salt" (which is deadly), and the sodium and other mineral salts that occur naturally and abundantly in whole plant foods (which are vitally important nutrients needed by every cell of our bodies). Eating a variety of vegetables, especially celery and tomatoes, provides all the organic salts and other minerals our bodies need in just the right amounts and combinations we require.

Our cells rely on a delicately regulated ratio of sodium and potassium, with sodium residing outside the cells (extracellular) and potassium inside (intracellular). If the potassium/sodium ratio is at all out of balance, cellular dehydration or super saturation result. Either of these conditions seriously compromises cellular function.

If we lose too much sodium through exercise or any other effort that results in perspiration, potassium is "pulled" out of the cell to maintain the proper ratio. Attempting to compensate by consuming salt simply stresses the body even more, like trying to make up for lack of sleep by drinking coffee. The potassium within the cell must be replaced in order for the cell to "hold" sodium extracellularly again.

The salt in seawater causes dehydration regardless of how it is consumed. Ocean water is caustic and irritating, tastes vile, and causes people to vomit. In quantity, drinking seawater causes death within days, even though it is diluted by a lot of water.

When we extract salt and ingest it with our meals, we head in the same direction, only at a different speed. Removing the salt from seawater gives us sea salt, the very substance that causes death by dehydration. Consuming sodium chloride of any kind—including sea salts and other highly marketed, pricey specialty salts—is a self-destructive practice. Specialty salt producers expend great effort to convince you that you "need" the extracted minerals in their products to offset a grave nutritional imbalance common in modern society. (Such deficiency may indeed exist, but in any case it can be healthfully remedied only by eating an abundance of low-fat raw plant foods. To do otherwise only creates more nutritional imbalances.)

True, we need minerals but we need to ingest them in the quantities and the form in which they occur in whole plant foods. Eating a highly mineralized form of poison makes no logical sense whatsoever.

Salt eaters who cease the practice can often take years to expel all of the retained salt from their bodies. But take heart, as the bulk of salt (and cravings) diminish significantly within just a few short weeks of total abstinence. I cannot overemphasize the importance of making the commitment to wean yourself from this ubiquitous poison.

## Can I use vinegar in my salad dressing?

All forms of vinegar, including apple cider and balsamic, are highly toxic to the human body. Vinegar is made by diluting one part acetic acid (a common poison found in any chemistry laboratory ... in a bottle with a skull and crossbones) with 19 parts water.

Vinegar excessively stimulates the thyroid gland, leading to hyperthyroidism and eventually hypothyroidism and concomitant health issues such as endocrine disorders, calcium metabolic disorders, metabolic rate disorders, fat metabolism problems, body-weight issues, lethargy, headaches, and the classic bulging of the eyes. This stimulation also accelerates the aging process.

The body pulls phosphorus from the adrenal glands to negate the effects of acetic acid in the system. Depleted phosphorus results in impaired function of the adrenal glands and thus, again, the entire endocrine system. The outcome of all this can include body odor, pains in the heart, rapid pulse, increased mucus production, chronic fatigue, and headaches. Repetitive use of vinegar will also result in hardening of the liver. Vinegar should not be considered "food."

## Is it okay to eat frozen produce?

Some damage to living foods occurs when they are frozen. Freezing can expand and burst cell walls, and the resulting oxidation diminishes the nutritional value of the food. However, nuts and seeds, which are designed to survive through cold winters, are less damaged by being frozen. Generally, the lower the water and the higher the fat content of a whole, fresh food, the better it will take to freezing.

As for fruits and vegetables, the practice of freezing should be minimized but not necessarily eliminated, as it is one of the least-damaging ways to preserve foods (especially when a chest freezer is used instead of the frost-free variety). One advantage of freezing food relative to other forms of preservation is that freezing introduces no known toxins.

You should be aware that eating frozen and ice-cold foods damages the essential bacterial colonies that live in your gut and may be harmful to the bacteria that produce vitamin $B_{12}$. Once again, we see that eating foods as we find them in nature proves to be the most healthful ... it is true every time.

## Are dehydrated foods OK to eat?

Dehydrated foods are not whole foods; they have had their water removed. Unfortunately, we have not been taught to recognize the vital value of water as it comes packaged in fresh plant foods. Fruits and vegetables are nature's most pristine water filters, and the water we cook and dehydrate out of them can never be adequately replaced. Drinking water, no matter how purified, alkalized, or "structured," just doesn't compare.

Dehydrated foods can never be as nutritious as the whole, fresh foods they started as. Nutrient damage has been shown to occur, even if the water is replaced. The use of dehydrates is a personal decision, but dried foods should always be considered at best a compromise, second in quality to whole, fresh, ripe, raw, organic fruits and vegetables.

Current research indicates that vitamin $B_{12}$ changes to an analog and unusable form where it is found in dehydrated foods. This appears to be true, by the way, for spirulina, chlorella, algaes, and other pills and powders made from ocean plants.

## What about spices and condiments?

In Natural Hygiene, there is a saying, "If you can't make a meal of it, it likely is not people food." When people hear this statement, they often view it as draconian and idealistic, for it rules out the consumption of virtually all spices, seasonings, and condiments. Yet, think about it: no creatures in nature season their foods, nor even generally combine more than one food in a meal (at least not for purposes of gustatory pleasure).

Yes, humans are undoubtedly different than the "lower" animals. We have the dexterity and the equipment to mix up grand concoctions ("combo-abombosa-bombs," as R.C. Dini so aptly dubbed them), and we have the ingenuity to create gloriously seasoned taste treats. But I promise you, our digestive systems have not kept up with our creativity—not by a long shot. In fact, they are virtually identical to those of our ancient ancestors, as well as those of modern-day frugivorous anthropoid primates. By design, we are meant to eat one whole plant food at a time, unadorned, until we have made a meal of it.

Herbs and spices like garlic, onion, curry, cumin, ginger, cayenne, chili powder, and oregano contain alkaloids and other toxic chemicals. These seasonings stimulate our taste buds and nerves while delivering toxins to our nervous systems. Their use should be avoided, or at least minimized. They act as irritants in the digestive tract, often causing the body to produce mucus for protection. They also function to disguise the bland or noxious taste of cooked foods and seduce us into consuming foods that would not attract us on their own.

Like salt, spices provide such an intense "flavor hit" that our taste buds lose their ability to recognize the natural but more subtle tastes of fruits and vegetables. The same holds true for the use of all condiments, including mustard and ketchup.

## Can I drink coffee on the raw diet?

The beans in coffee are roasted, making them no longer a raw food item. The fatal dose of caffeine is 10 grams, the amount in approximately 70 cups of coffee. Caffeine is considered such a powerful drug that just three cups of coffee supplies enough caffeine to disqualify an athlete from competing in the Olympic games.

Many people take one tenth of the lethal dose every day. I had one patient who drank over thirty cups of coffee per day. His health was failing, but it was regained when he stopped this noxious habit, which he did overnight.

Moreover, caffeine decreases the amount of pepsin in your body. Pepsin is used in the digestion of protein. Ironically, many coffee drinkers on the standard American diet criticize the raw diet because they believe they would not receive "enough" protein every day, while their daily intake of coffee impedes their absorption of the very protein they claim they need.

Caffeine is also known to deplete the body of water, calcium, potassium, manganese, and the vitamin B complex. Caffeine is just one of many toxic substances that can be found in coffee.

## Should I continue taking my medications?

The medical profession and its supporting industry, the medico pharmaceutical cartel, operate from the theory that thousands of separate illnesses exist whose symptoms can be treated or suppressed by ingesting synthetic chemical compounds. The Natural Hygiene approach is entirely different.

We recognize that genetically inherited abnormalities exist, usually arising from generations of poor dietary and lifestyle choices, and that very little can be done about these. Otherwise, however, we propose that there is only one illness: toxemia. This is a condition of unclean blood and tissues, caused primarily by improper diet and lifestyle. Unchecked, toxemia and its attendant enervation (nervous exhaustion) get progressively worse over the years, leading to all manner of symptoms.

People find this very difficult to comprehend, but we must remember that the symptoms are not the disease. Rather, symptoms are actually the body's methods of coping with toxemia. In order to "cure" a disease condition, such as diabetes, cancer, or cardiovascular disease, one must eliminate the underlying toxemia of which the "disease" is only a manifestation.

As you begin to eat a healthy 80/10/10 raw diet, you will no longer overload your body on a daily basis with toxic residue from food. Your body will begin to clean your blood, tissues, and organs of their toxicity, and the medical condition(s) for which you are taking the pharmaceutical medicine(s) will fade away. Check with your doctor as your health improves, in time he or she will likely agree that your need to medicate will become obsolete.

Generally, the younger you are and the less time the body has spent in the toxic state, the more rapidly it will clean itself. An older person with more accompanying degeneration and accumulated toxicity may take longer to cleanse and return to a healthy state. Nevertheless, limited only by its vitality level, the body will respond positively to cessation of the daily insult of cooked foods and high-fat raw foods and to their replacement with whole, fresh, ripe, raw fruits and vegetables. Still, food is only one part of healthful living, and proper eating will never result in health in and of itself.

Pharmaceutical medicines are toxic substances that you introduce into your system at your own peril. Rarely are any claims made that a drug will cure any particular chronic disease. At best, they usually profess only to substitute one set of symptoms for another.

### The Myth of the "Cure"

The very notion that "cure" is possible is preposterous. Healing, on the other hand is not only possible but is ongoing. The inborn healing intelligence of the body is always at work, repairing us and compensating for the challenges we subject it to. This healing occurs as quickly and efficiently as possible given our level of vital energy—and in a priority order we cannot comprehend. All attempts (both conventional and "alternative") to aid this process through outside interventions or treatments or ingestion of any external substances only shift symptoms and create greater problems for the body in the long run.

Healing comes through cessation of cause. We are never cured from a disease or symptom, for if we once again participate in its cause the body again begins the process of generating the symptoms in response.

The fact that pharmaceutical drugs are sold legally over the counter or are prescribed by licensed physicians does not make them any less dangerous to health than street drugs. Over 100,000 people die each year from the side effects of these patented medicines. No one has ever died from eating an adequate supply of fruits and vegetables.

The advice to continue or curtail a particular medication is beyond the scope of this book. However, any reputable physician should encourage his or her patients to improve their underlying health so as to make the continued reliance on pharmaceutical medications unnecessary.

## How can I stay raw in the winter cold?

Fortunately, most folks who live in colder climates have homes in which to eat, sleep, work, and live. We maintain our homes at comfortable temperatures. People continue to drink cold beer and eat ice cream in the winter. They eat hot food in the heat of summer. Neither geography nor the seasons are valid reasons for us to change our diet from 80/10/10.

If in cold weather a person finds that they need more food, it is perfectly acceptable to increase consumption. The caloronutrient percentages should not change appreciably, however, just as it does not change whether a person consumes 1,500 calories per day or 4,500 calories per day. Of course, it is almost always a healthy idea to take a winter vacation to a warm-weather climate if you live in a location where this season is particularly harsh.

## Is there such a thing as foods that heal?

It is important to understand that foods don't heal us; the body does all the healing. Foods, cooked or raw, simply supply the materials the body uses to perform its various functions. However, low-fat raw vegan foods provide the widest range of high-quality nutrients and are, therefore, more likely to furnish the perfect proportion of raw materials needed by the body for healing.

Beyond that, no specific raw food is better for "healing" than any other. Each supplies a form of raw material that the body may need and use. Unlike cooked foods, raw foods do this without leaving a toxic residue that can overwhelm the body's ability to maintain a healthy, balanced state.

A good variety of low-fat raw vegan foods in the diet is more than adequate to attain, regain, or maintain health. It is always healthiest and most economical to emphasize in-season foods that are grown locally, as these will likely be the freshest. It is best to seek out variety over the course of the year, rather than combining foods at every meal, every day, or even every week.

## Is it all right to juice fruits and vegetables?

With a few exceptions, it is preferable to consume the whole foods rather than to extract and drink part of them. Drinking fruit or vegetable juice without the pulp being present to slow the absorption rate of the nutrients can spike the blood sugar and throw your blood chemistry out of balance.

One exception is fresh-squeezed citrus fruits, since a significant portion of the pulp is generally retained with the juice. The other "exceptions" are to blend fruits such as melons into a watery slush or to make fruit smoothies out of fruits like bananas, strawberries, peaches, or mangos. Liquefying a blender full of whole fruit turns it into a thick smoothie, while keeping the entire nutritional package together. Blending whole tomato, celery, and orange makes a thick, tasty, salad dressing.

## Do I need to take supplements?

You have no need for supplements if you are eating a calorically adequate low-fat plant-based raw diet, engaging in frequent vigorous activity, and otherwise living a healthful lifestyle. All the vitamins, minerals and nutrients any body needs are amply supplied through the variety of fruits, vegetables, and leafy greens found in a healthful diet.

That said, the health of each individual always takes priority over any philosophical position. In individual cases, it may be necessary to supplement the diet nutritionally during the initial phases of lifestyle change rather than risk potential health damage. One example of this is a possible need to supplement $B_{12}$. If you experience extended periods of extreme stress, are nursing, eating too much frozen food, are in transition, or your food is not grown in healthy soil, supplementing this nutrient for a short period of time may be beneficial. Supplementation would be done solely to allow time for the benefits of correct living to accrue or for extenuating circumstances to pass.

Nonetheless, the amount of nutrients that we require, across the board, is far less than conventional guidelines would have us believe. When the body is in a fit and healthy state and all systems are working optimally, we experience superior absorption and utilization and overall greater efficiency in every aspect of cellular function. When we slow down and gum up the works with fat, however, it's a different story. And supplement vendors capitalize on this fact to your detriment.

People have come to equate nutrition with pills, powders, and potions, rather than with whole foods from nature. Ironically, you generally won't find a single food of any kind in most "health-food" stores. Their products, no matter how "whole" or "natural" the ingredients, may shift symptoms but do not and cannot create true health.

If "health foods" were truly whole and natural, they would contain all of the water, fiber, and other vital components that nature provides them with, and their sale would require no packaging or labels. (The profit margins would also dwindle, as whole produce doesn't carry the markup of "nutritional" products.)

No pill or powder that has had any of its water removed can properly be called a "whole-food" supplement, and anyone who markets their dehydrated product as such is kidding themselves, as well as you. The water in our plant foods is simply too critical for our cellular health to be compromised, and no drinking water of any kind can ever adequately make up the difference. When the water is removed, the oxidative process that occurs has a degrading impact on the nutrients that remain, leaving supplements far less nutritious than their whole-food counterparts.

When people follow the nutritionally unsound advice of supplement salesmen selling fractional, isolated "foods," they shouldn't be surprised when they end up not feeling their best, with a nagging sense that "something" is wrong. This opens the door wide for the salesman to then sell supplements to "correct" the dietary and nutritional insufficiencies their own advice occasioned.

I'm always dumbfounded when I hear about the money people spend on nutritional supplements. It seems there is no high-end limit to the amount of product recommended by supplement salesmen. In conveyor-belt fashion, they roll out a bewildering array of "newly discovered" miracle "foods," while at the same time replacing older products with newly reformulated versions. Such antics essentially amount to an open admission that yesterday's silver bullet, which they touted so highly, really didn't work as well as their sales pitch had promised.

Most of what comes from the world of nutrition these days is no more than slick marketing disguised as education, in the form of infomercials and edutisements. The marketer informs the audience that some nutrient is good for a particular condition and then follows up with a strong push to convince the audience to buy lots of it.

Of course, the marketers neglect to mention that too much of that nutrient is harmful in a variety of ways, not the least of which is the inevitable imbalances that result when we consume supplements of any kind. Most supplements are concentrated from plant foods, and despite our American "more is better" mindset, the body does not appreciate these unnatural concentrates and has to work to expel them similarly to the way it has to eliminate toxic residue from cooked foods.

Like an amateur barber who finds himself trimming each side of the hair to make things "even" until his client is bald, a person who supplements with single nutrients (or any formulation or combination of extracted nutrients) inevitably creates greater and more confounding imbalances, whether or not the cause and effect are discernible in the short term. It is always better to correct the diet than to supplement it. On a healthy diet, supplements are not needed. On a less-than-healthy diet, supplements do not make up for the nutrition that is lacking.

## Is the raw food concept flawed?

Every creature on this planet has a specific diet for which it is designed. All animals get their nourishment exclusively from the foods present in their natural environment—one food at a time, when they are hungry, until they are full. Simplicity at meals ensures optimum digestion and nutrition. Animals do not use or demonstrate any need for supplements or condiments. Nature provides adequately for all life forms, and humans are not an exception.

Like all other primates, we were made to function perfectly on the amount of nutrients found in fruits and vegetables, in the quantities that we would eat those foods whole. Juicing, dehydrating, concentrating, and refining those foods introduces excesses and nutritional imbalances that our bodies were not designed to deal with.

I maintain that the optimal raw food diet consists of whole, fresh, ripe, raw, organic plants—in the 80/10/10 caloronutrient ratio—period. The raw food kitchen need not include jars, bottles, boxes, cans, bags, capsules, powders, remedies, potions, pills, or tinctures of any kind.

So many eager new raw fooders find themselves in the unfortunate situation where some nutritional "guru" guides them to "the world's most nutritious diet" and then convinces them that the diet is inadequate and requires supplementation. The ultimate promotion strategy, this ploy is as old as marketing itself: First you create a problem, then you sell the solution. How many mom-and-pop grocery stores were vandalized by the very men who were there to sell them "security"? How many people became patients for life by following the advice of their medical doctors?

The problem, in the case of raw foods, is that people do not feel great when they eat insufficient carbohydrates or when they continually under consume total calories. They experience voracious hunger, and they binge, falling off the "raw food wagon" repeatedly. They develop uncomfortable and unhealthy relationships with food. Their health deteriorates as their diet becomes erratic.

I choose to acquire my learning on any topic from organizations and individuals whose clear and explicit intention is to educate me. I steer away from information sources that include an obvious and motivated "back-of-the-room" sales table filled with consumables and repeat products that will, if they have it their way, have me coming back for more … for years to come.

If the only way to be truly well nourished is to consume vitamins, minerals, oils, enzymes, medicinal herbs, white powdered pharmaceuticals such as MSM, refined isolates such as lecithin, "super" foods such as algae and sea vegetables, and other purportedly "nutrition-enhancing" substances, then the raw food concept is flawed.

# Appendix C.
# Personal Success Stories with 80/10/10

## *Table of Contents*

## Mark Squire, St. Petersburg, Florida

Back a few years ago, a struggling raw food friend of mine referred me to the work of a guy named Doug Graham. I had never heard of him before, so I began to educate myself a bit on the message he brought to the table. My first reaction? "This guy is a damned fool!" However, I had become so frustrated with my current raw food program (which was about 50% fat) that I was willing to give anything a shot.

I started eating larger and larger portions of fruit, but still neglected other important aspects of healthy living. Now my initial stance was solidified: "This guy IS a fool and his suggestions are insane!" Yet, for some reason, I continued on. Why, I do not know.

Slowly but surely, Doug's teachings made more and more sense. The more consistently I applied Doug's program (with a little dash of Squire mixed in) I began to notice miraculous things happening. Not only was my health improving dramatically, but I was also getting stronger and faster, and my endurance was skyrocketing. I had been lifting weights on a raw food diet for three years prior to 811 and had nothing to show for it. Roughly one full year later, being 100% dedicated to keeping my fruit intake high, I was nearly 30 lbs. heavier, all of which was muscle. Over the next year, I added an additional 10 lbs. of muscle, bringing my total up to 40 lbs.

The added muscle isn't the main benefit of being on a raw food diet. The best part of the whole journey has been my childlike energy levels, my blissful state of joy, and my ability to tune into nature, all of which were amplified measurably. When I was about to give up on raw foods once and for all, Doug steered me back on the right track.

The program isn't easy, but with enough inner strength and persistence, you will undoubtedly experience a radical transformation in every aspect of your life. As much trash as I talked about Doug in my learning process, it's because this 811 program was changing me down to the core. My belief system was threatened, and I fired off about him, as a defense mechanism. It was quite a struggle getting to the point I'm at now, but now I see as clear as day that Doug is an amazing person, and I have nothing but the utmost respect for him and what he does. My stamp of approval is all over this book, and all over Dr. D. himself. Thanks a million, brother!

## Cyrus Khambatta, San Francisco, California

I'll never forget the first time I exercised with Dr. Graham. I was half his age, in the prime of my athletic life, fueled by a combination of years of soccer training and an ever-growing dose of athletic hubris. I thought to myself, "I'll show this guy what it really means to work out." It took only fifteen minutes to realize that I had completely underestimated Dr. Graham.

I was so wrong, in fact, that there was nothing I could do that Dr. Graham couldn't. I was flabbergasted that a man as old as my father could jump higher, run faster, balance longer, react quicker, push harder, lift more, breathe slower, and still have more energy at the end of the day. What was accounting for an athletic ability that I had witnessed in only a handful of other athletes in my life? How could he recover faster than me when he was more than fifty years old? What was he fueling his body with that I wasn't?

The truth is, at the age of twenty-two I was diagnosed with Type 1 diabetes, a life-changing condition that not only changed my relationship with food, but was silently crippling my body. Having implemented the recommended Atkins-esque "low-carb" diet, I had reduced my insulin intake by 25%. I thought that I had taken steps to ensure my long-term health. Instead, I was taking steps in the wrong direction, further exacerbating the autoimmune reaction by consuming grossly high levels of animal protein and fat.

I did exactly what the cookbooks instructed me to do: I eliminated breads and pastas, routinely consumed more fish, and increased my consumption of chicken, beef, eggs, and dairy. A few times a week I snacked on fruits and vegetables, but only when the dairy and meat drawers in the fridge were empty. The low carb approach seemed quite logical; if carbohydrates are responsible for spikes in blood sugar, limiting their intake should regulate blood-sugar levels throughout the day. I bragged to my friends and family about how I had "figured out" diabetes, and how I was able to control my blood sugar better than most.

Despite this, I failed to make the connection between the low-carb diet and my ailing athletic health. I rationalized that because I was past my eighteen-year-old athletic prime it was normal to be constantly fighting injury. I settled for the explanation that my physical health was on a course for the worse. After all, I was in constant receipt of a pessimistic outlook from medical professionals.

I learned of the 80/10/10 philosophy through a fortunate series of events involving a friend in the San Francisco area who had unsuccessfully tried a raw food diet. Because his diet was high in nuts and avocados, and thus high in fat, he did not gain long-term benefit from his raw food experience. Having listened to his troubles, I was curious about how to make a raw food diet work, especially in the context of improving diabetic health.

A few days into learning about 80/10/10 from Dr. Graham himself, I remember thinking to myself, "eating fruits and vegetables—what a novel idea." Why had it never occurred to me before that the answer to my ailing health could simply be in the food that I wasn't consuming? I always knew that fruits and vegetables were good for you, but as far as I knew, athletes were unable to sustain themselves without animal protein. From the first time I was taught the food pyramid in second grade to the depths of the varsity soccer locker room, it was always reinforced that animal protein was a necessity for developing musculature, speed, and athletic endurance. After all, how can you perform without protein?

My first inclination was to reject the 80/10/10 philosophy as a lifestyle that only sedentary people could maintain successfully. Only because I was desperate to find a better solution to overall health, I decided to give Dr. Graham and the 80/10/10 idea a shot. If anything, his lifestyle had instant credibility based solely on his athletic prowess.

At the moment I officially adopted the 80/10/10 regimen, I decided that I would give up meat. I also decided that I would give up grains and dairy. It would be hard, but perhaps there was a benefit in this radical approach to nutrition. I was told by family and friends to "be careful," that giving up meat could have severe ramifications for my health. People understood my desperation, but few were truly accepting of the low-fat raw foods approach.

It has been more than two years now, and I can safely say that the benefits of being on the 80/10/10 diet are more numerous than I could have ever imagined. My body has completely changed. My skin is softer, my fingernails look normal for once in my life, I am almost always well hydrated, my gums don't bleed when I brush my teeth, and I sleep more efficiently. For the first time in my life I am able to compete in endurance athletics, supported by an enhanced ability to uptake, transport, and utilize oxygen. On long bicycle rides, my heart rate stays unusually low, which allows me to push harder than I previously could, and for longer periods of time.

Most important, I am able to consume more calories during the day on a fraction of the insulin I was previously taking. The formula I use to monitor my progress is the ratio of the number of grams of carbohydrates to the number of units of insulin. On the Atkins-esque approach I had maximized this ratio at 16 grams of carbohydrates per unit of insulin. By eating 80/10/10, I am now capable of eating 68 grams of carbohydrates per unit of insulin when I partake in regular periods of endurance training. This means that I am now able to eat larger quantities of food, use less insulin, and free myself physically and psychologically from an insulin pump.

One unexpected benefit of the 80/10/10 diet that I have welcomed with open arms is a seeming inability to get sick. Having transitioned to this form of nutrition at the end of the autumn season, I was unknowingly providing my body with an influx of vitamins, minerals, enzymes, sugars, fiber, coenzymes, phytonutrients, etc. that (in combination with regular exercise and other elements of healthful living) would help build an immune response capable of mounting an arsenal against a collection of the worst maladies in years.

I live in an apartment with three other people, and work in an office building with over one hundred and fifty others. The winter months brought a series of illnesses that absolutely crippled my household, stopping each housemate in their tracks for at least one three-day period each. One of my housemates suffered from three colds and/or bouts of influenza, not only infecting my remaining housemates, but touching bowls, cups, plates and silverware with almost no regard for common hygiene. At work, a number of coworkers suffered from sicknesses that kept them from the office for a number of days at a time. Without exception, almost every colleague produced symptoms at some point between the months of November and March.

During this extended winter season the symptoms I produced were as follows: I coughed on one occasion for about a minute, and sneezed a grand total of four times. That's it. Nothing more. Never once did I feel groggy, run down, suffer from a headache, or feel nauseous. I surprised even myself. And because I am playfully competitive by nature, I challenged my family and friends to a contest in trying to get me sick. So far no one has succeeded, and quite frankly I don't believe that anyone will.

Before becoming an 80/10/10 raw foodist, I had heard numerous allegations that eliminating grains could increase mental clarity and create a heightened sense of consciousness. I remained skeptical, wary about the change in mental perception that could be brought about by a change in diet. I failed to make the connection between food and systemic human health, ignorantly asserting that food has a limited capacity to affect any more than the function of the digestive system. I didn't believe that nutrition possessed the power to change the way I think. I didn't believe that the 80/10/10 diet could change my emotional state. Simply stated, I didn't believe that eating differently could change any part of my consciousness. I was always taught to believe that consciousness was governed by my genetic blueprint, and that it could only be affected by either a drastic change in environmental conditions or an intensely traumatic experience.

Once again, I was proven incorrect. Within the first month of eating 80/10/10, I began to experience the ability to remember people's names and faces, recall events from several years back, and revisit playful ideas that I thought had escaped forever. Throughout college my friends had labeled me as "the guy who has too much going on to remember anything." I used to invite friends to come and dine with me, forget about the invitation, and be surprised when they showed up only a few hours later. I used to tell people the same stories while they pretended to listen for the first time. A few times I seriously believed that I suffered from a mild form of anterograde amnesia, a condition in which an individual wanders through life unable to form new memories. In the same way that I rationalized an athletic decline, I reasoned that it was normal to experience mental deterioration in life, and that perhaps I was experiencing it earlier in life simply because I was diabetic.

Now, however, I have a significantly improved memory. I can recall people's names after only a single brief meeting. I rarely forget an appointment or a commitment. I am more productive in my job, and can work for longer periods of time in a single stretch. I realize that I now have a memory more closely resembling that which I'm supposed to have at my age—one that works, and one that works well. My days of using diabetes as the generic scapegoat for any mental or physical health symptom are officially over.

Learning the 80/10/10 philosophy has helped me develop a holistic understanding of nutrition that opposes the basic desire to obsess about the intake of a subset of nutrients. Nutrition education in this country makes it almost impossible to know where to look for essential fatty acids, vitamins and minerals, and calcium, to name a few. It is also difficult to know how much of each nutrient one should aim to consume on a daily basis. After all, the recommended daily allowance values change almost every year, and intake values seem to change constantly, in a seemingly arbitrary fashion. There seems to be little logic to this system.

Many Americans ponder about what the best source of omega-3 fatty acids is, whether it's necessary to consume bran flakes to keep "regular," whether organic produce is really worth the price differential, whether dairy products are the best source of calcium, and whether supplementation is really necessary. One day you read an article in the newspaper that claims one point of view; the next day you read an article in a magazine that contradicts it completely. The information comes from hundreds of sources, most of it is confusing, and almost nobody knows what to believe.

It wasn't until learning the 80/10/10 philosophy that I finally learned how to filter mainstream nutrition information to achieve optimal health. Dr. Graham's coined statement, "Increase the percentage of whole, fresh, ripe, raw, organic fruits and vegetables in your diet" was so simple and so sensible that I felt like a fool for not understanding it previously. In fact, after feeling the difference that whole fresh, ripe, raw, organic fruits and vegetables made in my body, I never stopped to question my nutrient intake. I stopped obsessing about individual nutrients and started focusing on creating holistic health.

The message that I've taken from the 80/10/10 lifestyle is simple: eating a low-fat vegan raw foods diet makes me feel like a natural human being. Besides feeling like a million dollars every time I awake from deep slumber, I enjoy a feeling of simplicity that was never present in my life on a cooked food diet. My perception of the world has changed for the better, and I am more at peace with my friends, family, and daily routine.

At first I thought that in order to become a raw food vegan you had to have a reason, an ailment, or a condition. I thought that you had to be a cancer patient, a diabetic, or someone suffering from chronic fatigue syndrome. After all, why else would anyone want to deprive him- or herself of the good food they grew up loving?

Today, however, I realize that the only reason you need to adopt the 80/10/10 lifestyle is that you want to feel like a natural human being. If you're already athletic, be prepared to experience increased performance and a shockingly efficient ability to recover. If you've lost track of what's important in your life, be prepared to experience the simplicity of all that life has to offer. If you suffer from a clouded mental state, be prepared to experience a new sense of clarity. And if you're like me, and have a condition like diabetes, be prepared to look to the future with an overwhelming sense of hope, a gift that both the 80/10/10 nutritional philosophy and Dr. Graham have taught me to never give up.

## Justin Lelia, Miami, Florida

Dr. Graham is the strongest, most humane and effective health educators I know. His level of happiness and his high-energy diet inspired my turnaround. Before Dr. Graham's program, I weighed 190 pounds, had chronic joint pain, worked in a fast-food restaurant, and experienced dangerous levels of depression. Now, I play tennis and basketball, have ridden my bike over 6,000 miles in three years, have lost close to fifty pounds, and I work at an outdoor organic farmer's market.

Dr. Graham's emphasis on practicing a low-fat dietary regimen is particularly noteworthy. Raw fats may be healthier than their cooked counterparts, but high-fat diets remain unhealthy no matter how we slice, dice, or soak them.

The standard of health Dr. Graham upholds is humbling; indeed, it's incredibly challenging, and for this he remains unpopular with medically minded raw fooders. They overestimate the power of food, and can often be heard giving others prescriptions, treating foods as if they were drugs.

Doug refuses to promote fragmented nutrition, superfoods, supplements, flushes, and other concepts designed to compensate for people's lack of willpower, persistence, and responsibility; he refuses to encourage the medically brainwashed. He has taught me that the best way to help others heal is through friendship and attention, and by inspiring them with outstanding levels of performance.

Dr. Graham is in a league of his own … another stratosphere. His humanity is alien-like in a world that is often categorized by greed and impatience. The amount of time and energy Doug has graciously and patiently volunteered in order to help me and others climb out of the hole we've dug ourselves into blows my mind. Sometimes I think he's too human for the world.

## Janie Gardener, Kauai, Hawaii

I first came into contact with Dr. Graham through his VegSource online discussion board about raw foods and sports nutrition. My visit there was prompted by my decision to eat raw again.

The first time I tried going raw I did it a differently—high fat, low fruit with ferments, condiments, oils, and the like. It worked better than any other diet I'd tried, but my body wanted me to do what Dr. Graham's program is all about, even though I did not know Dr. Graham or his program back then.

Too bad I didn't have the guts to just go with it like he did. I'm glad I found my way back. Thank goodness I came across that discussion board and found out about Dr. Graham's 80/10/10 low-fat raw vegan diet. It has made all the difference in the improvement of my health, well-being, and life. The differences are radically beyond anything I had experienced before, beyond my hopes and expectations, and into a whole new realm of health and vitality.

### *Autoimmune Disease*

Prior to starting back on raw, I could see my health rapidly deteriorating before my eyes. In the summer of 2001, I was diagnosed with antiphospholipid antibody syndrome. This autoimmune condition literally means that you have antibodies that are attacking your own phosphorus fats. Symptoms are mostly related to a tendency of the blood to clot and/or bleed excessively but also include heart attack, stroke, and easily bruised and sunburned skin, as well as miscarriages. The condition is found in lupus patients, but does not always develop into lupus or in all lupus patients.

I had at least four miscarriages and a host of other health problems before it was diagnosed. I spent some time following my MD's suggestions (aspirin), then my chiropractor's suggestions (fish oil), and a mix of alternating between the two, but it was just getting worse—and I had the side effects of the "medicine" to deal with as well. I tried eating more EFA-rich foods like salmon, flaxseed oil, walnuts, etc., but that didn't help either.

When I switched to Dr. Graham's program, I decided to stop all of the fish and fish oil, flaxseed oil, and aspirin I had been taking. I started working on eating the 80/10/10 raw vegan way in June of 2002. At first I misunderstood the 10% (or lower) fat recommendation, thinking it referred to overt fats, not all fats, as I couldn't imagine not eating much overt fat. I had been eating a very high-fat diet all of my life, including when I ate raw/living foods the last time around.

Thus, I started out by keeping my overt fat intake down to not more than 10% of calories (about 20% overall), which isn't quite 80/10/10. This intermediate step allowed me to get things going well enough to experience fantastic results and inspired me to keep on going. About six months into it, I discovered my mistake and adjusted my diet and activity level so that I was able to meet the recommendations soon afterwards. I don't think I could have done 80/10/10 without this transition, even if I had understood it from the beginning.

I had enormous improvements in my first six months, even with my 20%-ish fat intake. The improvements were way beyond those I had experienced eating any other way (including other variants of the raw/living-food diet). I am now doing 80/10/10 fully, have taken no supplements or medications of any kind since the beginning, and I feel great! All of my symptoms have improved and in some cases, disappeared! I am wonderfully pleased with the results!

### *Four Miscarriages*

Backing up a bit, in college I became a vegetarian, and eventually a vegan, trying various versions of both. At the age of twenty-three, on a cooked vegan diet, I gave birth to my son and raised him on cooked vegan food. I discovered Natural Hygiene and living foods when he was a toddler and worked toward eating a vegan raw/living-food diet.

When my son was about seven years old, my husband and I decided to birth another child. It took a few years before I became pregnant. Unfortunately, I miscarried. My family and I had been following the living-food diet for about a year and a half. During that time, I was eating for nutrients and even created a custom Microsoft Access database to track my nutrient intake. This enabled me to compare my intake with the requirements for a pregnant woman, and assure myself that I was meeting all of the RDAs.

Some people, including my midwife, blamed my diet, assuming a lack of protein or "something," although my OB/GYN (an MD), upon seeing my diet, did not think it was diet related. Even though my database indicated I was getting plenty of protein, I was unsure, as my husband was concerned about protein overall, and we had a friend who'd failed on raw claiming lack of protein as the culprit. (We now realize it was due to other conditions.)

I also was not listening to my body's desire for a diet like 80/10/10, as I was surrounded by fruit-fearing, living-food misinformation. I was eating for nutrients rather than health, and I was not feeling as vital as I could have on raw, as a result. Since I had my son while eating a vegan diet (including cooked), I decided to temporarily go back to cooked vegan (with raw) in order to have another child, and planned to go back to raw afterwards. Too bad I didn't know Dr. Graham then. I could have saved a lot of time and heartache.

Going back to cooked vegan, of course, did not work, and I ended up having another miscarriage a year later. I decided to add in dairy and eggs and had another miscarriage the year after that. In the meantime I saw people who ate all sorts of diets and lived unhealthy lifestyles having children left and right. From my farmer's perspective, I figured that maybe it was similar to the way plants go to seed when stressed, in order to continue their genetics before they die. I thought that perhaps I'd have a baby more easily if I was less healthy, and then I could regain my health afterwards. I was grasping at straws, trying whatever I could to have a baby.

During that third miscarriage I tried adding in poultry and fish and stayed on that diet to try again. I didn't get pregnant for some time and thought, maybe I just couldn't anymore. Years later, at the age of thirty six, I became pregnant again—unexpectedly—and again miscarried.

It wasn't until this fourth confirmed miscarriage that additional blood work led to a diagnosis of antiphospholipid antibody syndrome. I gave up on birthing another child, because I did not want to take the drugs or risks involved, nor subject a child to them, either. In retrospect, it seems clear to me that my high-fat diet caused this condition and/or greatly contributed to it. After following Dr. Graham's raw vegan program, including the reduced fat, which I feel is key, my observable symptoms of the autoimmune condition have either reduced or completely disappeared. And that is amazing.

Since our son is now an adult, we are not sure if we will attempt to birth any more children at this point. But at least I feel like it is a viable option again. Now that I am enjoying the best health and vitality of my life, I am confident that I would have a successful pregnancy and a healthy child, if I were to become pregnant while following the 80/10/10 plan.

### *Symptoms Gone Since 80/10/10*

My condition tended to make my blood clot more readily, which affected my periods (and also caused the miscarriages). I no longer get the clots with my periods, nor the weird hormonal "off" feelings I'd get from ovulation through menstruation.

I no longer bruise mysteriously and easily with the littlest of bumps or pressure. In fact, it's hard to get a bruise these days, even if I have some pretty major thing happen. Lesser events gave me major hematomas before. I also don't get the "restless leg syndrome" all night anymore, or that pain in the veins and arteries of my legs that felt like a clot was forming (that got worse with aspirin or fish oil taken too late in the day).

I don't know if it's all gone yet, but I definitely know my condition isn't getting worse (as it was when following the instructions of my MD and chiropractor). I do plan to get my blood tested when I can for the numerical proof; however, I don't really think I need it anymore. I am fairly convinced that the condition is gone, or lowered to such a degree that it is not a problem anymore.

### Unexpected Gains and Benefits

Dr. Graham's program has improved my life not only in the ways I had hoped for, but also in ways I never imagined were possible. I have eaten 100% raw, low-fat vegan for more than four years so far, and things are still getting better every day. It's amazing—absolutely amazing.

When I first read about Dr. Graham's program, it made total sense to me and had the "ring" of truth. I had some questions about the volume and frequency of food at first, but soon learned (from my body) that my body agreed with even those recommendations. Admittedly, I tend to lean toward Natural Hygiene, and Dr. Graham's recommendations are about the simplest and most efficient way of following Natural Hygiene I've found.

With every other diet change, my results were much more subtle than this. I've eaten variations of the standard American diet (SAD), SAD with no red meat, lacto-ovo vegetarian, lacto-vegetarian, vegan, vegan macrobiotic, vegan Natural Hygiene, and even raw (the living foods way), and others. I felt improvements with each diet change in different ways, but nothing came close to what I've experienced with Dr. Graham's low-fat 80/10/10 diet. It's worlds—no, universes—no, even more than that—different, and better.

I just can't begin to describe the difference. My health has far surpassed the condition it has ever been in for as far back as I can remember. I have experienced improvements in my energy, vitality, abilities, attitude, and appearance that I never even imagined were possible. I don't get so worn out at the end of the day anymore, and I sleep much more restfully. I have a new level of joy in my life, and I experience daily the plain enjoyment of being alive. I'm feeling less shy and more adventurous socially as well, so I'm more outgoing.

I am back to the clothing sizes I wore once I reached my adult height at the age of thirteen, yet am firmer and stronger than I was then. The stretch marks from the pregnancy of my now eighteen-year-old son have become firmer and less saggy—even when I'm on my hands and knees. I now get regular and varied exercise and plenty of recreation. I have greater strength, power, agility, muscle, and overall physical and mental abilities than ever before.

I recently broke a toe 90 minutes into a terrific Ashtanga yoga practice session, while I was doing a jump-through on a cement floor and didn't quite lift enough (as I'm still a beginner)—oops! I had broken that toe on the other foot before 80/10/10 and had such a rough time with it back then. This time, even though it took a lot more to break the toe, it hardly swelled up, so it didn't really hurt afterward. I am also more in touch with my body, so the toe healed much more quickly and smoothly than before. Last time I had to tape the toes together, wear a special shoe to walk, and keep it up for several weeks, in pain. This time my toe "said" it didn't want taping. It was not painful, though it still wanted to be put up—but not as desperately, and it simply wanted mainly sleep for the first two weeks. I still had to work and walk at the farmer's markets and in our garden, resulting in more time on the foot this time, yet it hurt less and healed faster.

At three weeks, my toe was what I would have considered completely healed before, as I could do everything I did before 80/10/10. That's less than a third of the time it took the first time. Since I'm more active now than at any other time in my life, it took a few more weeks before I could do everything I was doing again—still less than half the time it took for a less-severe break that occurred before going low-fat raw vegan. My foot feels as good as new now and doesn't give me any trouble in any of my activities, even with the contortions and stresses I put it through in the process. Nice.

### *Now I Love to Exercise!*

The first thing that I noticed when switching from approximately 20% of calories from fat to 10% or less was that I felt better. My body seemed to get down to deeper repair work. My legs suddenly felt lighter and stronger, too, like they could jump really high more easily—and they wanted to, so I did. My husband was simultaneously amused and amazed.

When I first started eating low-fat raw vegan, I used to have to get my son or husband to carry the watermelons I got at the market. Now, not only do I carry them myself with ease, I can even carry two of them at a time—and they're each twice as big, too!

For the first time in my life I actually truly want to exercise. I find myself looking for excuses to move my body, which is very foreign to me indeed. I had always been one to find excuses to sit where I was and not exercise. Never before have I experienced looking forward to my free time in order to exercise! As a result, I'm starting to look more athletic. People now think I'm a dancer or a gymnast.

I feel so physically adventurous now—loads more than I ever was before. I'm no daredevil or anything—I'm not skydiving or bungee jumping—but I have become more athletic, and I'm willing to try new things that require physical activity, purely for the fun of it or just to see if I can. (It's not hard to be more willing than I used to be … heck, I wasn't at all willing before.) I'm no bodybuilder, although my body's been building itself quite nicely. I have been gaining strength, endurance, and muscle weight while eating this way—once I got rid of most of my excess fat, that is.

I discovered new physical abilities, as well. My balance, coordination, and dexterity dramatically improved somehow, even at the beginning, before I had been active much at all. My aerobic exercise had always been limited by my breathing capacity, because I would lose my breath long before my muscles would get enough of a workout to work out my heart.

Now, in retrospect and in comparison, it was like I had been running on dirty fuel when I exercised before. Suddenly, aerobic workouts felt so "clean" and "crisp." I felt like I could go forever (but my heart wasn't used to it, so I took it gradually). I could breathe really deeply and not have that sick and dirty feeling at the beginning. It was and still is great! Now when I'm exercising, I feel happy and my body feels happy, which makes me happier, which gives me more energy and motivation to keep exercising, which makes me even happier, and so on … I love it! I've never felt like this before.

Until I was following Dr. Graham's program for a while, I never was able to do full-on push ups, even though I used to bodybuild a bit in college and could do hundreds of bent-knee push-ups in various hand arrangements when doing martial arts in high school. I discovered that I could do a full push-up after eating this way for a time, and I worked on them to see how many I could do. I got up to 23 in a row before I moved onto something else.

I later went back to push-ups, going airborne this time by quickly powering the pushing so that at the top of my full push-up my hands and toes hop off the ground while keeping my full body tight and straight! I got up to 15 in a row before I got sidetracked with pull-ups.

I got a pull-up/chin-up bar for myself and couldn't even pull myself up enough to make a movement at first—as had been the case all my life. My husband showed me how to help myself with a step stool and after a month, I could lift myself halfway up. Exciting! It wasn't much longer before one day I pulled myself all the way up—without the step stool. My chin was all the way above that bar on my own—not just above but high above, so the bar was at my chest and my chin was above the door! Not long after that, I became hooked on Ashtanga yoga practice, so I haven't continued with the chin-ups much since. I'm having so much fun!

I went surfing for the first time ever about a year into the 80/10/10 lifestyle. I did pretty darn well, especially for a then thirty-eight-year-old mom who had only ridden a skateboard a few times (for only a few feet each time), a boogie board once, and a surfboard not at all. I stood up and rode the very first wave! I was catching little waves on my own and riding after only about 45 minutes. Cool!

I belonged to a health club for a while about a year into 80/10/10 and was surprised to find myself, a petite 5'2", then 98 pound woman, lifting about the same weight or more than the businessmen there, without effort. I was more surprised to find that some days I could just keep adding more and more weight, seemingly to no end. I would go with small increments, so on those days, I usually ended up getting tired from the number of reps before the weight ever got to be too heavy.

Big guys were always there lifting tons of weight in order to build more muscle and get more "cut"...and then there's little old me lifting relatively minute amounts of weight while my muscles just burst out. I can actually feel my muscles growing during my "off" time, and they don't get sore if I eat fruit afterwards like Dr. Graham suggests. It makes me feel bad for them—if only they would do their exercises properly and follow Dr. Graham's program, they'd get much better results for their time and effort.

These days, I no longer go to the health club, as I've gotten more into bodyweight exercises, Ashtanga yoga, aerial fabric, dance, and other things. I also have free weights at home and at work, if I decide that I want to use them. The machines are fun, but they aren't "calling" me right now.

### *This Is Eeeeeasy ...*

I have found this way of eating is much, much, much easier, quicker, and more efficient than any other I've tried. Life itself has also become easier overall. Not only do I have greater peace of mind, increased physical abilities, increased energy, and greater health and happiness, but my personal needs are so much simpler and easier to meet than before. I have more time and resources to spend on other things. My life is very full of activities and responsibilities, so this improvement really helps.

I know that there is no way I could have done all that I have done and all that I am doing, if I were still eating any other way. Since beginning Dr. Graham's program, I started homeschooling my gifted and dyslexic son with self-created custom curricula, started two corporations with my husband, organized a local branch of our church, was ordained as one of the clergy, and counseled members of our congregation. I have also started a homeschooling support group, araw food support group, and organized regular raw food potlucks, all with corresponding websites.

I am still doing all of these things now, and I am also writing two books, filming a video/TV series, working on building up my fitness level, doing occasional work for long-standing clients from my old consultancy, and of course, continuing to maintain terrific and loving relationships with both my husband and my son.

Now I find it much easier to go places for the day, or even a few days. I have less stuff to take with me. I no longer need to walk around with a water bottle on a shoulder strap so I always have water. I don't even use it during the day now. I still drink water in the morning and after intense exercise, but I don't find the need for it otherwise. My body regulates its temperature better, so I don't need to take as many clothing options with me when going out, either.

Because of my autoimmune condition, I used to get sunburned almost in minutes, at times even in the shade, whereas now I can stay in the sun without a burn ten times longer than I used to. My skin is not tan yet, but it's not pasty anymore. I don't need to desperately seek out the shade at the beach, or figure out which hat will stay on and give me adequate protection. I can actually take walks on the beach without all the cover-up gear and out of the shade. I only use a sun hat if I'm out in the full sun during midday. For the first time, I can go to the farmer's market in the afternoon without a hat and no burn!

My hair is just getting silkier and better looking—without shampoo or conditioner! Wow! My skin, teeth, and nails have never looked or felt better either. Amazing, because while I brush and floss my teeth and bathe daily with water, I haven't used shampoo, conditioner, face soap, body soap, toothpaste, deodorant, makeup, lotion, sunscreen, bug repellant, or anything but water on my body (except dish soap on my hands) for over two and a half years now. Funny—just some scrubbing and water. Who'd have thought?

My skin has never been smoother or more lovely than it is now, and I am virtually free of the acne that I've had ever since puberty. People comment frequently now on how my skin "glows," how healthy I look, and how pretty my hair is, wanting to touch it and do things with it. I haven't had people wanting to do that with my hair since I was a very young child.

Eating this way requires little food preparation. All I have to do is put my fruit for the day in a box, and maybe grab some salad and tomatoes if I don't have enough at work already, and go. No need to slice, spread, arrange, layer, bag, or cook, transfer, clean, etc., as with cooked food. Of course, you can make the 80/10/10rv food fancy enough for any gourmet undertaking if you want, but you don't have to go through all that every day just to eat.

If I don't have enough with me or get caught out at mealtime, I can go into practically any grocery store and get fruit. No more shakiness, spaciness, and low blood sugar if I have to skip or delay a meal. Instead I feel fine and still perform well mentally and physically until I refuel.

If I know I'm going to have a busy day, I'll throw some fruit and possibly greens or celery in a blender with water in the morning before I leave, to take with me to drink while working. I take a bit of this, watered down, to Ashtanga as my sports drink and often drink the full smoothie afterwards on my drive back to work. I have a blender at work too, in case I decide to exercise or have a smoothie or dressing while there, as I am often at the office for over twelve hours at a time. But in truth, I rarely need or want to use it at work.

I use less trash, and have more compost with which I can grow more food. At the end of the day, I have only a salad bowl, occasionally a smoothie container, and a compost container to wash for the whole day. You can do that with just water, too, if you do it right away.

The day we got rid of our stove was such a wonderful day. It was such a freeing experience, and it made the whole kitchen seem so much cleaner somehow. I have no need for pots, pans, ovens, or other cooking appliances and accessories. In fact, I could get away without any food-preparation utensils or dishes at all if I wanted to. I don't need spices, herbs, medications, vitamins, minerals, or other supplements, either. It's just so much simpler and more natural—less expensive too.

### *Finally, I'm at Peace*

Prior to going raw, I had been close to a nervous breakdown as a result of living in a high state of stress for several years. I knew I needed to de-stress, but I couldn't see how, without conditions changing in my life. I couldn't exercise or do other stress-relieving activities, because I would just feel like I was getting further behind on things, which would stress me out even more (counterproductive to say the least).

Now I am far less prone to stress and emotional baggage issues. My emotions are more even and at a higher level than before. I still attend to things, but I don't feel stressed about them. I feel too good to bother, actually. It is not my life that changed, it's me. I simply am not as stressed about things anymore. In fact, I have had even more stressful things happen in my life than before, yet I have felt less stressed during these times.

It's kind of hard to describe … I guess the best way is to say that I'm at peace, more so than ever before—at peace with who I am, who everyone else is, and with what is going on in my life and around me. From my experience, good health truly is happiness and peace of mind. I just plain feel good, and it's hard to get too down when you feel so darned good all the time, you know? My body tells me it wants to play, and I follow!

### *Learning to Eat Enough Food*

Once I started on Dr. Graham's program, I started really liking my food again. It is yummy, and I look forward to it. I don't put off my meals until I get ravenous anymore. I used to be so disinterested in and uninspired by my food that I'd wait until I was so hungry I would just grab whatever was closest and quickest—which was almost never a healthy food choice. My body just wasn't interested in the food I was giving it. Now that I'm providing healthy food for my body, it loves my food, and so do I.

I find it fairly easy to get enough calories now, but it took a while to get to the level of eating this much. When I started out, I wasn't eating enough calories, although I felt fine. I think my body just didn't want that much food back then, because it wanted to clear out old stuff. I figured out that I was only eating as many calories as would support an 80-pound person, but I also realized I had some fat to live off of to help my transition.

Over time, it did work out. Initially, I only lost weight because I had excess fat. Eventually I lost most of the fat, gained some new muscle (and weight along with it), and gradually started eating more calories naturally as my body adjusted to things. Currently, I probably eat more calories than some would think I should and many think I could. It works out anyway, as I am getting stronger, gaining weight while keeping a healthy body-fat level, and I am feeling quite well.

### *Don't Live a Little ... Live a Lot!*

If you're looking to save time and effort in finding what works, look no further. Dr. Graham's method works. I used to "live a little" from passing pleasures like non-optimum food, sacrificing my health and well-being in the process. Now I "live a lot." I don't feel badly about my food choices or feel like I'm giving up anything. I'm choosing better health and more lasting pleasure, and I am all the more happy as a result. I feel so much better and see so many results that I am inspired to keep going and don't want to go back to cooked food or even high-fat raw. The fleeting satisfaction just isn't worth the risk of losing all that I've gained.

This raw stuff is amazing. Not raw any way—but this low-fat vegan way—that's what's making the difference! The more I follow all of Dr. Graham's recommendations (which incorporate other lifestyle factors besides diet: exercise, rest, pure water, pure air, sunshine, sleep, recreation, etc.), the easier it is to stay on the 80/10/10 raw vegan diet, and the better I feel. In fact, eating this way has enabled me to joyfully and naturally make improvements in many other areas of my life, which I was unable to do before, no matter how hard I tried.

To sum it all up, I just feel so alive! I want to tell the world! It's so simple, and it works so well! I feel like my body is celebrating life on a cellular level—it is happy to be alive and wants to move to celebrate. I gladly oblige. Happy happy, joy joy, happy happy, joy!

Reading my praise of Dr. Graham and his program, you may not realize that I am actually exceedingly cautious and conservative about recommending any products or services, as I take this responsibility seriously. That said, I highly recommend that you read and reread this book as many times as necessary, until you are able to try this program and discover for yourself just how life-enhancing it is. Give it a good chance though, and follow everything as much as possible. Like any generic guideline, the program described in this book may need adjusting for your individual situation. The general method has worked wonders for me. I wholeheartedly recommend a private consultation with Dr. Graham to clarify or address special health issues, if you need to. You won't be sorry.

Janie has a website, www.ringlet.org, which documents her first six months of following Dr. Graham's program and includes a photo history of her as well. She is currently writing two 80/10/10 raw vegan-related books: Ready for Raw, due out in Summer 2005, and A Fruit Lover's Guide to Edible Fruit, to be released later. She also stars in a video/TV series on similar subjects due to be released in late 2005 or early 2006.

## Richard ("Ribs") Friedland, Malibu, California

I became a vegetarian in 1967, because I heard it would heighten my consciousness. It all made sense to me right away, especially when I realized that the way I had been eating was contributing to the death of innocent animals, and that I could eat in a way that might be healthier, raise my awareness, and not harm other creatures that lived on the earth.

I went through a lot of changes during the first four years on a vegetarian diet. I ate a lot of junk food in the beginning, as long as it wasn't meat, fish, or eggs, and that made it easy for me to stick with the diet. Then I started to switch from regular commercial sweets to organic health-food sweets and organic goat's milk ice cream. I tried macrobiotics in those years, which was interesting but very hard for me to stay on.

Against the advice of three doctors who said they would put their reputation on the line that I couldn't survive for more than 18 months, I became a fruitarian in 1971 for a lot of the same reasons that I became a vegetarian. I ate only raw fruit, which didn't include nuts or seeds or dried, frozen, of dehydrated fruit. I followed this diet very strictly for eight years.

I didn't know anything about the fat content of the avocados and olives I picked and ate raw from the trees. (Yes, I did actually like the taste of one particular type of olive. If I allowed the smooth green ones to ripen on the tree until they were black and shriveled, I enjoyed their taste and ate quite a few at a time). I also had never heard of food combining, so I generally mixed anything that was available on a given day. For example, I might eat avocados, dates, tomatoes, and citrus within a few hours of each other, although I didn't do that often.

I read a few books about fruitarianism, like Arnold Ehret's Mucusless-Diet Healing System, and then I waited to see if I would have experiences like they described in the book: almost unlimited energy, and incredible strength and endurance. I did not get the results I was hoping for after eight years. I still had sinus problems, along with gas and mucus.

For the next couple years, I ate raw foods, with mostly fruit. I went to see a lot of alternative doctors, including ayurvedic practitioners and others in the next few years. I had a lot of tests and a lot of dental work done. A number of these alternative and ayurvedic doctors suggested very strongly that animal products would be beneficial for me, as well as spicier foods, because I was too yin or cold, and I needed yang, heating foods.

I did try chicken, fish, and eggs, with cayenne pepper and very little fruit, for about six months in the winter of 1985. I didn't feel much worse when I ate those foods, but I really didn't like the idea of consuming innocent animals, and I didn't feel stronger and healthier like all the doctors said I would. So I started eating sweet fruits again.

In 1992 I met a Natural Hygienist who explained to me about food combining. I bought Dr. Shelton's book and started eating raw fruits and vegetables at certain times in certain combinations, as described in his book.

I did this for about eight years until one night after eating some cherimoyas and sapotes I woke up after about two hours of sleep and couldn't fall back to sleep. I was very uncomfortable the whole night, trying to relax, massaging myself, and attempting to stretch. Finally, I did an enema at around 4 am and felt a little better. I couldn't figure out what had caused this, and I thought it might be a fluke. Well, the same thing happened the next night. That was much more difficult, because I only got an hour of sleep both nights, and I was exhausted. It was hard to think and figure out what to do next.

I was eating all raw fruits and vegetables in combination, which included daily nuts, seeds, and avocados, and I was eating a late last meal of sweet fruit around 10 pm, which was pretty close to when I went to sleep. The main reason I ate that late was that I found it impossible to sleep if I didn't. So I figured I would eat some raw sweet fruit, which was my favorite food. I didn't sleep for four nights straight, and on the fourth night I started to panic. I called the paramedics and told them I might be having a heart attack. I couldn't tell what was going on. They took me to St. John's hospital, where I was tested for hours. Doctors there finally told me that my heart and cholesterol were perfect. The only problem they could find in all their extensive testing was that I had a $B_{12}$ deficiency.

I left St. John's in the morning and went to the Westside Alternative Center, which did a lot more very expensive testing. The tests cost me as much as the hospital bills from St. John's, which came to a few thousand dollars. After about a week, I received the results from the tests from the alternative clinic, and they said I had a $B_{12}$/folic acid deficiency. I took $B_{12}$ injections in my butt for a few days, and then they put me on folic acid supplements.

I started asking everyone I knew for help and information, because I still didn't know what had caused my inability to sleep. I also wasn't sure what I should be eating, because I had been eating the same way for 20 years straight. I knew a 30-year raw food chiropractor who told me not to eat any sweet fruits and to get my $B_{12}$ from Standard Process Labs. I felt a lot better for a while. That chiropractor died in a bicycle accident, and I went back to eating sweet fruit.

I tried different cleanses, including the Arise and Shine one-month cleanse, which I followed to the letter. I got really weak during the final week of the cleanse, where you don't eat any food. I called the company to ask about it, and they thought it was some type of parasite like candida. I went to a doctor, who said that I could send a stool sample to the Great Smokies laboratory if I wanted to know for sure whether I had candida. The test results showed that I had two strains of candida at the highest level. All my symptoms made sense to the doctor, because she had recovered from candida and had written a book about it.

They say with candida that fruit feeds it, and I ate a lot of fruit. I went on a long, expensive candida cleanse for six months and felt pretty lousy the whole time. I ate nothing sweet for six months, not even carrots or lemons, and I had to rotate my foods every four days. I took a lot of supplements, including Super Garlic, Primal Defense, some expensive flora from England, and many others.

I had a really difficult time during those six months. I found it hard to get any work done, because all my symptoms had gotten more extreme. I was so uncomfortable. I stayed with it for the full six months and then took another stool test, which showed that I still had candida albicans at the highest level. The doctor suggested taking prescription drugs, and I started back on a diet with sweet fruits.

I tried numerous other diets, supplements, and cleanses during the next few years, until I heard Doug Graham and Rozi Gruben speak at an event called Raw Passion. Rozi talked about what happens to the blood when we eat certain foods. Doug said that it isn't the sugar in fruits, but rather the fat that people with candida consume that inhibits the body's ability to get the sugar out of the blood.

I didn't know whether what they were saying was absolutely what was happening with me, but I knew I liked both of them immediately. They seemed to have a lot of conviction about what they were saying, and they definitely had done extensive research and discovered a lot of information.

I started to reflect on my situation. No one, out of the many, many doctors I had consulted with over the years had helped me make any health improvements. I thought I was on the best diet I could think of, but I wasn't feeling well. These two people looked very healthy. It seemed obvious they had extensive knowledge about health and had already worked with people in a similar situation to mine, with improvements. If I didn't like the way it was working, I could always go back to the way I was eating now. I didn't have anything to lose by cutting out fats except my illness. There wasn't really much of a decision left to make.

I started eliminating fat from my diet that very day, and I began experiencing some very heavy elimination. I didn't eat any overt fats for six months, because I didn't know about 80/10/10, and I thought the idea was to eat as little fat as possible, so I did. This meant no avocado, olives, or durian, and of course no nuts or seeds.

Also, I didn't know about Doug's VegSource board, so I went back to eating a raw diet with fat in it. The elimination slowed way down. I ate that way for the next six months, even though I felt terrible again, until I saw Doug speak at the Living Light House in Santa Monica. I got to ask him some questions, which he was very willing to answer, and I cut the fat again. Except this time I ate an 811 diet, which meant that I ate a little fat once in a while.

I had so many wonderful improvements, but I still didn't have the full health picture. So I saved up a little cash and had a private consultation with Dr. Graham. During the consultation, we sat down face to face within two feet of each other. This was really helpful to me, because I got a sense of what he was all about. I found a genuine, caring individual who was absolutely interested in improving my health. It was hard to imagine what he would come up with to help me, because I was following the diet to a T. At the time, I thought that was what it was all about.

What I didn't realize, is that diet is only one part of a healthy lifestyle, and that you're only as strong as your weakest link. Those were only words to me at the time, but after he found an aspect of my life that needed some work and I worked on it, my health improved dramatically. That means I felt better. What greater gift could anyone give to me? I felt more energy, and I enjoyed living more. That's the best gift you can get!

One of the topics we covered in the consultation was Doug's sports camp, called Health and Fitness Week. He thought it was important for me to attend, and he asked me what he could do to make it possible. I didn't see how I could ever work it out at the time, because I had just spent all my extra money on this consultation, and I had so little time. But I took a risk, because it seemed like I needed so much to happen. I told him all the conditions it would take to make it possible for me to come, and he helped me work it all out! I was just amazed by the honesty, sincerity, knowledge, and dedication of this person standing right in front of me, along with his sincere desire to help me with my personal health issues.

I attended the sports camp, and it was the best thing I could have done. It was so helpful and beneficial that I ended up signing up for the following year's sports camp before I left. This was the jump-start I needed to get headed down the road to true health. If you can figure out any way to make the next camp, I recommend that you do it, whatever it takes!

I've been on the 80/10/10 diet for a year now and have had the most remarkable success with it! I just want to share this with people. When you start to feel really good after not feeling so good for a long time, you want to let other people know that they can feel better, too.

People sometimes ask me what I typically eat in a day, so I will share it with you. I usually eat three meals a day, once in a while only two. I normally eat my breakfast at around 10 a.m. Yesterday (April 2005), I ate 12 ounces of blueberries, 8 ounces of raspberries, 8 ounces of boysenberries, and about 4 green baskets of strawberries. I ate lunch at 2:30 p.m., which consisted of 6 cherimoyas and 4 sapotes. I ate supper at 7:30 p.m.—about 8 pickling cucumbers, 1½ heads of red butter lettuce, about 5 lbs. of tomatoes, and a couple of celery stalks.

Today as I write, it's 10:30 a.m. After I do my last set of 100 stomach crunches and maybe some push-ups, I will eat breakfast, which will be 12 ounces of blueberries and about 4 or 5 baskets of strawberries. If I'm still hungry, I'll eat a papaya. For lunch I will eat at least 4 or 5 more cherimoyas, because I already felt them and they are perfectly ripe! I'll also eat some sapotes and 2 or 3 mangos. I'll probably have a similar supper, but I might have some avocado if it ripens up or some sugar snap peas, depending on how I feel at suppertime and what exercise I've done today.

The first benefit I noticed from 80/10/10 was that I didn't feel spacey or bloated when I ate sweet fruit. That was a great relief to me, because I loved to eat sweet fruits, but getting bloated and spacey made it very difficult to work, exercise, or focus on projects. The next amazing benefit I experienced was that I started to be able to exercise without all the pain and discomfort that had made it next to impossible for me to exercise more than one day a week. The pain has improved to the point now that I can exercise every day, which is wonderful, because I get a lot of very good benefits from exercising. The third improvement was that I didn't need to eat late at night in order to fall asleep. This helped me not to wake up as groggy and out of it in the morning. Now I can get going earlier and start doing things I need to do, like work or exercise or take care of the kids. I've had other side benefits, like my body getting more toned and looking better. Also, being stronger overall is nice, too.

It's hard to explain how much better my life is now as compared to the way it was before I was following 811. It's like I'm a new person who is not horribly sick with candida and whatever other problems I might have had. Not only has my life improved tremendously, but I continue to get better daily. This is fantastic beyond anything I could have imagined the day I first heard Doug and Rozi speak about food during the Raw Passion event.

Not only have these two people dedicated their lives to sharing health with as many people as possible, but they have also identified some of the most important keys to achieving and maintaining ideal health.

If anyone is interested in health, they should start following the 811 way of life. I can't imagine anything that a person could possibly do that would be anywhere near as important—or as helpful. 811 is a healthy way to live life, and there's so much more to it than just diet. Food is only one part of the whole picture of health.

One of the things that really impressed me about the 811 lifestyle is that emotional stability is considered just as important as diet or any other factor of healthful living. Emotional work has been the main focus of my life for the last 35 years. When I heard Rozi explain that we need to feel all our feelings no matter what they are, I realized that she understood feelings in the same way I did, and I consider feelings to be what I know most about in the world.

So there you have it: Doug and Rozi have developed a system of living that incorporates all of the important factors to achieve optimal health for human beings on this planet. I plan on following this lifestyle and learning more and more about myself and about health every day. I wish everyone who reads my story the best of luck on their path to better health.

## Laurie Masters, San Jose, California

During my first five or so years of eating a substantially raw diet, I blew through at least one 32-ounce bottle of flax oil each month. I ate an avocado most every day and night, and I ate plenty of prepared nut and seed dishes. For about a year, I brought an almond/raisin torte (with my special lemon-date-spearmint frosting) to every raw potluck.

Like my raw friends, I was eating a ton of fat and didn't know it. I thought I was eating a fantastically healthful diet. I ate dishes like raw granola, oat groats blended with soaked almonds, or bananas and almond butter for breakfast. These probably averaged 250 fat calories. Lunch was usually a salad with one avocado (and that addictive lemon/oil/Bragg/garlic dressing). Between my lunch and dinner salads, I would down ¼ cup of flax oil each and every day … that's 480 calories of pure fat right there! I often ate a second avocado at dinner, the two of them probably totaling about 450 fat calories. The nut/seed concoctions I made for dinner (mock tuna, salmon nori, etc.), contributed another 400 calories of fat. That's 1,580 calories of overt fat in my day. My total calories probably ran about 2,000 per day—which meant that I was eating about 79% fat! WOW!!

My "healthy" eating was somewhat legendary within my own little world. Goodness! The salads I would concoct in the lunchroom at my Silicon Valley offices … It was the company joke. On the way out to local restaurants for lunch each day, the analysts I worked with would take a field trip past the lunchroom to see what "shrubbery" Laurie was eating today! They called my salad bowl "the trough." At 88 pounds and five feet tall (I've been that size since I was 14; it has nothing to do with raw food), I could pound down a lot of salad. Or at least it looked that way to mainstream eaters.

I spent an ungodly amount of time in the kitchen each day, even buying a second food processor, blender, and juicer to keep in my office so that I could now also whip up mock tuna and other such concoctions for lunch if I wanted … which did nothing for my caloronutrient ratio, let me tell you!

I enjoyed my food (who wouldn't, with all that fat and salt), and I enjoyed the attention I received ("Where is a tiny person like you putting all that FOOD!?"). But I had one problem: my longstanding fatigue and lifelong recurring bronchial infections were NOT getting any better than they were when I ate cooked food. It was maddening!

As a child, I recall having a cold at least once every two months. Without fail, I'd get swollen glands a day or two before the full-on bronchial affront would begin. Next, I'd get a croupy cough, a sore throat, and sometimes earaches. I'd always hope that the cold would stay in my head this time, but darned if it didn't "go down to my lungs" every single time. These "colds" never lasted less than 8 or 10 days.

I lived on antibiotics. Mom would have us stop them early when our symptoms went away, so we could "save" some antibiotics. That way, we would have some on hand and wouldn't have to wait for a doctor's appointment the next time. At the slightest indication of swollen glands, I'd pop the pills ... "to nip it in the bud," you know? We were smart consumers!

It's a wonder I got through school at all. I was often absent a full week of school in a month. I'd do my schoolwork from home, my bedroom desk stocked with antibiotics, throat lozenges, vitamin C, and expectorant cough syrup. I spent a good portion of each winter "under the vaporizer," as we called it. The bedroom walls and windows would be wet with condensation from the mentholated vaporizer steam mom used to try to keep me breathing.

Somehow, though, I managed never to manifest a diagnosable disease ... mainly just those incessant chest colds. They continued unabated through my young adult life. Chronically underslept and overstressed, I worked ridiculously long hours at my college studies and at my jobs, living on adrenaline and working right through my ongoing illnesses. I'd come to work with no voice. I'd take work home and work from bed. I'm quite sure I exhausted my body to a devastating degree.

By 1990, newly married and still working crazy hours as operations manager at a small electronics company, I was diagnosed with Epstein-Barr virus. Regularly sick, and dragging myself to work each day, I continued the downward spiral of ignoring my body and pushing through the colds, flus, episodes of strep throat and bronchitis, and occasional cases of pneumonia. I remember nearly falling asleep on the road driving home from work just about every day that summer. Sometimes I'd pull over and nap for awhile, but mostly I'd talk or sing or scream out loud, slap my own face, and blast the music while I drove, trying to push my exhausted body another 20 minutes until I could get home.

In the eighties I worked for a wealthy stockbroker who took us on incentive bonus trips to places like New Orleans, where we would eat at five-star restaurants night after night. I learned to love rich, gourmet foods and ate more than my share of prime rib and creamy risotto. After nine years of working for this broker and her husband, I could no longer afford my own taste in food.

Always interested in what I believed to be health and nutrition, however, I tended more toward grilled vegetables and fish, rarely if ever eating fast food. I pored over magazines for "healthy" recipes. At home I would broil oil-coated vegetables and pour them over corkscrew pasta topped with pine nuts and herbs, sure that I was eating a supremely healthful meal.

Then at age 34 (1997), I learned about raw foods from Pam Masters, a light-filled soul who taught hundreds of people in the San Francisco Bay Area to eat raw food and heal their bodies as she had done herself. Pam shared with us dozens of hand-written recipes that she had learned to make at Hippocrates Health Institute years before. Wow! This rich, salty, fatty "health food" was right up my alley! I loved what I was learning, and my taste buds loved it even more.

Yet it never added up: I ate all this healthy food but still had endless severe head colds. Instead of getting better, it seemed as if my colds were coming more frequently and were increasingly more virulent. They never lasted less than three weeks, usually dragging on a month or more at a time. I would lose my voice completely, every time. I would cough violently. I would still work right through it all. In the late 1990s, it seemed I spent more of the year with a cold than I spent feeling good.

Finally one day in total desperation, I phoned Doug Graham in Florida. I still have the audiotape of that phone conversation. We were friends by then, so he knew of my history of chest colds … but I had never asked him for help, so he hadn't laid it on the line to me. Now I was asking, and I was in tears. First, he asked me to list for him what I ate on an average day. He listened patiently, then he told me what he tells nearly every raw fooder who consults with him: "Laurie, you're eating way too much fat and not nearly enough fruit."

Never having had a weight problem, I had no concept of how many calories or how much fat was in the foods I ate. I didn't believe that my diet could be as full of fat as he claimed, but I started investigating. Over the past half-dozen years, I have delved deeply into caloronutrient calculations, verifying for myself the tremendous amounts of fat that raw fooders are eating. I learned that nuts and seeds average about 75% fat. (Who was the rocket scientist who told us these were protein foods?) This kind of information gave me motivation to make some serious changes!

Now, I have learned to eat pretty darned close to an 80/10/10 diet (cooked and raw, not the rv version). A lot of people fall over when they hear the quantity of fruit I eat each day. Together with my partner, Tim Trader, I buy bananas by the case—we go through about 250 a week. We frequent farmer's markets, and our kitchen counter is a beautiful cornucopia of dozens and dozens of colorful fresh fruits at all times. I start every day with a 12-banana smoothie to which I add about a pound of one or two other types of fruit: pears, strawberries, mangos, stone fruits … whatever catches my eye. (Yes, all that plus a couple cups of distilled water does fit into one Vita-Mix container; it makes nearly three quarts.) Or I'll eat a banana/celery smoothie, sometimes adding parsley or kale or cilantro or other greens to it. Most days I continue eating fruit in the afternoon (grapes, mangos, watermelon, nectarines, etc.) and then eat a salad for dinner, usually with cooked vegetables as well. I am working on incorporating more whole foods and fewer smoothies … but for now this is what works for me.

My fat consumption has dwindled dramatically. These days when I eat at home, I eat about 2 avocados a week and virtually no nuts or seeds, except some ground flax on my salads. I am just not attracted to heavy foods anymore. My salad dressing is often a Mexican salsa, or sometimes just fresh-squeezed orange juice or blended fruit. About once a month I blend fruit and nuts for dressing (six strawberries, one orange, and eight mac nuts, for example, or 2 oranges and 2 tablespoons of tahini). Rarely, I still have a salad with ½ tablespoon of olive oil, but a small bottle of oil these days would last me years.

Here is a list of what I actually ate one day in July of 2004:

- 9 bananas (900 grams/32 ounces)
- 1 apple (200 grams/7 ounces)
- 4 khadrawy dates
- 2 navel oranges (200 grams/7 ounces)
- 16 strawberries (250 grams/9 ounces)
- 1 nectarine (120 grams/4.2 ounces)
- 3 figs (100 grams/3.5 ounces)
- 10 cherries (60 grams/2 ounces)
- 3 small tomatoes (250 grams, 8.5 ounces)

- ½ large head of lettuce (225 grams/9 ounces)
- a little cabbage (100 grams/3.5 ounces)
- a few sugar snap peas (25 grams/1 ounce)
- ½ ear of white corn (35 grams/1.25 ounces)
- lemon juice
- ½ tablespoon olive oil
- The verdict? 1,740 calories, 87% carbs, 6% protein, 7% fat. Not bad!

At potlucks and other events (maybe six times per year), I still usually eat at least a small portion of those gut-bomb combinations I used to consume daily. I still enjoy the taste of the high-fat dishes, but they're almost always far too heavy and salty for me anymore—which is no small statement, as salt for me has been a lifetime addiction!

Life is getting better and better. Slowly but surely I am learning to move this body. For decades, I used to think to myself with resignation that I would never feel good enough to exercise in this lifetime. I do have a lifetime of adrenal exhaustion to undo ... so it's not happening as quickly as I'd like. But the fact that I get motivated to move at all is an unforeseen miracle.

I get lots and lots of sunshine. My skin never used to tan, but now it's brown all summer long. I know that the sun is nature's disinfectant and that the sun nourishes me. The toxins that cause skin cancer live inside of acidic bodies filled with fat, and the sun merely draws the poisons to the surface, like a poultice ... but research shows that the sun does not cause cancer in people who eat a low-fat diet. Don't let anyone tell you that it does.

My colds are coming far less often now. In fact, the last one was two years ago. This may not sound like a big thing, but for me it's a miracle—and a direct result of my low-fat diet. Naturally, I always thought of myself as "perfectly healthy, except for these colds." But the truth is, I spent a great deal of my life in misery, and I missed out on lots of life.

One more thing: since I've been raw, I keep nothing medicinal or supplemental in my house, period. Except for a couple of daily vitamins I took as a kid, a bottle or two of Shaklee vitamins in my twenties, and the enzyme tablets I bought in my first year of eating raw foods, I pretty much haven't touched herbs, algaes, minerals, powdered greens, or other such refined, dehydrated, encapsulated nonfood items of any kind. Thankfully, that's one part of the high-fat raw regimen I managed to steer clear of!

If I hadn't learned about the low-fat (raw) vegan diet, I'm sure that my forties would have been a downward spiral of evermore frequent, ever-worsening chronic illness. Instead, I have a new life to look forward to. For me, whole-food 80/10/10 is the way to eat as Nature intended ... it's far easier, lighter, and healthier than all those fatty, salty, dehydrated, taste bud-pleasing "transitional" foods I began this journey with.

I am deeply grateful to Doug (and Rozi Gruben and Tim Trader) for helping me learn how to eat high-fruit raw! Finally, after a lifetime of increasingly debilitating chest colds that lasted a minimum of three weeks at a time and came three to six times a year, I am feeling better all the time... and even exercising! Yes!! All is, most certainly, well!

## Lisa Oborne, Toronto, Ontario, Canada

As a child, I spent numerous days in the hospital and often missed school due to asthma and allergies, among other maladies. In an average year, I would miss 70 days of school. At age 12, a severe asthma attack put me in the hospital for more than a week, where I had to be in an oxygen tent. Even so, I turned blue many times.

After leaving the hospital, I instinctively began changing my eating habits and I became a vegetarian. In my childhood years, cheese, eggs, and fish were the only "meats" I ate. This change in diet helped, and my health began to improve. I believed I was doing the best I could for my health.

At age 24, I was in a major car accident. With no feeling in my body from the neck down, I was told by my doctor that I would be in a wheelchair, probably for the rest of my life. After he left the room, something amazing happened: an electrical current came from within, starting in my head and working its way down to my toes. I immediately sat up and walked out of the hospital. This was the turning point in my life. I knew that my body was capable of amazing things, although I did not know how or why. With new respect, I began to listen to my body's messages.

Wanting to learn more about my body's functions, and sensing that I needed to trust more fully in its capabilities, I began reading widely in the area of natural health. My curiosity only grew the more I learned. I have since taken many classes/courses in Natural Hygiene, including those offered by Dr. Doug Graham and Dr. Robert Sniadach.

More than four years ago, after attempting to resolve some of my lingering health problems, I went to a naturopath, who informed me that I had very weak kidneys and was a Type 2 diabetic. I could not understand. I had changed my diet, I had been vegan for over 12 years at this time, and tried to live a simple life ... what more could I do? I did notice that I did not have a lot of energy, and although I slept nine to ten hours a night, I still woke up tired. I decided I needed to take action.

On December 1, 2000, I began a 30-day juice diet. It was not nearly as difficult as I thought it would be. Upon completion of the 30 days, my kidneys had rebuilt themselves and the signs of diabetes were gone, as well as 30 pounds. That was an added bonus. Then I was faced with the question of what to do next. During my studies, I had read a lot of books by Dr. Shelton, and I asked myself if the raw diet was for me. The response was a resounding "YES!"

I tried the raw diet, beginning very simply. Not yet understanding the variety of ways that people eat raw, I ate a very low-fruit diet for more than 12 months, with a lot of greens and nuts & seeds. After about six months, the initial energy I received from this new diet started to dwindle, and I was feeling very weak. I promised myself I would do this for 12 months, so I continued, and unfortunately, my health did not improve at all. Everyone I saw asked me what was wrong with me. I looked very thin and my skin tone was grey. I had become a skinny fat person. I had dropped down to 116 lbs., but what I did not know was that my body fat was over 35%. My muscle tone was terrible, and I did not have the energy to exercise. My asthma was getting worse, so even if I wanted to exercise I could not.

One day, my husband was searching the Internet and discovered Dr. Doug Graham's website. I signed up to attend Healthful Living International's first symposium in 2002. I tried to do Dr. D.'s diet based on what was on the Web, immediately increasing my fruit consumption and dropping the quantity of nuts and seeds in my diet. Although my energy started to pick up, my asthma symptoms were still there.

I did not realize how much in my life would change after attending the symposium. I spoke one-on-one with Dr. D. and received a lot of fantastic advice. I immediately started putting his advice into play and saw changes very quickly. Now my energy really started picking up. I got more productive sleep at night, and my skin tone started to improve.

It took until June of the following year for my asthma symptoms to be reduced to the point that I no longer needed my meds, which I had been on for over 30 years. I finally had the energy to begin exercising, and my lungs were now able to handle the extra load.

I began going to a gym and started bodybuilding. Still holding over 30% body fat, I could not believe the strength I had ... it was incredible! Needless to say, my progress was huge in a very short period of time. I put on 35 lbs. of muscle in less than one year and reduced my body fat by more than 10%.

When I started on the 80/10/10 diet 12 months ago, my recovery time was approximately 2 weeks per body part. The weight that I am lifting now has increased substantially, a minimum of 300% on any body part. My recovery time is now approximately three to five days per body part without overtraining.

My plans now are to enter either a bodybuilding contest or a strongwoman competition. I want to have one more year of training before entering to improve my strength and muscle density. This is somewhat amazing, coming from a person who, until I met Dr. D., was not able to do any exercise because of my illnesses and weaknesses.

My exercise regimen now consists of weight training, martial arts, kickboxing, yoga, jogging with my dogs, and running at dog agility classes. Without Dr. D., I would never have been able to do any form of exercise, let alone progressed to the level of amateur competition. Thank you, Dr. D.

## Ireland Lawrence, Mission Viejo, California

At 22 years of age, I was up to 300 pounds and had to work hard to maintain that weight, speed walking six to nine miles a day and eating no more than 1,500 calories a day. I also had my hair falling out in clumps, no menstruation, acne, and lethargy. In addition, I had autism, hyper dyslexia, and attention deficit disorder. I had to rehearse my speech for hours to make a simple phone call and spontaneous speech was not something I could do. I had difficulty in school and stressed out over writing, often spending several hours on writing just one single paragraph.

For my weight and hair loss, I went to doctors who told me to lose weight by exercising and going on a diet. I cut my calories down to 500 calories a day for a few months and lost a half pound a week. But I found it an impractical lifestyle, as I felt depressed and even more lethargic. I was desperate for a useful solution.

I started by going to the health-food store and reading every book they carried on diet. I found a short book on raw foods. It made sense to me, and the next day I began the diet. I had been a vegetarian for about six years prior, but raw foods was much easier. At the time, I understood raw foods to be fruits and vegetables and greens that were not cooked. I went to the market and bought all the different fruits, celery, and coconuts. I put them all in a bin in the refrigerator and ate whenever I was hungry.

I lost five pounds the first day and twenty pounds the first month. I found that counting calories and undereating no longer worked; for the more I ate raw foods, the louder my body screamed when I was going against it. Also, I could feel my body becoming worn out and exhausted. I stopped exercising and rested, taking sunbaths and slow walks during the day and attending class for five hours at night. I did this for about six months, at the end of which I lost about 80 pounds, had regular periods, and no more acne. Then I transferred to a new university and led a stressful lifestyle studying until late at night, living in a building full of mold and lead paint, and drinking lots of orange juice, which I later learned was pasteurized.

The health improvements I noticed dwindled and I went to a doctor. I was diagnosed with hypothyroidism, hypoglycemia, insulin resistance, and polycystic ovarian syndrome, which included cysts all over my ovaries and no ovulation. These were all conditions I had prior to the raw foods diet, but they had been undiagnosed. The doctor recommended a low-carbohydrate diet. I decided to try a vegetarian version of it and did not feel much better. I stayed on this for two years. I often thought about how great I felt on raw foods when I first tried it and wondered why that process stopped.

Eventually, more raw food books came out, and I realized that the "fresh-squeezed" orange juice I had been drinking was pasteurized and may have adversely impacted my health, along with the stress I was under. I decided to try raw foods again. The first several months I ate raw foods as before—fruits, vegetables, and greens. I noticed even more health improvements: I menstruated regularly, after three months the cysts on my ovaries were gone, I began to ovulate, I had no clinical evidence of insulin resistance, and after a year, my thyroid was healthy and I lost five pounds a month, getting down to 150 pounds. Reading and writing were no longer difficult, and I could speak without rehearsing.

After I had spent about six months back into raw foods, the diet started to pick up in popularity in my area. There was a family that came to town and gave a talk and dinner on raw foods. They included nuts and seeds (which I previously did not include as raw foods) and gave recipes for foods like raw veggie burgers, raw un-chocolate cake, and raw ice cream made with spices, salt, honey, flavoring extracts, frozen fruits, and nut milks. They introduced me to the "eat anything as long as it is raw" diet. Soon, I added all these items to my diet. I then hit a plateau where for about two years, I noticed no health improvements, although my health did not deteriorate either.

I started investigating what changes I could make to again experience health improvements. I began practicing Ashtanga yoga daily and noticed improvements in strength and vigor. Also, I did some consultations with some of the raw foodists whose books I had read. One told me that my liver was severely damaged from all the weight I lost and that I needed to do 12 liver flushes with 1 cup of olive oil and lemon juice. I did them but did not notice a difference.

Another told me that fruit was causing my body to be taken over by fungus, so I cut out all sweet fruit. I ate avocados—up to 5 a day—as well as greens, sea weeds, and vegetables. I did that for one month, at which point I began to have bruises all over my body. I added low-sweet fruits for two months and did not get any more bruises but did not feel better either.

Then I went back to the "eat anything as long as it is raw" diet. Soon after, I injured my back in yoga. I kept going to practice but made modifications. After a month, my back still had not healed. I added MSM, thinking it was the missing link that would heal my back. I had what I thought was more energy and slept five hours a night, but I also had heart palpitations, and my back stayed the same.

Eventually, I cut out the MSM and experienced mononucleosis. I think taking the MSM led to excess stimulation, resulting in a lack of sleep and subsequent weakened immune system; mono was one of the consequences. I stopped taking the MSM and was so lethargic for months that walking upstairs was a big event. I stopped practicing yoga and I eventually recovered—both from the back injury and mono.

I still did not feel right though. So I added raw dairy mainly in the form of raw goat milk cheese, thinking I had some sort of protein deficiency. I became addicted to it and ate it every day for two months. I felt worse at this point but did not realize it. Then I went camping for a month.

One morning, some wild turkeys were outside my tent eating breakfast. I opened my tent and said, "Good morning turkeys!" They did not answer. They just ignored me. It occurred to me that I am not here for their purposes, and they are not here for mine. I thought about goats and the goat cheese I was eating and decided not to eat it any more. I went two days without eating it. I was craving it though, so I had some. I watched my mood change as anger and hatred engulfed my body. I realized the impact eating the goat cheese had. After that, I made a commitment not to eat it anymore. It took several weeks until I no longer thought about it.

I started to read the VegSource website where Dr. Graham has a discussion board. I had lurked there before. I even tried eating lots of fruit and low fat, but I felt groggy and addicted to fruit when I did that. But this time I kept lurking and reading. Eventually, I read a post where Dr. Graham talked about chasing your fruits with greens. Then I realized a change I could make—eating more greens. Until then, my greens consisted of the salad I ate each week and the occasional glass of green juice. But I was not eating green leafy vegetables regularly. Also, I thought greens had to be kale, collards, dandelion—dark greens—otherwise they were not nutritious; but I did not care for the taste of them.

I gave Dr. Graham's 80/10/10 raw vegan diet a try. I began eating fruit and following it with mild greens like celery or romaine. I started with a leaf or stick and worked up to two bunches of celery and/or two heads of romaine each day, along with a very large quantity (at least a dozen) of one or two types of fruit each day. Also, I cut out all supplements, spices, oils, frozen fruit, juices, salt, dehydrated foods, raw dairy, honey, green powders, and seaweeds. I started losing weight again. I began craving movement again and took up running and went back to practicing yoga. Most days I now average two hours of yoga, one hour of pranayama, 1 hour of running, and 25 to 50 handstands.

I also started to let go of bottled-up emotions. Now, they just flow out. I think that when I was eating heavier raw foods and spices and juices, there were a lot of emotions like anger and hurt that were right at the surface, but they kept getting shoved down with the foods I was eating. Now there is a channel opened for them to freely float out.

I no longer overeat or binge on foods. I am in touch with my body and feel full and know what my body needs. For example, shortly after I began running, I pulled a muscle in my back on the right side. I could not roll over on that side. I knew that if I rested, it would heal. I did that and after two days, it was back to normal. There was a time when I would have ignored my body and gone running anyway, but my body speaks so loudly now, it is hard to go against it and effortless to work with it.

I have been following Dr. Graham's 80/10/10 raw vegan lifestyle guidelines for four months now and have noticed more improvements in those four months than in four years on the "eat anything as long as it is raw" diet. The simplicity of the raw food diet is what was first attractive. After reading a simple book on raw foods, I instinctively followed a plan similar to the 80/10/10 raw vegan diet. It is only when I read more books and listened to others that I veered from what I knew worked for me and stopped doing what I knew was useful to me.

I have learned that if given the right conditions, my body will let me know what it needs and the key is to go with what I know works and tune out all the chatter—both my own and that of others. Dr. Graham is the only example I have come across in the raw food movement of what works for the long term.

## Roen Horn, Sacramento, California

Looking back, I definitely could have avoided a lot of troubles if I had known about the 80/10/10 diet at the start of my raw journey. At age 15, I became convinced by my brother and also Internet sites I visited, that fruitarianism was the ultimate ideal, because it avoided "killing the plant." I had already advanced through the stages of vegetarianism and veganism, which had caused me to lose some weight. After becoming a fruitarian, I immediately started to lose more weight, and I was already very thin!

My mother was concerned and sent me to get a checkup. From that point on, because of my low weight (111 lbs. at 6'1" tall), the doctor's scary threats of antipsychotic drugs and hospitalization lingered over me. I was scheduled for weekly checkups to ensure that I gained weight—or else!

Believe it or not, my psychologist told me that I was mentally ill/obsessive compulsive, because I wouldn't eat hot dogs, hamburgers, ice cream, donuts, etc. like "normal kids." He also ignorantly claimed that no one eating only nuts, seeds, fruits and vegetables could possibly sustain his life, and that I would die from malnutrition if I persisted! Furthermore, he said that if I would not take his word for it, I was "delusional."

With the pressure from both the doctors and my mother, I gave up my raw fruitarian diet. I began eating a cooked diet that included a lot of grain dishes, such as spaghetti, couscous, and rice, but I insisted on taking my oatmeal raw. This heavy-grain diet caused me to be the most constipated I've been in my entire life, and it exacerbated my acne problem. It did, however, increase my weight from 111 to 125 lbs.

Fed up with the loss of control over my diet, I decided that I would once again eat only raw fruits, vegetable fruits, nuts, and seeds. Doing so, I felt better, but again I began losing weight. So I started to trick my mom and the doctors with weights on my ankles and in my pants. Admittedly, I wasn't concerned that this change caused my weight to drop to 107 lbs., because I felt great, was strong, and my blood tests came out fine. In fact, fruitarians were telling me that I had to lose weight to "detox." After this phase, they insisted that the weight would naturally come back on the same diet.

Well, as you will see as this story progresses, I nearly starved myself to death waiting nine months for that to happen, and I don't recommend it!

I loved avocados, so I often ate meals of them. I did not know better, and as a result, I continued to break out and was extremely constipated, even as a raw fruitarian. Here I was, on what I thought to be the ultimate diet, still contending with many health challenges. Even though I stopped eating cooked grains, which I assumed were to blame for my problems, and despite eating a ton of fruit, my bowel movements were infrequent, very small, hard as rocks, and painful to pass. It was so bad that many times I had to strain to get anything to come out! I was confused, thinking that a raw diet should be the last thing to cause constipation. Later I would discover that not all raw diets are the same, and the variations certainly produce different results.

It wasn't long until the weights were discovered. Soon, Child Protective Services (CPS) arrived at my house with a warrant to seize me for a psychological evaluation and possibly put me into a mental illness lockdown facility! In the kitchen (while peeling the first orange for my breakfast meal), I heard the argument between my parents and the officers, and I shot out the back door. With the help of my brother and my cousin, who understood that I was not mentally ill but just wanted to be healthy, I ran away to Canada, accompanied by my brother.

My brother and I made up fake names and identities, and we became known as the "Wild Bush Boys of BC." I was forced into this fugitive role, having been told that if the American authorities got their hands on me they were going to make me eat "normal" food and force-feed me Ensure (a "liquid meal replacement" drink that is extremely loaded with refined sugar and artificial additives—designed to "ensure" proper nutrition) through a tube if I refused to drink it!

Still dealing with constipation, when I got to Canada, I went for a colonic irrigation. After studying my eyes, the colon hydrotherapist (who also happened to be an iridologist) told me that my bowels had been left with no options other than to balloon out and form "pockets." If she was right, then I may have to deal with these pockets for the rest of my life. If I had read Dr. Graham's book Grain Damage, I would have known better!!!

On the road, and with limited funds, I didn't have access to all the fruit I wanted, so I started losing even more weight. Eventually I was put into a Canadian hospital through the efforts of a very concerned woman who helped and befriended us. My body had unwittingly wasted, losing mass until my weight plummeted to only 84 pounds. Even I was shocked!

At first I was absolutely panic stricken with the thought that they were going to make me eat cooked processed hospital food, but to my utter relief, this hospital let my brother go to the health-food store daily and bring me the raw organic foods that I requested!

Having lost faith in the fruitarian diet that had failed me, and being in such a vulnerable state, I was completely open to new ideas. Following the advice of many raw food books, I decided to gain weight "the healthy way." In addition to the green leafy vegetables, I began eating TONS of fat. Some days I was wolfing down 6 or 7 avocados a day, not to mention all the nuts, seeds, nut butters, and oil I used in my dressings. Having abandoned some of my previous dietary dogma, I felt that I had opened a window and had "seen the light." I thought that I had finally found what worked for me. Little did I know what I was getting into!

Because I was already in a hospital (just as the American doctors had wanted), and because I thought I had nothing to lose, I agreed to risk blowing my cover to be filmed by the Canadian media. Sure enough, this event led to my discovery, and nine months after I ran away, my family finally found out where I was.

When my parents came to visit me, I told my mother that I wasn't a fruitarian anymore, but now I was a raw foodist. With some prodding from my mom, I completely gave up the fruitarian ideology by adding some cruciferous vegetables and roots (eating roots requires the death of the plant) to my diet. With this new identity of being a raw foodist, I tried to prove to everyone that I was flexible in my eating habits. At this point I subscribed to the "ism" of raw, pretty much eating anything as long as it was "raw."

Hempseed butter ... tahini ... cacao ... "Is it raw?" became the ultimate question. Everything so far was in accordance with the raw books that I was reading. However, my mother encouraged me to eat sushi, raw eggs, and raw dairy, which were forbidden by many raw foodists.

Although I agreed in theory to eat these foods, it was more of a put-on than anything else. There was no raw dairy to be had, and the hospital wouldn't allow raw eggs (or raw milk for that matter). My mom got me some raw smoked salmon, but I gladly used the excuse that it contained table salt as my reason not to eat it. However, despite my aversion to animal foods, I did include some fresh raw egg yolks when I got home, because some raw food authors approved of them, and because they seemed to be less of a taboo in my own mind.

Despite gaining weight very rapidly in the Canadian hospital (in only a couple of months I was up to 110 lbs. and rising), and in spite of how far I had come from being a fruitarian, those meddling American doctors had me flown to America in an emergency supersonic jet (flown in from Japan), where they unjustly locked me in a mental institution and tried to coerce and trick me into eating cooked hospital foods!

My mom adamantly warned them what a raw food expert told her—that raw foodist's bodies have a tough time adjusting cold turkey to a standard diet. Since they have less of a mucosal lining as a barrier from allergens and toxins, they need to gradually introduce cooked foods, starting first with lightly steamed vegetables, and should also avoid glutinous grains. Her words were utterly disregarded!

I could fill pages expressing the horrors of my experience with this lockdown facility. As soon as I got there, I was offered a plate of chicken, milk, greasy rice, canned green beans, and chocolate cake! The nurses led me to believe I had to eat what was on my plate or drink Ensure. Faced with these options, both of which were wretched nutritional abominations, I started to panic. Thinking that all my previous attempts at eating healthy and my running away to avoid the hospital and its food may have been in vain, I almost had a nervous breakdown.

Now under the control of CPS, I felt vulnerable without the protection of my parents. But I didn't lose my wits and give in. Seeing as how this American hospital was much different from the Canadian one, I realized that I would have to be persistent. Eventually, after much persuasion, I was given raw food.

How did I finagle myself out of cooked food and Ensure? My guess is that my weight wasn't low enough to warrant force feeding, and I was willing to eat what little variety of raw foods the hospital offered (mainly walnuts and some poorly ripened bananas, apples, and oranges).

Much to the disappointment of the psychiatrist who was in charge of me and was planning to starve me into submission, a judge ordered that she must let my parents bring me more variety of what I would eat. Finally, the psychiatrist realized that her plans to control me and make me eat cooked food were futile, so I was released under many conditions.

Having achieved one victory, I was soon faced with a new challenge. Not long after I was released from the hospital, I had my body-fat percentage tested, and it was 25%!!! (Conventional "wisdom" considers body fat in the mid-teens to be healthy for men; however, I later learned from Dr. Graham that single digits—under 10%, ideally about 4 to 8% for an athletic male—is a truly healthful level of body fat.)

The lady who tested me was shocked that such a skinny person could be so fat! She said I was looking at increased chances of heart disease and many other health challenges as I got older. It looks as though my weight-gaining strategy was working all too well!

During a visit to the doctor who was appointed to oversee my weight gain, my mother expressed deep concern about my 25% body fat and the substantial abdominal cellulite I had developed. But my doctor showed no concern and even told us that it was "anorexic thinking" for us to be concerned with my body-fat percentage!

I'm not surprised that I became fat, considering that neither hospital would let me exercise. The American hospital even went so far as to tell me to sit down if I was caught idly standing!!! This is why I blame the doctors for my exceptionally high body-fat percentage. For the second time, they had blatantly ignored my mom's reasoning—she had forewarned the doctors what she had read—that it was vitally important for emaciated people to exercise while they gain weight or they would only gain fat—not muscle.

Even knowing that my body-fat percentage was high, I forced myself to gain more weight every day, to meet the demands of the doctors (they wanted me to be in the 10th percentile of BMI charts—where 10% of males my height and age weigh the same as I do—even though the 5th percentile is normally considered acceptable). This was absurd, since I didn't have enough muscle for my age to meet this requirement without having an excessively high body-fat percentage.

I always feared being put back in the mental facility, because one of the conditions of my release had been that if I went four weeks without weight gain they could put me back ... only next time I would have to cooperate and eat hospital food!

They should have known that this was unreasonable, because muscle is slow to gain. I heard that even the best bodybuilders rarely gain more than a pound of muscle a month. I felt trapped, and I continued to eat unhealthy amounts of avocados, nuts, seeds, and oils to gain this weight within deadlines the doctors had set for me. In the back of my mind, I was scared by the thought that every pound I gained would even further add to my already-too-high body-fat percentage. I knew that I should be exercising to gain muscle, but I was not in the best of shape, and I didn't have enough energy to motivate vigorous exercise.

Further adding to the problem, I became introduced to raw potlucks. The dishes there mimicked all my favorite cooked foods, only this time, they were "healthy" (… not!) Luckily, I was too lazy to make them at home, or else I probably would have eaten nothing else! I had completely forgotten my hygienic background of mono fruit meals, and I had lost the euphoric joyful feeling of simple eating.

Many raw food books had it so backward, even as to proclaim fruits as the enemy because they had too much sugar. Thank goodness I was never strict enough to exclude fruits, but I did limit them, which even further added to the number of calories I consumed from fat. I felt heavy, had lots of extremely foul-smelling gas, my acne returned in full force, and I once again suffered from constipation. I didn't feel healthy anymore.

So, what did I do? I turned to superfoods. I thought that I wasn't getting enough minerals or that I must be deficient in some nutrient. Raw food books told me that organic food wasn't enough, and that I must have wild food, and more variety, including the full array of superfood products they sold. So I ordered jars of powdered wild vegetables, bags of cacao beans, and many other "extreme" foods that were supposed to solve all my problems. But none of them could offset the effects of my poorly combined, high-fat diet.

It wasn't until I met Tim Trader and Laurie Masters at the National Essene Gathering in July of 2004 that I got my first dose of 811. Laurie told me that she was editing Dr. Doug Graham's book entitled The 80/10/10 Diet. The two of them described for me the basic concept behind the book—that "Fruit or Fat?" are really the only two choices for getting calories as a raw fooder. I immediately knew that I was on the extreme fat side of "Fruit or Fat?" I told them about my situation, and they showed a genuine concern for my health.

At Tim and Laurie's urging, I got myself to Dr. Graham's lectures at the International Festival of Raw and Living Foods in Portland later that summer. Though the event left me feeling more informed, it was eye-opening to see all the different opinions and conflicting advice among the speakers.

To my relief, it seemed as though Dr. Graham had sorted all this confusing mess of information into a clear, sensible plan. Especially convincing, was his description of how blood-sugar problems, commonly blamed on fruit, are actually caused by the impaired function of insulin due to excess fat consumption. I knew I had to make some changes if I was going to be healthy. If I was going to succeed as a raw foodist, I would have to be more discerning in my food choices. I would have to ask more than, "Is it raw?"

Even after hearing Dr. Graham's compelling speeches, I continually struggled with 811. I must admit, that it was at that very same festival that I left with a CASE of cacao beans! Let me tell you, it is HARD to get over addictions.

I would be lying to say that I didn't attend the very next local raw food potluck after my return home from the Portland Festival. But something had changed. I was no longer ignorant. Now I knew that this fat-laden, "combo-abombo" gourmet food was not furthering my goal of ideal health. There's no way I could enjoy my raw pizza as I had before after hearing Doug's "if it looks like pizza, and tastes like pizza, you can be sure its going to digest like pizza" speech! Now I knew what I should be doing, and if I did slip up, at least I knew it was a slipup.

At the end of August, I attended Raw stock for the first time, and it was a blast. Seeing 811 being practiced up close and personal was so inspiring! I was reminded of how natural and fun it was to eat simply. Knowledge is empowering, and it really does inspire change. After Raw stock, 811 really hit home for me. Now, it was only a matter of correcting bad habits, battling past addictions, and striving for 811 every day.

Whenever I have a question about 811 or other related topics, I can refer to Dr. Graham's VegSource message boards. Dr. Graham himself takes out of his own time to offer his best advice. Many people on the boards offer expert advice and truly speak out of experience. People there are friendly; no matter how silly or trivial the question seems, usually someone can relate or offer their piece of useful insight. This board continually inspires me to continue with my goals, teaching me new information and equipping me with the knowledge to solve my own health challenges.

Knowing what I know now, neither my psychologist nor my mother was right about why I couldn't maintain my weight. I didn't need grains, and I certainly didn't need hot dogs, hamburgers, ice cream, and donuts! All I needed was a little understanding, and a LOT more calories! I just assumed that because I always ate when I was hungry, I was getting enough calories. However, Dr. Graham pointed out that on the standard American diet, the food is dense, high in calories, and doesn't take up a lot of room in the stomach compared to lower-calorie, water-rich fruits and vegetables. He explained that in order to get enough calories on 811, you need to expand the stomach back to its natural size and elasticity in order to fit in a lot more fruit. Not having this little piece of information was, perhaps, the primary cause of my downfall as a fruitarian, second to not including greens.

I thank Laurie Masters, Tim Trader, and Dr. Graham for empowering me to make the right choices. Because of their help, I am no longer ignorant of the consequences of my actions. 811 taught me how to manage my calories without overeating fat, so I have no problem keeping on the weight.

The more fruit and less fat I eat, the more energy I have, and the more I feel like exercising, which is precisely what I need to convert my high body-fat percentage into lean muscular weight. The closer I eat to 811, the more all of my health challenges fade. Clearer skin, better-functioning bowels, and increased energy are a great payoff for my efforts.

It feels good to eat simply, and I LOVE fruit! Unfortunately, I LOVE fat too! I am still struggling, but I am doing my best, and my best gets better every day. At least now I can see where I am going, and I am not walking around with a blindfold on.

Because of past experiences of letting other people influence my decisions and consequently falling into many traps, I have learned to become a very independent thinker. My grandma used to get mad that my parents paid for so many avocados when I could have saved them some money by using olive oil instead. Now, after being a fan of 811 for quite some time, my mom just told me that my grandma says that I'm "mentally ill" because I eat such an abundance of fruits, because I avoid grains, and because I believe Doug Graham.

I just have to smile.☺

## Theresa Remley, Sacramento, California

Finally, I can hear what my body is telling me after a lifetime of confusion and pain. After first experiencing trauma-induced illness at about age five and my health spiraling downward into debilitating physical and mental disorders, I searched diligently for answers. I saw psychologists as a child and psychiatrists as an adult who could never pinpoint the reason for my depression and anxiety because my underdeveloped mind as a child suppressed what happened to me. I was often ill, eventually missing nearly one day out of every week of school in the tenth grade due to sore throat and fever, yet I still managed to excel academically.

In high school, I could not play soccer without having muscular-skeletal pain and spaciness the rest of the day, and chiropractor visits could not repair this continuing problem. At age seventeen, I awoke to severe pain in my lower chest over the course of several nights. An endoscopy located a preulcerous condition, and I received antacid pills as treatment instead of dietary advice, although I was already a vegetarian due to my own conviction.

My general tiredness and sore throat intensified into acute, mono-like symptoms when I was nineteen, so I went to yet another doctor and found out that I had an abnormally high Epstein-Barr lab result. However, this was not explained to me. I thought I had chronic fatigue syndrome, but this illness was widely misunderstood; thus, my symptoms were largely ignored. My college attendance plummeted because of insomnia, mental fogginess, and overwhelming fatigue and pain, and my depression intensified due to my increasing sense of helplessness.

In 1997, I saw a clinical immunologist who finally diagnosed my physical illnesses as chronic fatigue and immune dysfunction syndrome, fibromyalgia, and allergic rhinitis. He told me that I was an "extreme case" with a foreseeable future of having only chronic, disabling illness. I then applied for Social Security income because of his diagnosis which gave credence to my inability to work productively since I was nineteen, and after ongoing battles with the court system, I received the aid.

I never knew how I was supposed to get better, and by fate, I met a chiropractor two years ago who practices neuro-emotional technique, which involves muscle-testing to uncover subconscious thoughts. My childhood trauma finally came out after three months of twice-weekly sessions. The experience was draining, but I was relieved to find out the root to all of my problems. The experiences as a child were more than I ever could have imagined happening to me, so I understood why my once fragile mind could not deal with it all.

I realized then that I had post-traumatic stress disorder and dissociation, which gave me new focus in consequent emotional/ cognitive therapy and EEG brain-training sessions. It all makes sense now—all of my heightened senses, panic attacks, low self-esteem, difficulty concentrating, depression, anger, insomnia, and eating disorders—I can finally see that I reacted normally to something that was not my fault, and I am now taking care of myself out of love that I did not know how to have before.

To think that my doctor once wanted me to take intravenous AIDS medicine—No Way! As if more poison could heal me? I have learned that the band-aids that are put on illnesses do not make them really disappear.

I am extremely sensitive to any form of drug, even those in foods. During this time of illness in my adult life, my vegetarian diet transitioned toward vegan, and I frequented the VegSource.com website for general, vegan recipes. I then went to Dr. McDougall's low-fat whole foods forum and tried that diet, thinking this was the healthiest one for weight loss and vitality, although my body told me otherwise through its digestive upset. I did not understand that this was a big problem, since I had more pressing burdens in my life.

When I spent the time and emotional energy to seriously turn inward and peel away layers of toxic perceptions, I could see more about my eating habits. I saw that I needed sugars for energy, yet I could not eat enough fruits if I ate a cooked food diet because of my digestive troubles due to improper food combinations. I thus felt compelled to eat processed junk food or drink caffeinated tea for stimulation (which made me feel sick too).

After two years of eating that diet (which barely gave me benefit), and finding my identity, I was finally ready to take Dr. Graham's forum on that website seriously. His knowledge of exercise and food-combining principles that consist of low-fat, raw foods with emphasis on fruit fit wonderfully with my newly found focus on holistic health.

I researched the general raw food scene during my immersion into this new lifestyle over one year ago, and I made a few recipes from other leading raw foodists who limit fruit and increase fats and protein. I felt heavy and sick from nuts and oils as well as their improper food combinations, harsh flavorings, and unnecessary foods. I noticed how my candida also flourished while eating that way. Additionally, it was easy for me to overeat the dehydrated and "gourmet" meals, which is something that does not happen when I eat whole, raw fruits and vegetables.

Because I have such a sensitive body, shouldn't all "nutritionists" test their theories on someone like me who can best show if their diets cause harm?

Dr. Graham is the only raw food teacher I will heed because he teaches in accordance with my innate need to eat primarily fresh fruits and tender greens in proper combinations, or just one type of fruit for an entire meal. By eating this way, I obtain instant physical and mental energy that is sustained throughout the day—no more naps and no more aches and pains after eating!

Only by eating this diet can I exercise without stimulants, and my recovery time is much faster with much less pain than if I would eat overt, raw fats and cooked foods. I feel only healthful benefits, as though my body feels clear enough to start serious healing, and my throat and digestive tract began to feel amazingly better within the very first day of eating this way.

When I decide to turn to cooked, vegan food as a type of band-aid to numb my emotions and body, I instantly feel sluggish and dull-minded and have fibromyalgic pain and sinusitis. However, I still do this occasionally for my evening meal, knowing full well that this acts like a drug, because my emotional state is not the strongest. This need for temporary relief sometimes takes precedence over the part of me that "knows better," since cooked food definitely does not promote health for me. Dr. Graham also showed me the addictive power of cooked foods, and my heated supper can easily turn into an all-I-can-eat, vegan buffet unless I consciously plan my meal beforehand. However, even then I end up allowing more cooked food because of my addiction, which presents itself with the very first bite.

It is actually freeing to see this addiction. I am working to be strong enough to stop eating cooked foods entirely, for when I feel emotionally, spiritually, and mentally secure, I abhor the drugged effect that cooked foods, especially grains, give me. My goal is to be complete and connected, and the 100% low-fat, raw diet is an important truth in the big picture of health.

I emphatically believe from experience, that all of my physical symptoms, including candida, are secondary to the greater picture of my system originally shutting down because of the trauma I experienced when I was a young child. Our bodies are meant to heal when allowed to do so, and now is the time for me. I am happy to have finally found a teacher in Dr. Graham, who is a leader by example and an enthusiastic supporter of the intrinsic wisdom within all of us to heal.

## Jacky Dees, West Bend, Wisconsin

For many years, I had a candida overgrowth with severe symptoms. The symptoms were the classic ones—itching, burning, that "yeasty" feeling, digestive problems, constipation, acne, fatigue, depression, plus many, many more. In desperation, I tried everything I could think of to get rid of it. I read every book, pamphlet, article, and website I could find about candida. I spent gobs of money and time trying to cure myself.

I had tried conventional medicine, alternative medicine, supplements, therapies, homeopathics, cleanses, mini-fasts, "candida diets," naturopathy, and hypnosis, and I even had my mercury dental fillings replaced. You name it, I tried it. When nothing worked, I had basically resigned myself to the fact that the candida was here to stay. I would spend the rest of my days feeling like garbage, and I was only 33 years old. Depression set in, and my life turned darker and darker. On my darkest day of all, I decided to go raw, cold turkey. That was January 2002.

During my search for a cure, I had been reading about the raw food diet on the Internet. I started out using the high-fat raw diet, and over the course of the next year or so I lost 30 pounds and looked like a skeleton (I'm 5'3" and I was down to 85 pounds). About half of my hair had fallen out, my teeth hurt, and I was basically an empty, human-shaped shell walking around just trying to get through each day.

The amount of fat I was eating was incredibly high, but I had no idea that in reality, I was eating very few calories. During this time, on the advice of the high-fat raw diet promoters, I ended up on the "candida diet" for nearly a year (no fruit, only raw veggies and fat and tons of supplements). I was convinced that someday the candida overgrowth would just go away and all would be well again. But … that day didn't come.

One day I was reading a popular high-fat raw message board, and I kept seeing people there bad-mouthing Dr. Graham's high-fruit, low-fat diet. I became curious about this guy. I did a search, found his website, and eventually found my way to the VegSource message board hosted by Dr. Graham. I've been reading it daily ever since. I believe it has literally saved my life.

The thing I was struggling with on the high-fat, almost-no-fruit diet was that I desperately wanted to eat fruit but was frightened away from doing so. After reading some of Dr. Graham's VegSource messages on candida, I was absolutely thrilled to learn that I could eat fruit. Just reading that lifted my heart up to the skies. Also, when I read that my candida overgrowth could be gone within weeks on this diet, I could hardly believe it. Could it be? I had been fighting it for six years, and it could be gone literally within WEEKS?!

At this point, I figured that I had nothing to lose. Nothing else had worked, why not try this? I started to eat bananas. More and more bananas. I dropped the fats and ate tons of fruit. And guess what? It happened. Gone. Within weeks.

I had a consultation with Dr. Graham in June 2003 and what he taught me was incredibly enlightening. He educated me about 80/10/10rv and suggested healthy changes to my lifestyle. I began working on improving these aspects of my life.

... And then the bottom fell out from under my world. My father, who had been battling cancer for 14 years, was rapidly nearing the end. I was flying home every other month to see him "one last time." For comfort, I turned to eating cooked food—and not the "good" kind either. I mean junk, and lots of it. My father died a couple days after Christmas 2003; thankfully I was able to be with him during his final hours.

I'm happy to say that after I came home from the funeral, I picked myself up, dusted myself off, and began 80/10/10rv with a vengeance. I've stuck with it ever since, and each day is better than the last. My junk-food binge put the 30 pounds back on, plus more, so I'm working on getting fit and healthy again. One day at a time. I have a long way to go, but I haven't felt this good since I was in my mid-20s.

Today, I am a 37-year-old female, 5'3" tall, and about 120 pounds. I eat approximately 2,000 calories per day and exercise daily. Most days, my lunch consists of 11–12 bananas plus celery or lettuce, and for dinner I eat fruit in season and a large salad. I keep overt fats to only a couple of times a week. My goals are to lose the excess fat, build some muscle, and improve my overall fitness. Signs of improved health have returned—my hair grew back, my skin cleared up, my teeth stopped hurting, and my digestion is improving. I'm also working on getting more sleep, sunshine, and fresh air. It's been, and continues to be, a fantastic journey.

I thought it was worthwhile to tell my story to let people know that this diet and lifestyle do work to get rid of a candida overgrowth. I know firsthand. I was severely losing the battle against candida when I started the 80/10/10rv lifestyle. Now, I've not only beaten it, I've left it in the dust and gone on to win so many more battles.

The weapon to beat candida overgrowth is in the palm of your hand. If you decide to you use it, I promise you, you won't be disappointed.

## Valerie Mills Daly, Camp Hill, Pennsylvania

For the first forty years of my life, I was totally immersed in the standard American diet, depending a lot on processed foods and, as time went on, the fast food world as well. After the birth of my children in my mid-twenties, my body weight gradually increased, but my overall health was okay, at least to my way of thinking at that time. Sure, I would get colds and flu now and then, and yes, I wasn't as eager to run around in the park after my kids, and yes, the stairs seemed to be more of a challenge, but overall I saw myself as a fairly healthy person, even though the excess weight (at this time 70 pounds over my lowest adult weight) did not please me.

Just before turning 40, I married my second husband, and his children were attempting to be vegetarians, of the egg- and dairy-eating variety. As a way of connecting with the kids, I began to investigate this way of life, and decided it wouldn't really be that hard to change. So, for the next five years, we ate a mostly vegetarian diet, during which time I put on another 70 pounds. I also began to have problems with my health.

During this time, I also saw my husband dealing with several health issues which included high blood pressure, Type 2 diabetes, and gastric reflux. I also witnessed the severe side effects of the various medications he began to take to deal with these issues, and I found myself wanting to avoid the same kind of experience.

However, as time went on, my health problems began to multiply. I became asthmatic, which was very frightening. I also began to have problems with gastric reflux and a hiatal hernia. For the first time I had problems with blood pressure, and when I was 41 or 42, I was diagnosed with sleep apnea, and had to start using a CPAP (continuous positive airway pressure) machine at night to control my breathing. I had very little energy, began to have fairly regular anxiety attacks, and felt very low emotionally much of the time. I had perpetual head congestion, and I continuously cleared my throat. I began to have problems with dry skin and brittle nails, and then psoriasis began to appear. I began to break out with hives fairly regularly but could not find out what was causing them. My hair began to thin very noticeably.

Then about five years ago, there was a period of time when I had intense itching all over my body, but especially in the extremities, combined with intense swelling of my hands and feet. Then there was extreme joint pain in my knees and ankles. This went on for about a year. My doctor could not diagnose the problem and sent me to a rheumatologist who suggested that I might have something called psoriatic arthritis, and that I should try a certain medication. I can't remember what it was called, but I do remember that he said that it would require monthly visits for blood work, since the medication was highly toxic to the liver. So, I made a choice—I thought I could better deal with the itching and swelling than I could deal with not having a liver—so I just said, "No thanks!"

I began to seriously investigate the area of nutrition at this time, and some friends encouraged me to consider going vegan. I dropped the dairy and eggs that had continued to be part of my diet. I LOVED cheese, but I hated what was happening to my body, so I tried it out. I ate mostly fruits, veggies, grains, legumes, some raw and some cooked. I began to see some improvement almost immediately; the psoriasis began to fade away, I was able to use the CPAP less and less, and I began to lose some weight.

I was feeling pretty good about what was happening, and continued to do research in the area of vegan nutrition. That was good, but what was not good was that I began to increase my use of vegan processed foods, and I began to think I needed certain kinds of supplements. My cupboard began to fill with various powders, pills, etc., all guaranteed to be good for me. I also began to experience increased anxiety trying to find the "right way" to become healthy. I also gained another 20 pounds.

I then connected with some folks who were following a modified raw diet, averaging about 85% raw (15% fruit, the rest veggies, seeds and nuts) and 15% cooked. They used supplements, but minimally, and juicing was a large part of the diet, as well as making mock cooked foods, often with the help of a dehydrator. I was intrigued, and I gave it a try. I bought a juicer, I bought a dehydrator, I bought the books, I bought the special supplements.

I dropped processed foods entirely, drank a lot of juice, and ate a lot of salad. Cooked food portions would often be based on potatoes, brown rice, whole-grain pasta, or bread. I began to see improvement again: the weight began to come off, I had increased energy, I was able to get rid of the CPAP completely, and my gastric reflux disappeared. I still had problems with itching, but it had decreased.

The problem I ran into with this way of life, however, was that I began to have days of weakness and hunger, which I would assuage with nuts and dried fruits, or dense foods like hummus, other legumes, tahini, almond butter, etc. And I found I was beginning to feel some of the old heaviness and apathy that I remembered from my SAD days. I couldn't understand it, because I thought I was doing everything right. The other thing was, that I was simply tired of working so hard to make the right kind of food for me to eat, especially since I was still cooking SAD food for my husband.

Then, I became familiar with the world of the 100% raw foodists; initially, it was the writings of Victoria Boutenko and her family, Alissa Cohen, and Frederic Patenaude that opened the raw food door for me. Their enthusiasm, their stories, their sincerity—all of this inspired me to at least give it a try. So I bought books, milk bags, and slicers, got myself all ready to go … and ran into another wall.

The more I read, the more confused I got, because there were even more voices out there in the raw food world, and it was hard to find folks who would agree on the constituent parts of the optimal diet. And I was really afraid of not doing it "right." I might get sick, or I might fall apart. (Funny, how I didn't worry about this so much when I was eating Twinkies and Ding Dongs!) Again, anxiety was my friend.

Finally, through a friend, I became familiar with Dr. Doug Graham and his work in the area of raw food and Natural Hygiene. At first, I thought, "This is just way too extreme," but the more I read, the more I was attracted by the simplicity and common sense in his information. It was hard to imagine that eating mostly fruit could be good for me, and the whole 811 thing was pretty intimidating at first. (I am the Almond Butter Queen!) But I came to believe that it just might work for me. While some other paths had helped, I always seemed to come back to some basic problem with all of them.

Another part of his program that made a huge difference in my thinking was his list of the other elements of hygiene. As Dr. Doug says, you can eat all the right foods, but you are only as healthy as your weakest link—whether that be sleep, rest, water, sunshine, movement, etc. I could see that I was looking at what I was eating to heal me, and I was totally ignoring the other aspects of my health. I was trying to function on five hours of sleep each night, no rest during the day, not enough water, very little exercise or activity, no time outdoors in the sun at all (I didn't want to get cancer … go figure). I had never come across such a comprehensive program, and I decided to give it a try.

Well, it has been several months now. I am slowly losing weight (about a pound a week on average; I still have over a hundred pounds to lose, but I'm not worried … it's coming off). My skin has improved, I am more alert, and my mood is generally positive. I have no more anxiety attacks, no more swelling and itching of my hands and feet. I have no more gastric reflux at all, no more joint or neck pain, and my head congestion is minimal at worst (I can sing again without going into spasms of coughing, much to my relief).

I am trying to establish a more regular schedule of sleep, and I use my lunch hour for rest, sitting in my car and listening to soft music for an hour each day. I don't juice as much, and while I sometimes have monomeals, I still find myself depending on smoothies for a good portion of my food intake.

I am not 100% consistent, but I have come a lot closer to the 811 ideal for my intake, and it was easier than I thought. And it is definitely easier to eat a pile of clementines for dinner, than trying to make a raw vegan version of the cooked food I am preparing for my husband!

When we go visiting, I just pack a couple of boxes of fruit, and eat that wherever we go; most of my family and friends are used to this by now. If I go out for dinner, I just call the restaurant ahead of time. If they can accommodate me, great; if not, I eat before we go out and just go along for the company.

Things that I used to think would be hard about this way of life no longer seem that way to me. I am so tired of being so limited, so sick of having to deal with so much pain, that I am no longer willing to compromise in the name of "peace" with others; it is a false kind of peace that demands that I do something that will ultimately hurt me. I am going to turn 50 in 2005, and I hope to be even healthier and more energetic than I am now. Every day seems to be better than the day before, and I find even the hard things easier to handle. I would not go back for anything!

## Kathy Raine, Ithaca, New York

I went raw six years ago for chronic intense jaw pain, which subsided on the raw vegan diet when nothing else had helped. My husband and two young children went raw with me, but eventually we fell away from it. When my pain came back, we went raw again, and I researched a little bit more about the raw vegan diet through books and the Internet. I experienced initial improvement, but after a while I hit a plateau with my healing, and then started having health problems again. I felt I must be doing something wrong; I was sure that raw vegan was my best option, but I was starting to get frustrated.

All along my journey, I had been confronting and clearing up fears, misgivings, bad habits, and preconceptions about nutrition that were ingrained into me for years, and slowly but surely, I was making progress. I knew that the more simply I ate, the better I felt, but I wasn't ready to step into Dr. Graham's 80/10/10, low-fat diet until after I heard him speak at the raw festival in western New York state for the third year in a row. What he says about food and health makes a lot of sense. He also walks the talk about exercise and is very inspiring in that respect.

When we got home from the festival, my family and I went right to raw, fresh, whole, ripe, and organic fruits and vegetables. Our health started improving again right away, and it is slowly gaining every day. An added benefit is that life is much simpler now. I'm not spending hours prepping, dehydrating, and assembling fancy raw meals. I buy a wide variety of fruits and veggies, and now it's easier for my family to just look around the kitchen and see what it is their body wants for nourishment. We also make sure we exercise every day, and have fun doing it.

So in the last weeks that we've been eating this way, we're doing better than ever without all the nuts, oils, and dried "foods" we once relied on. We've also been doing very well without supplements and powders, thank you. Our energy, strength, stamina, and even mental attitude are improved. Our skin is healthier, our sleep better, and those little and not-so-little health problems that were sneaking back are now sneaking away. It's a great relief to have Dr. Graham's science and experience guiding my family and me.

## Carina Honga, Langley, B.C., Canada

In January 2005 my alarm clock went off. The time had been long coming, but now my health was deteriorating rapidly, and this time, my body wouldn't let me hit the snooze.

I was 22 years old, a full-time university student, and a professional model. It was crunch time. I had the biggest project of my academic career on my plate, no time for hiccups. However, amidst this external chaos was an invisible parallel crisis being waged inside my body.

Health had always been an issue for me; I had been given enough red flags in my youth to make a bed sheet. Every second bite of food I took seemed to bite back, increasingly so as time passed, and I quickly developed an unbalanced relationship with food. The bloating of my abdomen would often leave me appearing several months pregnant. I spent my adolescence hiding my inner pain, embarrassed by my symptoms. During this time, I was also very active as a competitive figure skater, and so my caloric intake was incredibly high, which only complicated my digestion further.

By 2005 I had long since abolished gluten and dairy from my diet of my own volition, and following the indications of "health care professionals," animal meat became the staple of my diet. I was told I needed it to build muscle for training. I was told I needed it because of my blood type (O–). I was told that I needed it for my candida, for calories, for this and that; in short, meat was the answer to all of my problems. I conceded, and reaped the consequences. My symptoms worsened.

So, when my digestion slowed even further in the fall of 2004, and ulcer symptoms mounted, I was not caught off guard. I listened to the suggestions of doctors and naturopaths and began to eat meat several times an hour to subdue the burning in my stomach. It was a stressful time, as I was heavily involved in a large-scale project that I was in charge of coordinating. Quickly, the anxiety attacks began. By now, my outward appearance evidenced my internal strife, to everyone but me. I maintained focus on school and ignored my health, modifying my involvement in projects only to the extent that I would pause for anxiety attacks. Life went on.

I made it through that semester with the help of family and friends. Come January however, the alarm was sounding so loudly that it became hard to ignore. My bowels were moving once every 10 days at best, and attempts to medicate my ulcer symptoms lead to mouth lesions. I was experiencing dizzy and fainting spells, as my blood pressure dropped and heart rate plummeted. I was forced to drop half of my school course load, as I was all but bedridden. Unable to care for myself sufficiently, I moved home.

The deciding factor came when my mother, a registered nurse, came home from work one day disturbed by a girl my age who had just been diagnosed with colon cancer. You're next, she thought. Everything I had been told by the medical community had led me to this.

I dropped everything and began my own research.

I soon happened upon information about raw food that changed my life. It didn't change my life because it was about raw—this is key—but because it described the natural, physiologically sound relationship that humans are meant to have with food, and with life. I first read David Klein's Self Healing Colitis and Crohn's, which lead me to Dr. Graham. In retrospect, had I found the wrong info on raw, I know that I would have continued to worsen. I was very lucky.

My diet changed overnight. Let me rephrase that, my life changed overnight. I stopped eating everything I had been eating and started to eat fruit. Within days, I had the first normal bowel movements I had ever experienced. However, my digestive system still on the mend, I followed my instincts and ate very small amounts of juicy fruit. This continued for about six weeks, after which I finally started to increase the quantity; somewhere between two and three months, I added in vegetables.

Also after six weeks, I noticed that my eyesight had normalized completely, after a decade of wearing glasses. Not just slightly improved, but entirely normal. My nails began to grow thick and strong, as did my hair, which thankfully stopped falling out. (I have since learned that this is a common occurrence among people switching to 811, predictably followed by a healthy regrowth of new hair.) My eyes shone bright, my previously puffy face deflated, and I looked the picture of health. So much so, in fact, that after a few short months on this program, my parents became so convinced, that they too began with 811. None of us have looked back.

I must stress that I did not only alter my diet; I altered my life. The school year ended for me, and I began a deep, extended rest. I was sedentary for nearly six months before I began vigorous exercise, and I avoided overt fats for this entire period. Each day I sought fresh air and sunlight. All of this was made possible by my family's love and valuable support.

This all began over a year ago. I have since been to Costa Rica as an intern for Dr. Graham at his fasting retreat, which inspired me to pursue health studies in order to prepare myself for a career in the field. My experiences there, and the leadership Dr. Graham has provided overall, have been influential beyond measure. Having found my calling, and my mentor, I can enthusiastically say that 80/10/10 was the turning point for the health of my family and me, and provided a foundation upon which I will pave my professional future.

## Ryan Earehart, Maui, Hawaii

The low-fat raw vegan diet has given me increased energy, more desire to perform physical activity, the best digestion I have ever had, and complete satisfaction with my pleasurable eating habits. Following a low-fat raw vegan diet has allowed me to achieve levels of health I never dreamed imaginable.

Overcoming chronic fatigue, severe allergies, annoying acne, and burdensome asthma were just the beginning. Over 3 ½ years ago, I virtually eliminated overt fats from my previous raw diet and adopted a diet of whole, fresh, ripe, raw, organic, delicious fruits and plants.

Now I can eat as much of anything I want so long as it passes my two tests: first it mustn't have a bar code, and second I have to be able to make a meal of it by itself. Eating mostly mono fruit meals with a nonfatty salad later in the day is my recipe for success. Eating this way is just so easy—hardly any dishes, no fat to clean out of my salad bowl, and hardly any time spent preparing my food.

Ten months ago, I changed my life dramatically and moved from the Arizona desert to the jungles of Hawaii. I was feeling great, excited to live off the land in a remote location without a vehicle. I soon discovered that I was unable to forage enough carbohydrates into my diet, so in order to get enough calories, I chose to eat what was raw, wild, fresh, and available. This included lots of veggies and garden greens, as wells as non-sweet fruits like tomatoes and cucumbers.

Yes, I was eating bananas, papayas, guavas, jackfruit, cherimoyas, oranges, and many other fruits, but not in sufficient quantities to meet my caloric needs. However, there were plenty of coconuts, avocados, and macadamia nuts all around, so I used these high-fat foods to meet my caloric needs. I was fine for about the first month, then I noticed some wounds not healing very fast and even getting worse with time.

I had developed a staph infection quite simply by eating lots of fats mixed with lots of sweet fruits, and my energy was drained. I was unable to perform intense physical activity, and my wounds were still not healing. After a month of trying to let my body heal itself while still eating the same way, I realized I was preventing my body from healing by eating the coconuts, avocados, and mac nuts. So I began a water fast that lasted nine days, during which I got lots of rest and completely healed all my wounds and gained back my vitality.

This demonstrated to me once and for all that the low-fat raw vegan diet was the only way for me. Since the fast, I have thrived each and every day by eating large quantities of sweet fruits and large nonfat salads in the evenings. I keep my fat percentage between 7 and 13%, and I have never felt better. Thanks, Doug, for teaching me the science that makes my body thrive.

## Julie Wandling, Akron, Ohio

Four years ago, I weighed 315 pounds, with high blood pressure of 199/100 and very high cholesterol. I was experiencing severe chest pains, ringing in the ears, dizziness, and overall body pain. I never slept well and was basically miserable in my own body. The doctor told me I was borderline diabetic, and I was living on muscle relaxers due to chronic lower-back pain—all at age 35!

In 2000, I discovered The Hallelujah Diet and from there Dr. Doug Graham. My mom and I adopted the raw food diet and immediately experienced physical benefits. After becoming Health Ministers, we started a support group and invited Dr. Graham to visit. After hearing him speak on the benefits of fruits over fats, I began limiting nuts, seeds, and oils and increasing fruits. I had always been told to avoid fruit because I was obese, so this was a bit scary at first. One doctor even told me never to eat bananas as they would cause me to become diabetic! Now I thrive on bananas. Needless to say, we've had Dr. Graham come back to speak for us several times now! Besides being a great lecturer, he is fun to play with.

My two boys, Corbin and Ryan, changed their diets along with me and have experienced awesome health ever since. Both love when Dr. Graham comes to visit because he plays tennis with them—soon they will be beating him! They eat cases of fruits every week along with plenty of salads and a few cooked vegan foods. They are training everyday and playing tournament-level tennis every weekend at ages 13 and 10 respectively. Ask them their favorite food and they will both reply, "Banana smoothies!"

Dr. Graham says something in his lectures that really prompted us to not just exercise but to play hard—he said we need to "earn our fruit." I am happy to report that four years later, I have lost 125 pounds, my blood pressure averages 110/70, and my cholesterol is 153! I play hard and live a full, pain-free life!

## Dr. Samuel Mielcarski, Roswell, Georgia

As a child, I loved to eat. I was never overweight, but I experienced a plethora of other problems, such as joint pain, lethargy, mood swings, gas and bloating, and feeling feverish, anxious, and sometimes really depressed.

As I moved into to my teenage years, I was informed that these issues were just part of being a teenager and that I would "grow out of it." When I hit my early twenties, I was still waiting to grow out of the problems I was having, but they persisted and eventually worsened instead.

I was always a competitive athlete growing up, and after college I decided to compete in an amateur body-building competition. In 1998, at the age of 25, I found myself on stage holding a second-place trophy at the Mr. Atlanta Body Building Competition in Atlanta, Georgia.

I appeared to look great to those watching the show, but this greatness was merely superficial. I did not look so great on the inside, as became evident in the weeks following the competition. It was then that my typical childhood and teenage symptoms began to worsen, compounded by significant intestinal pains and urogenital problems, including prostatitis.

Prostatitis is a condition where the prostate gland (the chestnut-like structure that sits below the bladder and surrounds the urethra in a male) becomes inflamed and irritated. This condition can lead to problems with urination and sexual functioning.

It became apparent to me that I had this condition when on several occasions I felt the need to urinate but was unable to do so. This was a most frightening experience at the time. I sought a professional opinion from a urologist, who confirmed the diagnosis of chronic prostatitis. When I asked him about the cause of this condition, he said, "We are not really sure, but it appears to be a cluster of infections that collect in the prostate region of the body." When I asked about a possible link between my diet and the intestinal pains, bowel irregularity, and prostate problems I was having, the doctor just said, "I suppose there could be a link."

I was determined to find the cause and rehabilitate it, and without drugs! Concurrently with rehabilitating myself from poor health, I discovered the science of Natural Hygiene. Implementing the principles of this true health-care system as part of my rehabilitation, I was somewhat successful in conquering the cause of the problem, as well as preventing other problems from developing. I had several signs and symptoms of cancer already, and I was in the prime age group for developing testicular cancer, despite being told by some medical doctors, "You are too young to have such problems."

A year after the competition, I was feeling better, but not 100% better. When it came to restoring my health, I wanted perfection. It was at this time that I met Dr. Doug Graham at a Raw Passion event. Dr. Graham provided me with profound dietary advice. He explained the concept of a raw vegan diet in simple terms, and it all made sense to me. I realized that although I had made many healthful changes in my life, my diet was still in need of some adjustment. The ways I ate as a child and during the body building competition were not truly healthful, as evidenced by the disease and distress I suffered while consuming such a diet.

After implementing the low-fat raw vegan dietary and lifestyle principles Dr. Graham shared with me, my body was finally restored back to optimal health and well-being. Dr. Graham showed me that bodily building was more important than just body building.

I still love to eat. The difference now is that I don't suffer the usual symptoms and distress I used to experience when doing so. From one doctor to another, thanks so much, Dr. Graham, for all your help!

## Laine Smithheisler, Nashville, Tennessee

I did not become raw because I had any noticeable illnesses, nor did I do it for animals' rights. I was young, in good shape, mentally stable, and was a member of a loving, albeit somewhat dysfunctional, family. I still can't put a finger on why I became raw. I just did, and much of the time that seems like an oddity in the raw community.

Yet, I have the feeling that a silent majority of people out there have had similar experiences of just happening to come into contact with the idea of raw foods. I want these people to know that a healthier lifestyle is indeed relevant to them. However, I don't want anyone to have to make the mistakes I did by following a high-fat raw diet supplemented with dehydrated foods. Because raw foods is much more widespread and mainstream today, everyone should be able to find the "right" sources; in effect, bypassing the hurdles that those of us who had no other knowledge ran straight into.

After two and a half years of eating completely raw (May 2002) and at the young age of eighteen, I began experiencing extreme fits of pain, which would endure for entire nights. It felt like someone was pressing down on the center of my chest while thrusting my stomach into my chest—like a heart attack mixed with acid reflux. For the next six or seven months, I let this continue, and continue it did—frequently (cycles of one or two nights a week followed by a few months of absence). However, I think the worst part was that slight pains, similar to acid reflux, would start early in the day before an entire night of full-blown pain. I often knew what was coming, imagining and dreading it.

In January of 2003, under the pressure of my family (who practice the standard American diet) and doctors, I allowed doctors to remove my unusually inflamed and infected gallbladder (which was even worse than that of a person on the standard American diet who has gallbladder problems, and certainly abnormal for someone so young).

Overwhelmed by a high-fat diet (and, yes, I was 100% raw), my gallbladder had fallen victim to gallstones, which are built from bile particles—in my case, mostly constituted from fats. Produced in the liver and secreted by the gallbladder, bile helps the small intestine digest fats and remove waste products. A gallstone can grow as liver bile passes through the gallbladder. Consequently, my high-fat diet multiplied this effect, meaning the more fatty foods I ate, the more bile was released and trapped.

Still, the pain failed to cease after doctors removed my gallstones. Near the end of that January, I developed jaundice—a symptom of a gall- bladder infection—which cast a yellow tint to my skin. It was at this point that the seriousness of what was happening hit me.

Imagine eating raw foods for so long and being confronted with this situation. A year of the most mind-numbing pain had deeply affected me, and I gave the doctors permission to operate on my body. Though I am thankful I do not suffer the pain any longer (though there are occasional pangs reminiscent of previous pains that continue to frighten me), I still experience mental grievances at the thought of what I permitted—no, not allowing doctors to remove a bodily organ, but rather, letting myself adopt the mindset that as long as I followed any raw diet, my worries were over.

Though I mostly avoided oils, at one point I had been consuming a small jar of almond butter a day for several months. I should have realized that eating two or three avocadoes a day wasn't the answer to Eden. Yet, my answer to high-fat was just as detrimental. Instead of focusing on fresh fruits and vegetables, I supplemented the stimulation and satiation I got from avocados and nuts with the quick fix of very high-sugar fruits. I would eat twenty or thirty dehydrated figs or dates daily. My payment consisted of dreaded trips to the dentist and multiple cavities.

I know one can be deficient on raw foods, and I struggle just as much as the next person. But, I also know that a sound diet can correlate with a sound mind. By learning to appreciate and reward my body by eating a low-fat, low-sodium diet (Doug Graham's 811rv), I have learned to love myself by realizing that health is much more than diet and exercise. For me, health can be as seemingly simple as proper sleep or the having a positive attitude, and as complex as intellectual stimulation or maintaining and repairing human relationships.

## Lori Williamson, Portland, Oregon

My name is Lori Williamson, and I am a licensed massage therapist. I have been eating raw food since 1997 and was building to an all-raw vegan diet. I finally leaped into 100% raw on August 25, 2003.

Before I started to eat raw food, I had a whole host of health problems that were terrible to live with. Vertigo, fatigue, depression, carpal tunnel syndrome, stomach aches, sciatica, neck pain, migraine headaches. Although raw food helped me get past these terrible ailments, changing to Dr. Doug Graham's 811 program took me beyond any diet I could imagine!

Still consuming lots of raw dehydrated products and raw fats, when I came across 811, I really started to notice some energetic differences. Even though I had been high raw for many years, I still had some problems. When I went 100% raw, the problems lessened a lot, but my teeth were very sensitive and were not doing as well as I would have hoped on all raw, because of the high nut content in my food. My back would be a little stiff from sleeping on a stomach filled with raw fat or dehydrated food. My periods were still slightly painful, and food did not digest well—until 811, that is.

Now when the I follow the 811 program, I have this boundless energy that tickles my stomach, and I get so excited I want to laugh and giggle. Maybe it's because I am so happy that I do not have to deal with health problems anymore.

When I think of Dr. Doug Graham's work, I think of the following quote from Albert Einstein: "Nothing will benefit health and increase the chances for survival of life on Earth as much as the evolution to a vegetarian diet."

As raw fooders, we thought we had it all, but when the 811 program came along, raw vegan truly evolved. I wish everyone could experience the way one feels on this diet. It is amazing!

Thank you, Dr. Graham, for your continued efforts to help people attain their optimum health.

## Petr Cech, Denmark

I have been incorporating Dr. Doug Graham's low-fat raw vegan plan into my life since 2003. At first I had my doubts, and I sometimes stepped aside from my path, making lifestyle choices that did not serve me so well. But I knew the 80/10/10 program was right for me, so I have stayed on this diet now for almost two years, learning and refining it more and more.

I used to struggle with my weight, undereating calories or overeating fat. I had no energy and was very thin. I have absolutely no problem gaining weight and muscles on 811. I have gained 20 pounds on this high-carb, low-fat diet, eating two to three meals each day. It takes some time to adjust the (unnatural) body to this (natural) diet, but it is undoubtedly worth it.

If I also meet the other needs of my body (sleep, rest, sunbath, exercise, spiritual needs), this diet plan allows me to focus fully on my daily activities, supporting my body's nutritional requirements and enabling short recovery time after training, better sleep, and better resistance to colds, sore muscles, and sunburn.

Dr. D. advises that we get "enough" calories in our main meal. For me, that is 1,500 kcal at lunch. Eating a large afternoon meal frees me to concentrate on things other than food during the day, leaving me satisfied for four to six hours after eating. Before, I was eating five meals a day; now it's usually two to three.

One thing is for sure, I would never make it without Dr. Graham. His wisdom, experience, honesty, and patience in answering questions have helped me through many dark times.

The most precious things I have learned from Dr. Graham's books and personal comments: Keep it simple and see the bigger picture of healthful living. I never met Dr. D., but my thoughts and love will ever be with him.

## Dave Klein, Sebastopol, California

Twenty years ago, after being very sick for eight years with ulcerative colitis, I saw the light and all at once changed my SAD diet to a 95% raw low-fat vegan diet of mostly fresh fruits. I healed up quickly and went on to experience robust dynamic health.

Over the past ten years, I have maintained a 100% raw low-fat vegan diet and my mental and physical energies have never been higher. I am age 46; a friend told me the other day that I look like I am 17. When I eat nuts, seeds and/or avocado more than once per week, my physical energy and mental clarity decrease, and I don't feel and look healthy and alive. Eating more fat than we can digest and utilize leads to toxemia and subpar health.

People forget that there is some fat in bananas and even lettuce, and I eat plenty of those. That is really sufficient, except during the winter. During the initial detoxification and rebuilding phases, a low-fat vegan diet may not seem sufficient, but if you stick with it and live a healthful lifestyle in a climate that is not too cold, it becomes apparent that the 80/10/10 diet is the optimum way to go.

## Robert Dyckman, New York, New York

Last year, I heard Dr. Graham speak about the 80/10/10 ratio of nutrients, and even though I'd been off the standard American diet (SAD) for three years, I still occasionally felt sluggish and a bit clogged up when I overconsumed nuts, seeds, and other fats. Now, while that was still better than the way I felt after a SAD meal, I prefer enjoying superior health, not just average or "standard."

So I made changes in my eating habits, vectoring my diet in the direction of 80/10/10, and in a very short period of time I felt more energetic during and after exercise, slept better, felt calmer and more at ease, saw better definition in my muscles, and perhaps best of all for me (an actor and singer), my singing voice was clearer and stronger! It also now takes a heck of a lot less time to warm up my voice before I perform.

This year has been amazingly healthful and I feel grateful for the bounty that awaits me every single day. Thanks Dr. Graham for your inspiration and wonderful knowledge!

## Sky Grealis, New Brunswick, New Jersey

I was so pleased with the results when I first transitioned to a raw diet, and I thought I could eat anything raw with abandon and maintain perfect health. When I found myself as tired as I had been before raw, I blamed it on "detox." Luckily, it was at that point that I found Dr. Graham and the 811 way of eating. Thanks to him and this program, I am energetic, have lost 35 pounds, and have been able to put on solid muscle for the first time in my life.

Dr. Graham is the most down-to-earth leader in the raw food movement—one who offers common-sense advice and speaks the truth even if the world doesn't seem ready to hear it. Hats off to Dr. Graham and low-fat raw veganism!

## Tera Warner, Montréal, Québec, Canada

I've spent 30 years feeling lost in my own skin. I've never suffered any significant health issues, and I always had tonnes of energy (relatively speaking), but I'd look in the mirror and think, "Those are my legs!? That's my skin!?" This morning I woke up feeling tearful appreciation for the fact that after 30 years of struggling with insecurity and self confidence, I'm finally starting to feel comfortable in my own skin. My skin is soft, water retention disappears more and more every day. I know my limits, I control my food (instead of it controlling me). This, the result of working relentlessly toward achieving 811rv.

I understand that health is more than nutrition, but for me, when proper nutrition has been applied, everything else sort of settles right into place naturally. I had no idea that 811 would have had such a tremendous effect on my life. I thought I was happy, high energy, active, and positive … I guess it's a matter of degree. I'm thrilled about plunging myself into this living adventure the most I can—and about reveling in this newfound liberty of thought. I look forward to meeting Dr. Graham next year and thanking him in person.

# Appendix D.
# Resources for Diet Analysis

A number of websites exist that can analyze the food you eat. Two of my favorites are **FitDay.com** and **Nutridiary.com**. They calculate your intake of various nutrients and help you make sure you are getting an appropriate number of calories each day. Most people do not realize just how little fat it takes in the diet to exceed 10%, given that even fruits and vegetables contain some fat. The automated calculators are very helpful in this regard.

You can also download a PC version of FitDay, which allows you to use the software without being on the Internet. Or you can download another excellent free program (I consider it the best), called **CRON-O-Meter**, from http://spaz.ca/cronometer. This tool yields results including a caloronutrient pie chart; a summary listing of calories, protein, carbohydrates, lipids, vitamins, and minerals; and a detailed breakdown of vitamins, minerals, amino acids, lipids, and more. You can view all of this data for any single ingredient or food, for any recipe you enter into the program, or for an entire day's intake.

Unfortunately, there are many variables in the caloronutrient equation, and you will find widely differing results among the various nutrition-analysis tools on the market (see sidebar, "Trying to Replicate the Numbers?" on page 337 ). Thus, your calculations may not correlate exactly (or even closely) with the ones in this book or with the numbers that others claim to have derived. At best, they are rough estimates. Use them accordingly.

## The USDA Nutrient Database

The above products and their competitors all use for their underlying data the USDA's National Nutrient Database for Standard Reference, a repository of nutritional information for more than 7,300 foods. Available on CD-ROM, as well as online at www.nal.usda.gov/fnic/foodcomp/Data, this database tracks more than 100 nutrients and is the foundation of virtually all public and commercial nutrient databases used in the United States and a number of foreign countries.

The database is a compilation of data derived from published scientific and technical literature as well as unpublished sources, such as the food industry, other government agencies, and research conducted under USDA contracts with universities and food testing laboratories. Unfortunately, less than 15 percent of its information comes from primary laboratory research.

The USDA periodically reviews and updates information for some portion of the foods it tracks and issues new releases of the database. For example, release SR-16 (its sixteenth major release) in January 2004, updated nutrient profiles for 28 raw fruits and 23 raw and cooked vegetables. At least nine fruits changed significantly in terms of caloronutrient ratio with that release. Therefore, it is a good idea to check that the software you choose for calculating your calorie and nutrient intake keeps up to date with the most recent data from the USDA. As of late 2010, the current release is SR-23.

### An Inexact Science at Best

Unfortunately, the information in the USDA database (though it is the best information available) is of questionable value. A 1993 General Accounting Office report criticized the Department of Agriculture for using lax methods to evaluate nutrients, citing (among other things) small sample sizes and "little or no supporting information on the testing and quality assurance procedures used to develop the data."[89]

Even under the best of circumstances, nutritional analysis is far from an exact science. The USDA attempts to address "physiological availability" of the caloronutrients in foods, but it does not consider in any meaningful way, whether the foods are cooked or raw, animal or plant. It does not begin to account for nutritional differences between conventional produce, organically grown produce, and produce grown in highly bioactive soils. At the micronutrient level, these cultivation methods would yield considerably different results. Sadly, Western science is generally ignorant of such issues at the level that raw nutritional science and Natural Hygiene understands them.

Nonetheless, the USDA database is the primary source of food nutrient data for this nation and beyond. Until some well-funded organization with a holistic health perspective and a different set of assumptions is able to undertake the nutrient analysis of fresh organic produce grown in nutrient-rich soils, the USDA database is all we have to analyze our nutritional intake.

## Trying to Replicate the Numbers?

If you are mathematically minded and attempt to deconstruct the numbers in this book or on the USDA website, you will have to do some serious digging. After years of working with these numbers, I have learned some things about their derivation.

### *Atwater Energy Factors: Not 4-4-9*

When assigning calories per gram values to each food item, the USDA does not simply multiply carbohydrate, protein, and fat by 4, 4, and 9, respectively. Instead, it uses the "Atwater system for determining energy values" for whole foods. The Atwater system uses specific energy factors that have been determined for basic food commodities. These factors purportedly take into account the physiological availability of the energy from these foods.[90]

The more general factors of 4-4-9 calories per gram (kcal/g) were derived from the specific calorie factors determined by Professor W. O. Atwater and his associates a little over a century ago. As evidenced in the "Food Description" table of the Microsoft Access version of the USDA database, Atwater's system is significantly more complex than one might expect, for its conversion factors vary widely among foods.

Here are some examples of the Atwater conversion factors for selected categories of whole plant foods which, with a few exceptions, are consistent for all foods within the category. (Multi-ingredient prepared foods listed by brand name in the database generally reflect industry practices of calculating calories based on the 4-4-9 formula).

| | | |
|---|---|---|
| Vegetables: | fat 8.37 | protein 2.44* |
| Fruit: | fat 8.37 | protein 3.36 |
| Nuts & seeds: | fat 8.37 | protein 3.47 |
| Flesh: | fat 9.02 | protein 4.27 |
| Oils: | fat 8.84 | (oils are 100% fat) |

Although the Atwater system does include conversion factors for carbohydrates, the USDA calculates carbohydrates by difference (100% – protein % – fat %), ensuring that the three caloronutrient percentages add up to 100.

Some of the nutrient analyses of recipes and foods in this book, as well as the food charts at the back of this book, use the Atwater numbers. However, we used Nutridiary for many of the calculations, which employs a slightly modified version of the 4-4-9 model.

### *Inaccuracies in Nutridiary and FitDay*

* The only instance where the Atwater factors and the general factors differ significantly is in the amount of protein contained in vegetables. In general, Nutridiary overstates the protein in vegetables by as much as 7 percentage points. FitDay's error (compounded by its use of an outdated version of the USDA database) is more significant, and the protein shown in vegetables can be overestimated by as much as 30 percentage points. Because of the extremely low caloric density of vegetables, however, these errors are unlikely to affect your overall caloronutrient ratio by more than 1%.

### *Varying Options for Common Portions*

In addition to differing conversion factors or outdated versions of the USDA data, another source of variance among popular nutrition-analysis software products is how differently they handle food portions. One calculator may give you lettuce choices that include "head," "ounces," and "cups shredded." Another may offer "grams" and "innerleaf." Nutridiary provides the most complete drop-down list of common servings for its food items that I have found, a very useful feature.

### *Operator Error*

Without a food scale, estimating portions can be highly unreliable. Neither guessing at weight nor choosing from highly subjective predetermined measurements like "1 medium fruit" or "2 small stalks" produces the best results.

If you are serious about taking on the 80/10/10 challenge, especially if you plan to analyze nutrition for others, I suggest purchasing a small digital kitchen scale. A useful model is the My Weigh KD 600, which has a 13.2 lb (6 kg) capacity with 0.1 oz (1 gram) increments, and features hold, tare, and automatic power off functions. The KD 600 is available through online auctions for about $50.

## Macronutrients in Common Plant Foods

My editor, colleague, and research assistant, Laurie Masters, created the content for this appendix, including the chart below, which lists the macronutrient and calorie content of a small collection of fruits, vegetables, and fats. Also included are a few starches and grains commonly eaten among raw fooders, even though they are not part of the 80/10/10 diet.

The charts include columns for:

- Calories
- Grams of water and fiber
- Percentage of calories from carbohydrates, protein, and fat
- Grams of carbohydrates, protein, and fat.

All food items are listed in 100-gram (3.5-ounce) portions—the size of a small 6-inch banana, a small 2.5-inch apple, or 2.5 medium stalks of celery. The information in these three charts is derived from the USDA Nutrient Database for Standard Reference, Release 18, available online at www.nal.usda.gov/fnic/foodcomp/Data.

### *More Extensive Charts Available at 811rv.com*

The table on the following pages is an abbreviated lists the macronutrient content of about a dozen common fruits, vegetables, and fats, as well as some cooked starches, for those who eat them. version of a Far more detailed data is larger set of charts available in a set of laminated charts available for purchase as full-color, double-sided laminated sheets through my website, (www.811rv.org.) The series includes a hand-picked list of dozens of common 80/10/10-compliant fruits, vegetables, and plant-based fats, as well as a selection of common complex carbohydrate and animal foods, provided for reference and comparison purposes only.

## Macronutrients in Common Plant Foods

| Fruits | Cal 100g | Water grams | Fiber grams | Carb % Cal | Pro % Cal | Fat % Cal | Carb grams | Pro grams | Fat grams |
|---|---|---|---|---|---|---|---|---|---|
| Apples | 52 | 86 | 2 | 95% | 2% | 3% | 13.8 | 0.3 | 0.2 |
| Bananas | 89 | 75 | 3 | 93% | 4% | 3% | 22.8 | 1.1 | 0.3 |
| Blackberry | 43 | 88 | 5 | 79% | 11% | 10% | 9.6 | 1.4 | 0.5 |
| Dates (medjool) | 277 | 21 | 7 | 97% | 2% | 1% | 75.0 | 1.8 | 0.2 |
| Figs | 74 | 79 | 3 | 93% | 4% | 3% | 19.2 | 0.8 | 0.3 |
| Grapes | 69 | 81 | 1 | 95% | 3% | 2% | 18.1 | 0.7 | 0.2 |
| Mangos | 65 | 82 | 2 | 93% | 3% | 4% | 17.0 | 0.5 | 0.3 |
| Nectarines | 44 | 88 | 2 | 86% | 8% | 6% | 10.6 | 1.1 | 0.3 |
| Oranges | 49 | 86 | 3 | 88% | 7% | 5% | 11.9 | 1.0 | 0.3 |
| Peaches | 39 | 89 | 2 | 86% | 8% | 6% | 9.5 | 0.9 | 0.3 |
| Pears | 58 | 84 | 3 | 97% | 2% | 1% | 15.5 | 0.4 | 0.1 |
| Strawberry | 32 | 91 | 2 | 85% | 7% | 8% | 7.7 | 0.7 | 0.3 |
| Watermelon | 30 | 91 | 0 | 87% | 7% | 6% | 7.6 | 0.6 | 0.2 |
| **Vegetables** | | | | | | | | | |
| Broccoli | 34 | 89 | 3 | 70% | 20% | 10% | 6.6 | 2.8 | 0.4 |
| Cabbage | 24 | 92 | 2 | 83% | 14% | 3% | 5.6 | 1.4 | 0.1 |
| Carrots | 41 | 88 | 3 | 90% | 6% | 4% | 9.6 | 0.9 | 0.2 |
| Cauliflower | 25 | 92 | 3 | 77% | 20% | 3% | 5.3 | 2.0 | 0.1 |
| Celery | 14 | 95 | 2 | 76% | 12% | 12% | 3.0 | 0.7 | 0.2 |
| Kale | 50 | 84 | 2 | 72% | 16% | 12% | 10.0 | 3.3 | 0.7 |
| Lettuce | 17 | 95 | 2 | 68% | 17% | 15% | 3.3 | 1.2 | 0.3 |
| Spinach | 23 | 91 | 2 | 54% | 31% | 15% | 3.6 | 2.9 | 0.4 |
| **Vegetable Fruits** (nonsweet fruits) | | | | | | | | | |
| Cucumber | 15 | 95 | 1 | 84% | 10% | 6% | 3.6 | 0.6 | 0.1 |
| Tomatoes (red) | 18 | 95 | 1 | 79% | 12% | 9% | 3.9 | 0.9 | 0.2 |
| Zucchini | 16 | 95 | 1 | 72% | 18% | 10% | 3.3 | 1.2 | 0.2 |

| | Cal 100g | Water grams | Fiber grams | Carb % Cal | Pro % Cal | Fat % Cal | Carb grams | Pro grams | Fat grams |
|---|---|---|---|---|---|---|---|---|---|
| **Starches & Grains** (only very young, sweet peas/corn) | | | | | | | | | |
| Buckwheat | 343 | 10 | 10 | 79% | 13% | 8% | 71.5 | 13.3 | 3.4 |
| Chickpeas | 364 | 12 | 17 | 68% | 18% | 14% | 60.7 | 19.3 | 6.0 |
| Corn | 86 | 76 | 3 | 78% | 10% | 12% | 19.0 | 3.2 | 1.2 |
| Peas, Edible-podded | 42 | 89 | 3 | 73% | 23% | 4% | 7.6 | 2.8 | 0.2 |
| Sweet Potato | 86 | 77 | 3 | 94% | 5% | 1% | 20.1 | 1.6 | 0.1 |
| Wheat | 331 | 12 | 13 | 85% | 11% | 4% | 74.2 | 10.4 | 1.6 |
| Wild Rice | 357 | 8 | 6 | 82% | 15% | 3% | 74.9 | 14.7 | 1.1 |
| **Fats** | | | | | | | | | |
| Almonds | 578 | 5 | 12 | 14% | 13% | 73% | 19.7 | 21.3 | 50.6 |
| Avocado | 167 | 72 | 7 | 19% | 4% | 77% | 8.6 | 2.0 | 15.4 |
| Cashews | 553 | 5 | 3 | 23% | 11% | 66% | 30.2 | 18.2 | 43.8 |
| Coconut Meat | 354 | 47 | 9 | 18% | 3% | 79% | 15.2 | 3.3 | 33.5 |
| Flaxseeds | 492 | 9 | 28 | 28% | 14% | 58% | 34.3 | 19.5 | 34.0 |
| Hemp Seeds | 533 | - | 3 | 17% | 27% | 56% | 23.0 | 37.0 | 33.0 |
| Macadamia Nuts | 718 | 1 | 9 | 8% | 4% | 88% | 13.8 | 7.9 | 75.8 |
| Olive, Canned | 115 | 80 | 3 | 20% | 2% | 78% | 6.3 | 0.8 | 10.7 |
| Pine Nuts | 673 | 2 | 4 | 8% | 7% | 85% | 13.1 | 13.7 | 68.4 |
| Walnuts | 654 | 4 | 7 | 9% | 8% | 83% | 13.7 | 15.2 | 65.2 |
| Sesame Seeds | 573 | 5 | 12 | 16% | 11% | 73% | 23.5 | 17.7 | 49.7 |
| Sunflower Seeds | 570 | 5 | 11 | 13% | 14% | 73% | 18.8 | 22.8 | 49.6 |
| Oil (all types) | 884 | 0 | 0 | 0% | 0% | 100% | 0 | 0 | 100 |

# About the Author

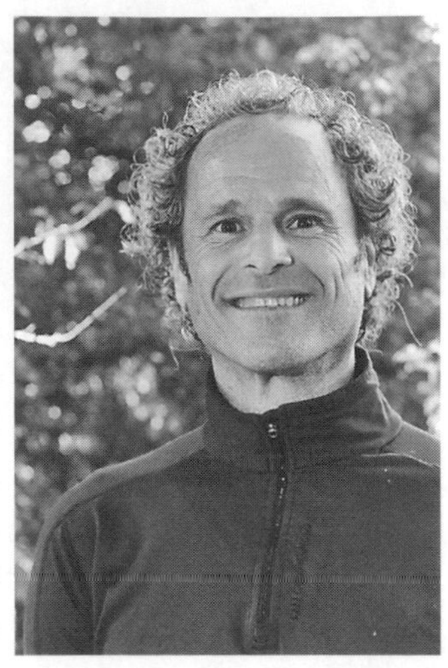

Dr. Douglas Graham, a lifetime athlete and twenty-seven-year raw fooder, is an advisor to world-class athletes and trainers from around the globe. He has worked professionally with top performers from almost every sport and field of entertainment, including such notables as tennis legend Martina Navratilova, NBA pro basketball player Ronnie Grandison, track Olympic sprinter Doug Dickinson, pro women's soccer player Callie Withers, championship bodybuilder Kenneth G. Williams, Chicken Soup for the Soul coauthor Mark Victor Hansen, and actress Demi Moore.

Dr. Graham is the author of several books on raw food and health, including The High Energy Diet Recipe Guide, Nutrition and Athletic Performance, and the forthcoming Prevention and Care of Athletic Injuries. He has shared his strategies for success with audiences at more than 4,000 presentations worldwide. Recognized as one of the fathers of the modern raw movement, Dr. Graham is the only lecturer to have attended and given keynote presentations at all of the major raw events in the world, from 1997 through 2005.

Dr. Graham is a founder of and is currently serving his third term as president of Healthful Living International, the world's premier Natural Hygiene organization. He is on the board of advisors of Voice for a Viable Future, the Vegetarian Union of North America, Living Light Films, and EarthSave International. He serves as nutrition advisor to the magazine Exercise, for Men Only and authors a column for Get Fresh! and Living Nutrition magazines.

Dr. Graham is the creator of "Simply Delicious" cuisine and director of Health & Fitness Weeks, which provide Olympic-class training and nutritional guidance to people of all fitness levels in beautiful settings around the world. He is living proof that eating whole, fresh, ripe, raw, organic food is the nutritional way to vibrant health and vitality.

# Endnotes

1. "Trends in Intake of Energy and Macronutrients—United States, 1971–2000," Morbidity and Mortality Weekly Report, February 6, 2004, pp. 80–82. Department of Health and Human Services, Centers for Disease Control and Prevention. Accessed at www.cdc.gov/mmwr/PDF/wk/mm5304.pdf.

2. U.C. Berkeley News press release by Sarah Yang, June 1, 2004, as quoted in U.C. Berkeley News, accessed at www.berkeley.edu/news/media/releases/2004/06/01_usdiet.shtml. Reprinted by permission.

3. Block, G. "Foods Contributing to Energy Intake in the US: Data From NHANES III and NHANES 1999–2000." J Food Composit Anal. 2004;17:439-447.

4. A widely publicized report from the Centers for Disease Control and Prevention lists obesity as the nation's second leading cause of preventable death, responsible for 320,000 to 400,000 annual deaths and predicted to soon overtake tobacco as the number-one cause. The number is being adjusted due to a statistical error, but regardless of the actual number, there is no doubt that obesity is a devastating health issue in our nation. See "CDC: Obesity Deaths Overstated," by the Center for Consumer Freedom, dated November 23, 2004, available online at www.consumerfreedom.com/news_detail.cfm?headline=2691.

5. Tanner, Lindsey. "Americans Eat Themselves to Death," Associated Press: March 9, 2004. Accessed at www.cbsnews.com/stories/2004/03/ 09/health/main604956.shtml.

6. "American Heart Disease," from the Franklin Institute Online website: http://sln.fi.edu/biosci/healthy/stats.html.

7. Arias, Elizabeth and Smith, Betty L. "Deaths: Preliminary Data for 2001," National Vital Statistics Reports. Vol. 51, No. 5, March 14, 2003. Accessed at www.cdc.gov/nchs/data/nvsr/nvsr51/nvsr51_05.pdf.

8. "Cancer Basics: What Is Cancer and Why Does It Occur?" May 13, 2004. Accessed at The Mayo Clinic website: www.mayoclinic.com/invoke.cfm?id=CA00003.

9. "Diabetes: Disabling, Deadly, and on the Rise," April 7, 2004. Centers for Disease Control and Prevention. Accessed at www.cdc.gov/nccdphp/aag/aag_ddt.htm.

10. Saxe, John Godfrey (1816–1887). "The Blind Men and the Elephant." This version of the famous Indian legend is in the public domain.

11. Greger, Michael. Atkins Facts. This 47-page eBook, which contains 487 source references, is available online at www.atkinsfacts.org. Quoted with permission.

12. For information on canine caloronutrient requirements, visit www.mercola.com/2005/feb/5/pets_grains.htm.

13. Visit www.pcrm.org/health/veginfo/dairy.html for a tremendous amount of information about the toxicity of animal milk for humans of any age.

14. If you wish to learn more about glycemic index versus glycemic load, visit www.mendosa.com/gilists.htm. The creator of this website, David Mendosa, is coauthor of What Makes My Blood Glucose Go Up...And Down? (New York: Marlowe & Co., August 2003).

15. "Evidence-Based Nutrition Principles and Recommendations for the Treatment and Prevention of Diabetes and Related Complications," Diabetes Care 25:202–212, 2002. Accessed at http://care.diabetesjournals.org/cgi/ content/full/25/1/202.

In addition to making a clear statement in favor of whole-fruit sugar for diabetics, this article from the American Diabetes Association recommends that Type 2 diabetics consume a "very large" amount of fiber—so much, in fact, that they predict most people will not enjoy consuming it. The 80/10/10 diet, which consists of essentially 100% high-fiber foods, aligns with this guideline perfectly. Here is the quote:

"In subjects with type 2 diabetes, it appears that ingestion of very large amounts of fiber are necessary to confer metabolic benefits on glycemic control, hyperinsulinemia, and plasma lipids. It is not clear whether the palatability and the gastro-intestinal side effects of fiber in this amount would be acceptable to most people."

16. The information in this table comes from an article entitled "Glycemic Values of Common American Foods," available at www.mendosa.com/com-

mon_foods.htm. It is based on data from the following publication: Foster-Powell, K. et al., "International Tables of Glycemic Index and Glycemic Load Values: 2002." Am J Clin Nutr 2002;76:5–56. Accessed at www.ajcn.org/cgi/content/full/76/1/5.

17. You can read more about the role of dietary fat in blood-sugar metabolic disorders in The Pritikin Program for Diet and Exercise (New York: Grosset and Dunlap, 1979), by Nathan Pritikin with Patrick M. McGrady, Jr.

I also recommend Health and *Survival in the 21st Century* by Ross Horne (Sydney, Australia: Harper Collins, 1997), an out-of-print Natural Hygiene book. It is now available only on the Web, at www.soilandhealth.org/02/02 01hyglibcat/020122horne.2 1stcentury/020122toc.html. "Chapter 6" on page 103, for information specific to fat and diabetes.

18. The information in this sidebar comes from Michael Greger's Atkins Facts. (See note 11.)

19. Dansinger, Michael L., et al. "One Year Effectiveness of the Atkins, Ornish, Weight Watchers, and Zone Diets in Decreasing Body Weight and Heart Disease Risk." Tufts University, New England Medical Center, Boston, Mass.

20. "Major Increase in Diabetes Among Adults Occurred Nationwide Between 1990 and 1998," press release dated August 23, 2000 from the Centers for Disease Control and Prevention. Accessed at www.cdc.gov/ diabetes/news/docs/000823.htm.

21. Joslin, EP. "Atherosclerosis and Diabetes." Ann Clin Med 1927;5:1061.

22. Breneman, Carol J. "Type II Diabetes…Self-Induced Disease?" Millersville University (1997). This article also cites studies by Felber, Anderson, Burkitt, and others, all demonstrating the correlation between dietary fat and diabetes. Accessed at http://home.judson.edu/academic/spinner/dia betes.html.

Also, a 2001 Science News article briefly describes Dr. I.M. Rabinowitch's work. Entitled "Diabetic Patients Can Eat Sugar If Fats Are Eliminated," the article can be found online at www.sciencenews.org/articles/ 20010915/timeline.asp.

23. Van Eck, W. "The Effect of a Low Fat Diet on the Serum Lipids in Diabetes and Its Significance in Diabetic Retinopathy. Am J Med. 1959; 27:196-211.

24. Anderson, J.W. and Ward, K. "High Carbohydrate, High Fiber Diets for insulin-Treated Men with Diabetes Mellitus. Am J Clin Nutr, 1979; 32:2312-21.

25. "Low-Fat Diet Alone Reversed Type 2 Diabetes in Mice," press release dated September 10, 1998 from the Duke University Medical center. Accessed at http://dukemednews.duke.edu/news/article.php?id=519.

26. Yiamouyiannis, John. Fluoride the Aging Factor: How to Recognize and Avoid the Devastating Effects of Fluoride. (Delaware, OH: Health Action Press, 1993).

27. For more information about Robert Koch, physician, bacteriologist and hygienist (1843–1910), visit www.zeiss.com/C12567A100537AB9/ContentsWWWIntern/D0C1165AA71F8BACC1256B45003DDE3D.

Interestingly, Koch's original version of postulate #3 did not contain the word "susceptible." In order to make germ theory consistent, the third postulate was changed to say that the germ had to produce the original disease in a "susceptible" new host.

Horne, Ross. Health and Survival in the 21st Century. (See note 17). In chapter 6, Horne relates, "With the addition of the single word "susceptible" the entire concept of the germ theory is changed. The accent is taken away from the germ and placed on the word susceptibility…in other words, for a germ to cause a disease in anybody, at any time, it can only do so if the person is susceptible. "

28. Horne, Ross. Health and Survival in the 21st Century. See note 17). The Pasteur story begins in chapter 2. Subsequent chapters, particularly 4 through 6, contain information specific to the fallacy of the germ theory of disease.

Another well-researched book on this subject is The Curse of Louis Pasteur: Why Medicine Is Not Healing a Diseased World, by Nancy Appleton, PhD. (Santa Monica, CA: Choice Publishing, 1997).

29. Wadley, Greg and Martin, Angus. "The Origins of Agriculture—a Biological Perspective and a New Hypothesis," Department of Zoology, University of Melbourne. Published in Australian Biologist 6: 96–105, June 1993. Accessed at www.acnem.org/journal/19-1_april_2000/origins_of_agriculture. htm.

30. "Trends in Intake of Energy and Macronutrients—United States, 1971–2000." (See note 1.)

31. Greger, Michael. Atkins Facts. (See note 11.)

32. Horne, Ross. Improving on Pritikin: You Can Do Better. (Australia: Happy Landings Pty. Ltd., 1988).

33. Horne, Ross. Improving on Pritikin: You Can Do Better (see note 32).

34. Technically, some form of gluten (a protein) is found in all grains, but "gluten-free" customarily means free of wheat, barley, or rye. Along with spelt, these are the primary grains that trigger an autoimmune response in people with gluten intolerance. However, gluten damages the small intestine in all of us and should be avoided regardless of whether we experience acute symptoms.

35. Coleman, John. "Opioids In Common Food Products—Addictive Peptides In Meat, Dairy and Grains." Accessed at www.vegan-straight-edge.org.uk/ opioids.htm.

36. To read more about excitotoxins, see "Not Just Another Scare: Toxin Additives in Your Food and Drink," by Russell L. Blaylock, MD. Accessed at www. aspartamekills.com/blayart1.htm.

37. I encourage you to print out the excellent list of dozens of disguised names for MSG, available at the "Say NO to MSG" website: http://www. saynotomsg.com/basics_list.php. Or better yet, say NO to all processed foods (anything with a label), and avoid the issue entirely.

38. "Trends in Intake of Energy and Macronutrients—United States, 1971–2000." (See note 1.)

39. "Diet, Nutrition and the Prevention of Chronic Diseases: Report of a Joint WHO/FAO Expert Consultation." World Health Organization Technical Report Series, No. 916 (2003). See section 5.1, "Population nutrient intake goals for preventing diet-related chronic diseases." Accessed at www.who.int/hpr/ NPH/docs/who_fao_expert_report.pdf.

40. "Report Offers New Eating and Physical Activity Targets to Reduce Chronic Disease Risk," press release dated September 5, 2002 from the National Academies' Institute of Medicine. Accessed at www4.national academies.org/ news.nsf/isbn/0309085373?OpenDocument.

41. National Research Council. Recommended Dietary Allowances: 10th

Edition, (Washington DC: National Academies Press, 1989) Accessed at http://books.nap.edu/books/0309046335/html/.

42. The USDA Nutrient Database for Standard Reference, Release 18 (available at www.nal.usda.gov/fnic/foodcomp/Data) shows the protein content for mature mother's milk to be 6.3% of calories, or 1.03% by weight.

43. Recommended Dietary Allowances: 10th Edition, pp. 58–59. (See note 41.)

44. Campbell, T. Colin. The China Study: Startling Implications for Diet, Weight Loss, and Long-Term Health. (Dallas, TX: BenBella Books, 2004), pp. 30–31.

45. Recommended Dietary Allowances: 10th Edition, pp. 70–71. (See note 41.)

46. USDA Nutrient Database for Standard Reference, Release 18. (See note 42.)

47. Campbell, T. Colin. The China Study. (See note 44.)

48. "Trends in Intake of Energy and Macronutrients—United States, 1971–2000." (See note 1.)

49. Recommended Dietary Allowances: 10th Edition, pp. 70–71. (See note 41.)

50. Campbell, T. Colin. The China Study. (See note 44.)

51. "But How Do You Get Enough Protein?," Vegetarian Society of Colorado brochure. Accessed at www.vsc.org/protein.htm.

52. Millward, D.J. "Optimal Intakes of Protein in the Human Diet." Proc Nutr Soc. 1999 May;58(2):403-13. Accessed at http://titania.ingentaselect. com/vl=1029643/cl=42/nw=1/rpsv/cgi-bin/cgi?body=linker&ini=nlm& reqidx=issn=0029-6651vl=58is=2yr=1999mn=Maypg=403.

53. Institute of Medicine. Dietary Reference Intakes for Energy, Carbohydrate, Fiber, Fat, Fatty Acids, Cholesterol, Protein, and Amino Acids (Macronutrients), p. 422.

(Washington DC: National Academies Press, 2005). Accessed at http://books.nap.edu/openbook.php?record_id=10490 &page=422.

54. Campbell, T. Colin. The China Study, p. 271. (See note 44.)

55. Erasmus, Udo. Fats That Heal, Fats That Kill. (Burnaby, Canada: Alive Publishing Group, 1993), p. 162.

56. Pritikin, Robert. The Pritikin Principle: The Calorie Density Solution. (Alexandria, Va.: Time-Life Books, 2000).

57. Ornish, Dean. Dr. Dean Ornish's Program for Reversing Heart Disease. (New York/Toronto: Random House, 1990), p. 255.

58. Esselstyn, Jr., Caldwell B. Prevent and Reverse Heart Disease. (New York: Penguin Books, 2008), p. 77.

59. Barnard, Neal. Dr. Neal Barnard's Program for Reversing Diabetes. (New York: Rodale, 2007), p. 51.

60. Williams, Clyde and Devlin, John T. (editors). Food, Nutrition and Sports Performance. (Van Nostrand Reinhold, 1992).

61. For an overview of the topic of essential fatty acids as they relate to the raw food diet, see the article "Essential Facts and the Organic Athlete," by Dr. Rick Dina, at www.organicathlete.org/index.php?option=com_content& task=view&id=119&Itemid=63.

62. See www.udoerasmus.com/articles/udo/fthftk6.htm.

63. "Interim Summary of Conclusions and Dietary Recommendations on Total Fat & Fatty Acids," from the Joint FAO/WHO Expert Consultation on Fats and Fatty Acids in Human Nutrition, 10-14 November, 2008, WHO, Geneva. Accessed at www.who.int/nutrition/topics/FFA_summary _rec_conclusion.pdf.

64. Dietary Reference Intakes for Energy, Carbohydrate, Fiber, Fat, Fatty Acids, Cholesterol, Protein, and Amino Acids (Macronutrients), p. 423. (See note 53.)

65. Jeff Novick, a superb registered dietitian and former nutrition director at the Pritikin Longevity Center, states the following on Dr. John McDougall's online discussion forum (you can view it at www.drmcdougall.com/ forums/viewtopic.php?t=6293):

"There is evidence that the actual minimum requirement [for ALA] may be as low as 0.5 gram a day … so, in regard to Omega 3s, even the 1.1 to 1.6 may be way more than we really need."

66. Nevin KG, Rajamohan T. "Beneficial Effects of Virgin Coconut Oil on Lipid Parameters and In Vitro LDL Oxidation. Clin Biochem. 2004 Sep;37(9):830-5.

For more information about the fallacy of popular health claims for coconut oil, see also Dr. John McDougall's article entitled " The Newest Food-Cure: Coconut Oil for Health and Vitality," in his May 2006 online newsletter, available at www.drmcdougall.com/misc/2006nl/may/coconut.htm.

67. Refer to chapters 2 and 3 of *Health and Survival in the 21st Century* (see note 17), which outline clearly the mechanisms by which the human body's innate intelligence—given a proper diet and other conditions—naturally and easily maintains homeostasis without the assistance of any drugs, herbs, "healing" foods, or interventions of any kind.

68. "Trends in Intake of Energy and Macronutrients—United States, 1971–2000." (See note 1.)

69. See "Nutrition and Well-Being A to Z" in the Internet FAQ Archives by Thomson Gale, accessed at www.faqs.org/nutrition/Smi-Z/Water.html. (Click "Water.") This Web page describes how body-water percentages fluctuate, with men and women hovering around 62% and 51% water, respectively. Physical activity increases this number as high as 70%, and overweight reduces it, down to 36% for the morbidly obese.

70. You can buy a bioimpedance-based body-fat monitor built into a bathroom scale, online or in drugstores, department stores, or sporting goods stores. I have used and recommended body-fat scales made by the Tanita Corporation for many years.

For information about bioimpedance and other methods of measuring body fat, see the online article entitled "Understanding Body Fat Analysis," excerpted from a 1999 Tanita pamphlet of the same name. Accessed at www.healthchecksystems.com/tbf.htm. Click "Bioelectrical Impedance (BIA)."

71. Volek, JS, Westman, EC. "Very-Low-Carbohydrate Weight-Loss Diets Revisited," Cleveland Clinic J. Med. 2002 Nov;69(11), 849-862. Accessed at www.ccjm.org/pdffiles/Volek1102.pdf. Low carbohydrate, high-fat dietary programs are shown to

result in weight loss due to appetite-suppressing high blood levels of hydroxybutyrate (a ketone satiety trigger).

72. The "conventional" body-fat percentage recommendations in this table come from a chart entitled, "Body Fat Ranges for Standard Adults," which you can access at www.tanita.com/MessageForWomen.shtml#, the website of Tanita Corporation of America, Inc. These numbers are based on NIH/WHO BMI guidelines, as reported by Gallagher, et. al, at the New York Obesity Research Center.

According to the National Health and Nutrition Examination Survey, an estimated 65% of the U.S. population is overweight and 30% is obese. Using my body-fat recommendations, these numbers would dramatically increase, since NHANES defines overweight and obesity as having a BMI of at least 25% and 30%, respectively.

I do not find BMI to be a useful measure, given that it attempts to suggest an ideal weight based on height alone and does not distinguish fat and lean mass. Therefore, I cannot provide a recommended number for comparison with the 25 and 30% guidelines quoted above.

73. Smith, N.J. "Gaining and Losing Weight in Athletics." JAMA. 1976;236: 149–151. "Muscle mass is increased only through muscle work supported by an appropriate increase in food intake. No food, vitamin, drug, or hormone will increase muscle mass."

74. See the article "Cabin Air Quality," on the Boeing website, accessed at www.boeing.com/commercial/cabinair/environment.html. Click "cabin pressure" or "air quality."

For more information on the significant relationship between altitude and dehydration see Quinn, Elizabeth, "High Altitude Vacations: How To Prepare," (2006), accessed at http://sportsmedicine.about.com/cs/altitude/ a/042004.htm.

75. See the Wikipedia entry for "Dehydration," accessed through http://en.wikipedia.org/wiki/Main_Page. Search "Dehydration," and click "Symptoms and Prognosis."

76. See a Medline Plus discussion of dehydration in the "skin turgor" entry at www.nlm.nih.gov/medlineplus/ency/article/003281.htm.

77. Tyls, Josef. "Are You Chronically Dehydrated?" Alive (#243) January 2003, Alive Publishing Group. Accessed at www.alive.com/index.php. Scroll

down to "alive index search" click on "Health and Disease." Then scroll down to "Health and Disease articles," and click "Are You Chronically Dehydrated?"

78. Rehrer, N.J. "The Maintenance of Fluid Balance during Exercise," Int. J. Sports Med. 15:122-125, 1994.

79. See www.vanaqua.org/education/aquafacts/seaotters.html.

80. See www.brookfieldzoo.org/pagegen/htm/fix/fg/fg_body. asp?sAnimal=Afric an+lion.

81. According to the Mayo Clinic, an adult stomach is capable of stretching at the sides to hold nearly a gallon of food and liquid. (See www.mayoclinic. com/health/stomach-cancer/DS00301/DSECTION=3.) The Indiana University School of Medicine, however, reports that the average adult stomach stretches to only about a quarter of its capacity, about two to three pints. (See http://medicine.iupui.edu/heartburn/anatomyfiles/notworking.htm.)

82. See www.nutramed.com/digestion.

83. In his book, Pain: It's Not All in Your Head (Trafford Publishing, 2003), physician assistant and clinical psychologist Jay Tracy explains how deficiencies cause us to crave the nutrients we lack, and this signal is misinterpreted as hunger and food cravings. See www.trafford.com/4dcgi/robots/02-0228.html.

84. Lucas, F., Sclafani A. "Differential Reinforcing and Satiating Effects of Intragastric Fat and Carbohydrate Infusions in Rats," Physiol Behav. 1999 May;66(3):381-8.

85. McArdle, William, Katch, Frank I., et al. Exercise Physiology: Energy, Nutrition and Human Performance, third edition. Malvern, PA: Lippincott Williams & Wilkins (1991). See chapter 9, "Human Energy Expenditure During Rest and Physical Activity, pp. 159–161.

86. "The Origins of Agriculture." (See note 29.)

87. "Bayer AG: A Corporate Profile," p. 39, by Corporate Watch UK, March 1, 2002. Accessed at http://archive.corporatewatch.org/profiles/bayer/bayer. rtf.

88. A good layman's article on the subject of acrylamide is "Acrylamide Angst: Another Annoying Distraction About Food Safety," by Dr. Allan S. Fel-

sot, an environmental toxicologist at Washington State University. Published in the October 2002 issue of Agrichemical and Environmental News, the article is available online at www.envirofacs.org/Acrylamide %20Angst.pdf.

You can learn more about the connection between acrylamide and herbicides at www.organicconsumers.org/monsanto/acrylamide.cfm.

89. "Food Nutrition: Better Guidance Needed to Improve Reliability of USDA's Food Composition Data." GAO report #RCED-94-30, October 25, 1993. Accessed at http://archive.gao.gov/t2pbat4/150400.pdf.

90. Some of the information in this sidebar comes from various USDA Web pages accessed through www.nal.usda.gov/fnic/foodcomp/, pages that document the National Nutrient Database for Standard Reference, or from the USDA publication, "Composition of Foods: Raw, Processed, Prepared," available at www.nal.usda.gov/fnic/foodcomp/Data/SR17/sr17_doc.pdf

For a full description of Atwater's work, see Agriculture Handbook 74 (Merrill and Watt, 1973. Energy Value of Foods...Basis and Derivation). U.S. Government Printing Office. Washington, DC. 105p. This reference is out of print, but a scanned copy is viewable at www.nal.usda.gov/fnic/ foodcomp/ Data/Classics/ah74.pdf.

# Index

# Notes

## Notes

## Notes

# *Notes*